# Prediction in Forensic and Neuropsychology

## Sound Statistical Practices

# Prediction in Forensic and Neuropsychology

## Sound Statistical Practices

*Edited by*

### Ronald D. Franklin
*St. Mary's Hospital
and Florida Atlantic University*

LAWRENCE ERLBAUM ASSOCIATES, PUBLISHERS

2003    Mahwah, New Jersey                    London

| | |
|---|---|
| Senior Consulting Editor: | Susan Milmoe |
| Editorial Assistant: | Kristen Depken |
| Cover Design: | Kathryn Houghtaling Lacey |
| Textbook Production Manager: | Paul Smolenski |
| Text and Cover Printer: | Sheridan Books, Inc. |

Camera ready copy for this book was provided by the author.

Lawrence Erlbaum Associates, Inc., Publishers
10 Industrial Avenue
Mahwah, New Jersey 07430

**Library of Congress Cataloging-in-Publication Data**

Prediction in forensic and neuropsychology : sound statistical practices / edited by Ronald D. Franklin.

    p. cm.

Includes bibliographical references and index.

ISBN 0-8058-3225-4 (cloth : alk. paper)
1. Clinical neuropsychology—Statistical methods. 2. Neuropsychological tests—Statistical methods. 3. Forensic neuropsychology—Statistical methods. I. Franklin, Ronald D.
RC473.N48 P74 2002
616.8'07'2—dc21

    2002071296
    CIP

Books published by Lawrence Erlbaum Associates are printed on acid-free paper, and their bindings are chosen for strength and durability.

Printed in the United States of America
10 9 8 7 6 5 4 3 2 1

# CONTENTS

# PREFACE

Considerable controversy exists between and within factions of neuropsychologists who hold any number of circumscribed views that they often attribute to the superiority of one training model over another. Differences include the number of tests to administer, which among the many available tests should be administered, and how administered tests should be interpreted. Some argue for a purely quantitative analysis where test scores are compared against established standards. Others demand inclusion of qualitative measures, such as a patient's approach to the test or the way a patient constructs a drawing. Both approaches demonstrate merit; both present limitations. Common to each approach is a reliance on the scientific method for the formation and testing of hypotheses. This work explores scientific methods common to neuropsychological approaches for establishing diagnosis and predicting future or prior performances. Particular emphasis is placed on statistical methods that are readily available to clinical practitioners.

Predictive statistics attempt to identify relationships between different data sets by using mathematical models for forecasting unknown behavior patterns from known patterns of behavior. Predictive statistics are distinguished from inferential statistics by their reliance on tests of association rather than test of differences between means. Inferential statistics concerned themselves with describing and interpreting differences occurring within or between data sets. In neuropsychological applications, these distinctions are often moot. For example, probability statements derived from inferential statistics are often used to test hypothetical differences between test scores presented by a patient and scores presented by others. From these data a diagnosis may be rendered. The rendering of a diagnosis is a form of prediction. This book explores ways that both inferential and predictive statistical models are helpful in answering clinical questions about individuals.

Most of the chapters were written for practicing professionals. An understanding of basic statistics is assumed by most authors. However, much of the work is within the grasp of practicing attorneys, physicians, and others who have practical experience working with psychological test data. Several sections were discussed in the hope that their inclusion in future neuropsychological research will produce greater clinical efficacy.

## ACKNOWLEDGMENTS

No work of this magnitude is completed without the assistance of many people. My admiration and appreciation is extended to each of the contributors, all of whom have been most patient during the conception and gestation of this collection. Perhaps no one has been more patient than the editorial liaison, Susan Milmoe. All of us are also indebted to Barbara Wieghaus for her excellent copy editing and Art Lizza for production.

Many others have offered advise, support, and criticism. The most vocal of these individuals follow here. Please think of them and the contributors when ideas in this work inspire you. Think of me when you are confused or disagree with content. The appreciation expressed to these individuals in no way implies their endorsement, approval, (or in some cases knowledge) of this work. Some disagree with the content, but all concerns they have expressed to me were carefully considered and often resulted in significant revisions of the work.

|  |  |
|---:|:---|
| Mary Acker, PhD* | Human Support Services, San Jose, CA |
| Hal Arkes, PhD* | The Ohio State University |
| Jeffrey T. Barth, PhD* | The University of Virginia |
| Brent Boerlage | Norsys Software Corporation |
| Odie Bracy, PhD | Psychological Software Services, Inc. |
| Thomas G. Burns, PsyD, ABPN* | Children's Healthcare of Atlanta |
| Sally Cameron | North Carolina Psychological Association |
| Robyn Dawes, PhD* | Carnegie-Mellon University |
| Ward Edwards, PhD | University of Southern California |

| | |
|---|---|
| Alan E. Friedman, JD | Tuttle & Taylor Law Corporation, Los Angeles |
| Shiela Cohen Furr, PhD* | Shiela Cohen Furr Associates |
| Charles Golden, PhD* | Lighthouse Point Fl |
| Bernie Gorman, PhD | Nassau Community College/SUNY |
| Michael Hayes, MA* | Marywood University |
| James Higgins, PhD | East Carolina University |
| A. E. House, PhD | Illinois State University |
| Morjorie Kyle, MA* | Our Lady of the Lake University |
| Penny Mangus, MA, JD* | Retired |
| Larry Means, PhD | East Carolina University |
| Susan Milmoe | Lawrence Erlbaum Associates |
| Wolfgang Neuwirth | Vienna Test System |
| Raymond Nickerson, PhD* | Tufts University |
| Win Noren | StatSoft, Inc. |
| Mark Oring, JD* | Professor of Law, University of West Los Angeles School of Law |
| Joseph Petrowski | Lawrence Erlbaum Associates |
| Margaret Petry, PhD* | Wasserman & Drucker, PA |
| Roy Poses, PhD* | Brown University |
| Cecil R. Reynolds, PhD, ABPP, ABPN | Texas A&M University |

| | |
|---|---|
| John D. Tinder, JD | Judge, US District Court Southern District of Indiana |
| Rodney D. Vanderploeg, PhD | University of South Florida |
| N. William Walker, PhD | James Madison University |
| Rebecca Hensley-Ward, MA* | Forest Institute of Professional Psychology |
| Theodore Wasserman, ABPP, ABPdN* | Richard and Pat Johnson Childrens' Hospital at Saint Mary's Medical Center Department of Child Development |

* We are indebted to those people who read and commented on various drafts.

# CONTRIBUTORS

Gordon J. Chelune, PhD, ABPP-CN
*Cleveland Clinic Foundation, Cleveland, Ohio*

Alan B. Fleming, PhD
*Horizon Psychological Services, Miami, Florida*

Ronald D. Franklin, PhD, FABPdN, (C. Psychol.), APA-CPP
*St. Mary's Hospital, West Palm Beach, Florida
and Florida Atlantic University, Boca Raton, Florida*

Selma De Jesus-Zayas, PhD
*Federal Correctional Institution, Miami, Florida*

Aarne Kivioja, MD, PhD, M Sci (Tech.)MD, PhD, Msci
*Helsinki University Central Hospital, Helsinki, Finland*

Joachim Krueger, PhD
*Brown University, Providence, RI*

L. Stephen Miller, PhD
*University of Georgia-Athens, Athens, Georgia*

Jennifer Langhinrichsen-Rohling, PhD
*University of South Alabama, Mobile, Alabama*

Martin Langhinrichsen Rohling, PhD
*University of South Alabama, Mobile, Aabama*

Michael J. Rovine, PhD
*The Pennsylvania State University, University Park, Pennsylvania*

Claude A. Ruffalo, PhD
*The Fielding Institute, Santa Barbara, California*

Christiane Spiel, PhD
*University of Graz, Graz, Austria*

Alexander von Eye, PhD
*Michigan State University, Lansing, Michigan*

# Prediction in Forensic and Neuropsychology

## Sound Statistical Practices

# Introduction

**Ronald D. Franklin**[1]

*St. Mary's Hospital, and Florida Atlantic University*

As a clinical practitioner, I am often asked by my patients, or family members of my patients, to tell them what is wrong, how a problem developed, and what can be done to "fix it." As a neuropsychologist who works with forensic patients, these questions take one of four forms. First, I am asked how much brain damage the patient has. In most circumstances some other doctor has already opined that the patient has brain damage and the referral is to establish degree of damage. Less often, I am asked to opine if the patient has brain damage. Second, the patient (or the patient's attorney) is eager to determine who was at fault, or who "caused" the brain damage. Third, patients and others want to know what kind of impact will the brain damage have on the future life of the patient, the family, or their interactions. Finally, patients or family members seek treatment recommendations. This book is written to provide clinicians with sound objective methods for developing and evaluating answers to these and other questions as they arise during the neuropsychological evaluation. I am guided by the observations of Robert Abelson (1995), who described properties of data that make data *MAGIC:* magnitude, articulation, generality, interestingness, and credibility. It is my view that neuropsychological assessment is so interdependent with data analysis methodologies, that attempts to make neuropsychological inference in the absence of considering statistical implications is malpractice.

In an effort to address statistical issues that aid in the development of inference and principled argument, I cover three topical areas in this book. In doing so, I realize that other topics could have been chosen.

---

[1]Please address correspondence to PO Box 246, Candor, NC, 27229 or rdfphd@yahoo.com

Those selected coincide with my work experiences during the previous quarter century. Because topical areas contain substantial overlap with one another, the contents of each area are disbursed within the work in order to limit redundancy and aid in overall readability. First, I review statistical methods that appear with some frequency in the neuropsychology literature. The discussion is largely limited to statistical methods that are used in developing inferences regarding specific patients rather than methods that are appropriate for research. Consequently some statistical methods, such as meta-analysis and nonlinear modeling, are beyond the scope of this work. Topical area 1 includes chapters addressing hypothesis testing, Bayesian inference, statistical evidence, and neuropsychological change. Second, I present several statistical models that are less well known in neuropsychology but have shown promise in other areas of science. Topical area 2 describes Bayesian belief networks, configural frequency analysis, and Rohling's interpretive method. Finally, I consider reviews of frequent referral concerns along with proposals for expanding the evaluation models offered in each chapter. Topical area 3 reviews patient advocacy, malingering, recovery of function, and prediction of violent behavior. I do not review several common problems such as prediction of premorbid function or evaluation of traumatic brain injuries. Although much has been written about the prediction of premorbid abilities[2], it seems to me that when demographic data are the default standard against which other prediction models are compared, then the value of using neuropsychology data in this way must be questioned. Instead, chapter 5 provides a model for evaluating differences between scores taken from earlier and later testings that can compare multiple data types[3]. Chapter 6 also discusses the topic, going into considerable detail using data appropriate to parametric analysis.

---

[2] As of September 10, 2001 *Psych Scan* listed 243 articles using a keyword of "premorbid," 146 with a keyword of "TBI," and 1,194 under "brain injury."

[3] Statistical data in psychology have four types: nominal, ordinal, interval, and ratio. Nominal consists of named categories such as male or female. Ordinal allows classification such as greater than or less than. Interval compares items that are measured in equal distances, such as inches or feet. Ratio refers to interval data that have a known starting point. Data types are important because they determine which, if any, statistical tests are appropriate in their analysis. See Glenberg (1996) for a complete description of data types and their uses.

I have ordered the chapters so that chapters 2–6 form a background that is helpful to developing an understanding of later chapters. Readers will better understand 7–11 by reading chapters 2–6, in order of presentation, first. The remaining chapters can be read in any order. The following chapter-by-chapter descriptions may help readers identify the sections most relevant to their concerns and interest.

"Advocacy in the Forensic Practice of Neuropsychology" (chap. 2) is an extremely important issue for both forensics and neuropsychology. The term advocacy typically evokes different beliefs among attorneys and other helping professionals. Dr. Ruffalo is a seasoned forensic psychologist who reviews the importance of differing views of the topic while providing a good overview of the litigation process.

"Neuropsychological Hypothesis Testing" (chap. 3) reviews models of hypothesis testing as they are used in statistical analysis within psychology. The chapter highlights essential components of each model, comparing their relative value in the neuropsychological decision-making process. Greatest emphasis is placed on variants of the null-hypothesis model as the most frequently used hypothesis-testing process in psychology. The chapter introduces the Bayesian model of hypothesis testing and its inclusion of prior probabilities in the statistical model.

"Bayesian Inference and Belief Networks" (chap. 4) expands the Bayesian model of hypothesis testing introduced earlier. Here, the rationale for the model is explored and discussed by example. Bayesian belief networks are introduced as a multifactorial extension of modeling beliefs such as diagnosis and recovery.

"Neuropsychological Evaluations as Statistical Evidence" (chap. 5) discusses differences between legal and statistical evidence. The chapter argues that exclusive reliance on findings from null-hypothesis models as the basis for professional opinions always produces impeached evidence. I describe a Bayesian model, likelihood ratios, as a better method for establishing neuropsychological findings as evidence.

"Assessing Reliable Neuropsychological Change" (chap. 6) presents Gordon Chelune's classical review of change analysis appropriate to parametric data sets. He discusses the importance moderator variables, such as regression toward the mean and intratest consistency, have on prediction accuracy. Included in the chapter are statistical corrections for the best understood moderator effects.

"Configural Frequency Analysis in the Practice of Neuropsychology" (chap. 7) introduces an analysis model that holds much promise for neuropsychology research. Drs. von Eye, Spiel, and Rovine have demonstrated many useful research applications for the technique. This chapter is the first to explore the model in neuropsychology.

"Actuarial Assessment of Malingering: Rohling's Interpretive Method" (chap. 8) is a variation on the null-hypothesis-testing model. RIM (Rohling's interpretive method) attempts to integrate and summarize large amounts of neuropsychological data into a quantifiable interpretive model. Rohling, Langhinrichsen-Rohling, and Miller present methods for data analysis that appear to update the model first proposed by Reitan. The chapter presents a review of the malingering assessment literature that is well thought out and concisely presented.

"Recovery of Function" (after traumatic brain injury) (chap. 9) offers readers a comprehensive review of the TBI (traumatic brain injury) literature from the perspectives of a trauma surgeon and a neuropsychologist. The chapter provides reviews of measurement instruments, considering their efficacy in predicting recovery. We also provide readers with a Bayesian network model for predicting recovery that is based on the studies presented.

"The Prediction of Violent Behavior" (chap. 10) offers readers a review of applied methods for assessing and predicting violence. Dr. De Jesus-Zayas presents personal views, developed through years of experience working in the federal correctional facilities. Dr. Fleming provides reviews reflecting public policies. As in all clinical application sections, there is a Bayesian network proposed from research findings.

## REFERENCES

Abelson, R., P. (1995). *Statistics as principled argument.* Mahwah, NJ: Lawrence Erlbaum Associates.

Glenberg, A., M. (1996). *Learning from data.* Mahwah, NJ: Lawrence Erlbaum Associates.

# Advocacy in the Forensic Practice of Neuropsychology

Claude A. Ruffalo[1]
*The Fielding Institute Neuropsychology Program*

## INTERPRETATIONS OF ADVOCACY

Any discussion of witnesses might best begin with the basic distinction between a percipient or lay witness and an expert witness (Bronstein, 1999). A percipient witness is a witness who testifies to facts and perceptions, and who is not permitted to provide opinions to the court. A psychologist could be called as a percipient witness. For example, the psychologist might be asked if a given person was, in fact, their patient and was that person in session with them at 3:00 *PM* on January 4, 1999. The psychologist, as a percept witness, would not be allowed to answer a question as to why that patient was in therapy with them because that would involve the psychologist providing an opinion, unless the psychologist was simply providing witness to the statement made by the patient as to why they said they were in therapy.

An expert witness is a witness who has special knowledge that the average person is presumed not to possess. An expert witness is permitted to testify as to their opinion and the basis for their opinions concerning special knowledge within the scope of their expertise. The expert may testify about that body of special knowledge or about the application of that special knowledge to the issues being addressed by the court. The present analysis addresses primarily the issue of the expert, not the percipient witness.

In the following sections, a number of different types or interpretations of advocacy are addressed: (a) scientific advocacy (evaluation-oriented advocacy), (b) case-oriented advocacy (side-oriented advocacy or collaborative bias), and (c) proposition advocacy (issue-oriented advocacy or issue bias).

---

[1] Please address correspondence to Claude A. Ruffalo, PhD, 2021 Santa Monica Boulevard, Suite 320E, Santa Monica, CA 90404, 310-306-6166.

## Scientific Interpretation of Advocacy

Scientific advocacy can be considered from the perspective of typical academic discourse. The wide range of typical arguments and analysis tools used in the assessment and evaluation of research and propositions in psychology are equally available in the analysis of the opinions of experts. It remains easy for those outside the adversarial system of justice to poke fun at the system and to sincerely believe that it is both preposterous and heinous. However, if one defines advocacy as the presenting of data and argument supportive of an opinion that one has, then a fair and objective look at research in general, whether academically based or otherwise, quickly uncovers the fact that some type and degree of advocacy is involved in all research activities and publications. Examination of the meaning of advocacy from this perspective of traditional research provides one way of approaching advocacy in a legal setting that may well satisfy both the needs of the legal system and the ethics of the professions. For example, a common approach to research is to provide the method of assessment of an issue, the data so acquired, a meaningful and appropriate analysis of that data, and to some degree an advocation of an interpretation of that data. An expert in a legal situation could be seen to be taking a similar approach.

Ziskin and Faust (1988) suggested that neuropsychology as a science was not sufficiently developed to offer accurate or useful information to aid the trier of fact. A challenge to this position was voiced by Barth, Ryan, Schear, and Puente (1992) and Giuliano, Barth, Hawk, and Ryan (1997), who described Ziskin and Faust as "method skeptics" because their position addresses general issues of the scientific method as the method applies to psychology.

## Case- or Side-Oriented Advocacy

One form of advocacy occurs when an expert provides or develops support for the side employing the expert; this can be termed case- or side-oriented advocacy. Though case- or side-oriented advocacy has consistently been criticized, it is generally recognized that such advocacy is prevalent and supported by marketplace economic factors. Some experts have argued that it is the work of the expert to be an advocate for the side that employs him or her. Kuvin (1986) responded to an article by Marcus (1986a) in the *American Journal of Forensic Psychiatry* by objecting to Marcus' position that a psychiatrist should become an advocate for his or her patient during litigation of the patient's injuries. Kuvin described an oppositional dichotomy between advocacy and honesty, and indicated that the court expects and depends on the psychiatrist to provide honesty to the court. Marcus originally (1983, 1985) asserted that the testimony of experts should not be taken at face value and that bias in medical testimony should be taken into account. Marcus (1986a, 1986b) presented plaintiff and defense perspectives on psychiatric disability evaluations and suggested that the psychiatrist becomes a client advocate when the client is examined for mental injury and compensation due to injury.

Although there are more sober, scientific, and less adversarial treatments of issues that finally boil down to addressing the matter of the case- or side-oriented expert such as those by presented by Huber (1991) and Foster and Huber (1997), currently some expositions attacking this type of advocacy have exploded into rather dramatic controversy with the introduction of such publications as Hagen's *Whores of the Court* (1997). Hagen barred no holds and dropped right into being about as intensely adversarial as one can be while attacking expert case- or side-oriented advocacy. She painted a very dark picture of the psychological experts in the legal arena. One could become entirely "swallowed " by the insufficiently informed and glibly presented arguments regarding psychologists' assistance in the legal system. Yet, Hagen's arguments are just as adversarial and misrepresentative as many others seen in the legal arena coming from experts who were acting with apparent side-oriented advocacy.

Case- or side-oriented advocacy can be well divided into two general categories: (a) advocacy for patients and (b) advocacy for nonpatients.

***Advocacy for Patients.*** Advocacy for patients should be considered separately because it involves some very strong biases that are built into the helping professions from which experts in psychology and neuropsychology originate. In fact, some authorities have argued that a division of roles is necessary between experts and treating doctors so that experts can be objective and independent and treating doctors can remain advocates for their patients (Moser & Barbrack, 2000). This issue is covered in greater detail in later section.

***Advocacy for Nonpatients.*** This is perhaps the most criticized of all forms of advocacy. It represents the use of psychological and/or neuropsychological expertise to deliberately provide expert evidence or argument regarding the position or condition of a "nonpatient" (someone with whom the expert does not have a doctor–patient relationship) that favors the position of the individual or institution that has hired the expert. Such experts are often referred to as "hired guns" and they are characterized as being experts who are willing to adopt whatever position most benefits their employer. These experts appear to receive the most dire and serious criticism when they are employed to attack the injury that is being claimed by a patient, and this may be because such a role is in complete contradiction to what it is that those in the helping professions are supposed to be committed to doing, that is, accurately diagnosing and appropriately treating people with diseases and disorders.

## Issue-Oriented Advocacy

There are many experts who may be called upon to testify because of their known or published positions on a particular issue or issues. Though issue-oriented advocacy can often amount to being specific examples of scientific advocacy, at times more may be involved, because there may be other motivations for the advocacy of certain issues than the simple pursuit of scientific truth. For instance, if an expert carefully sets out to provide data, research, evidence, or arguments to support a particular issue that is often litigated, then that expert may be involved in issue bias. Issue bias is addressed further in a later section of this chapter.

## Advocacy From a Clinical Practice Treatment Perspective

Moser and Barback (2000) provided some arguments in favor of separating the role of treating psychologists from that of expert witnesses in the legal arena. Moser and Barback asserted that treating psychologists should not answer questions in the legal arena that are directed to elicit new opinions, but that such answers should come from expert witnesses. It is their assertion that percipient or "fact" witnesses should testify only about past opinions that they had about their patient. An example of such a past opinion might be to answer the question, "Was it your opinion while treating the patient that the patient's anxiety was caused by the accident they sustained on July 15, 1995?" However, the treating doctor or "fact witness" should not answer questions like "Would it be your opinion now that the anxiety you observed in 1995 is related to the anxiety Mr. Smith is presently experiencing?"; instead this type of question should be answered by an expert witness.

It is not uncommon for a person with mild brain injury to seek out an "expert" in the field of neuropsychology to get an "expert" opinion as to what is wrong with them and to ask that "expert" to provide them some psychotherapy or rehabilitation related to their brain injury. Furthermore, it would be typical for many of such cases to later result in the patient's attorney requesting the expert to write a report concerning the results of their evaluation and to call the expert to testify as to their expert opinion in court when litigating the issue of compensation for the patient's injury. Imposing a requirement that the patient who goes on to litigation find another expert who has not treated them and who may never come to know the patient's condition as well as the initial evaluating/treating doctor is a considerable additional financial and emotional burden upon the patient in and of itself that must be given serious consideration before being recommended or implemented.

Another consideration in this matter is that it would certainly be more than reasonable for the injured person to ask the expert whom they have hired for litigation purposes to give them feedback concerning their test results and their diagnosis. Yet, how can this be handled without some consideration of the therapeutic impact of statements made to the patient? That is, even the simplest feedback must be seen as an educational procedure of a psychotherapeutic nature when the patient has come to be evaluated by that expert.

Hence, perhaps the statement that "treating psychologists are not expert witnesses" is too strong and absolute a statement and further examination of the subtleties of this issue is clearly indicated. It may be that in some cases, in some ways, and in some situations treating psychologists can be expert witnesses to some extent provided that proper guidelines are developed and followed.

## ETHICAL INTERPRETATIONS OF ADVOCACY

Behaviors of experts are greatly influenced by the behaviors of the courts and litigating attorneys, all of which can vary greatly from state to state. Some attorneys clearly express very ethical principles of practice such as those presented by Simkins (1997): "This is crucial and if a plaintiff is less than 100% honest and accurate about this, we decline to represent them, or if we find out about it during the course of representation, if appropriate, we seek permission of the court to withdraw from the case" (p. 281). All too often, however, appropriate ethical guidelines are ignored. Although the ethical practices of attorneys are beyond the scope of this work, revision proposals recommended for the APA Ethics Code (Jones, 2001) greatly expand ethical constraints for forensic practice in psychology. Important proposed changes permeate the text in both the introduction and specific sections. Principles B, C, and F contain important changes as do Standards 1.01, 3.01, 3.10, and 6.10. Standards 9 (Assessment) and 11 (Forensic Activities) hold particular salience.

## Assessment (APA Standard 9)

Historically this section of the ethics code required forensic examiners to conduct a forensic examination before forming opinions (§7.02). Additionally, conclusions and recommendations had to be based on examination data. Issues of competence in administering and interpreting data were loosely addressed (§2.02) as were test construction issues (§2.03). The 2001 revision proposes adding a category to include record review as a type of examination (§901(d)). Section 902 adds subsections with added documentation requirements when patients are tested in the absence of "appropriate tests" (§9.01(b)). Limitations on assessments using interpreters are added (§9.01(c)) with special caveats for delegating work to others, maintaining confidentiality, informed consent, and assessment by unqualified persons. New standards are proposed regarding informed consent, (§9.03(a)) and providing evaluations mandated by courts (§9.03(b)). Considerable revision of §9.04 provides for reduced requirements when test results are released to another professional. The section also limits release to courts, attorneys, and patients.

## Forensic Activities (Standard 11)

Two important new sections are proposed for this standard. For the first time, forensic activities are defined but methods for evaluating practitioners or specialists remain vague. The second important addition (§11.02) defines informed consent for forensic practice in more specific terms, requiring the evaluator to anticipate potential use of assessment results, implying that informed consent should be based on a philosophy of "avoiding harm." The section expands responsibilities for court–ordered evaluations: "When an evaluation is court ordered, the psychologist informs the individual and the individual's legal representative of the nature of the anticipated forensic service before proceeding with the evaluation" (§11.02(b)).

Cross-referenced are sections addressing third-party requests for services, avoiding harm, describing the nature and results of services, informed consent, boundaries of competence, and maintaining expertise. Once approved, revisions of the ethical standards have the force of law in many jurisdictions. More restrictive "clarifications" may prove problematic in states such as Florida where the standards become the basis for disciplinary actions and interpretations are made by nonpsychologists.

## PROBLEMS CAUSED BY THE EXPERTS AS ADVOCATES

### Misleading the Defense in Civil Litigation

The expert who is an advocate may mislead his or her employer by providing them with what they may want to hear, which is supportive of their positon, but that expert is failing them in another sense by not providing them with a more objective assessment of the situation they are being paid to "assess." If the expert provides a written opinion or testimonial opinion that is actually contrary to the "more objective" and "confidential" feedback that the expert may provide to the attorney directly, then, in effect, one would have to ask whether that expert has not thereby entered into a conspiracy with the attorney to undermine justice and the law.

### Blacklisting

Experts may feel forced to provide positions of advocacy because they believe that otherwise they significantly decrease the likelihood of their reemployment, a form of blacklisting. Many if not most of all insurance claims representatives have their lists (written or unwritten) of experts and know very well who will give them the opinion that they want to hear and who may not. Although I'm certain that a working claims representative would not publicly admit to such practices readily, I have been told in confidence by more than one claims representative from large and reputable insurance companies that this was in fact the case.

### Attorney–Expert Relationships

Although there are likely to be exceptions, the political reality of the attorney–expert relationship is generally that more often than not the expert who develops a good working relationship with an attorney is an expert who can be counted on to come through with an opinion of some degree of advocacy for the attorney's case and to be able to present that opinion in a professionally authoritative (i.e., convincing) manner.

At least two types of nonmutually exclusive bias can be distinguished. One might be called *collaborative bias* and the other *issue bias*.

*Collaborative Bias.* If an expert is judged to be a ready advocate for either side of an issue depending primarily on who has hired him or her, then he or she might have what is termed collaborative bias. During examination of an expert witness, the opposing counsel most often will carefully question the expert about the frequency with which he or she has provided evaluations for the insurance company or the attorney who is calling them as a witness because this type of underlying relationship (collaborative bias) is known to exist with notable frequency. For instance, when an expert is examined by the opposing attorney, that attorney usually asks how many times the expert has worked on a case handled by the particular attorney who has called the expert or who has hired the expert in the particular case in order to suggest to the trier of fact that the expert has a collaborative bias.

*Issue Bias.* It is customary for attorneys to question experts called by the other side as to what percentage of their cases are ones in which they are called by the defense or by the plaintiffs, attempting thereby to suggest to the jury or judge that a bias is present in the form of the expert having a general side-oriented bias. However, the expert might, in fact, not be a case- or side-oriented advocate at all. The expert could simply have a professional opinion about an issue that effectively biases that expert toward rendering a certain type of opinion. That is, the expert may have an issue bias that is favorable to either the defense or plaintiff side of certain types of injury cases. For instance, some experts may be more skeptical than others about the presence of posttraumatic stress disorder, brain injury, or some other particular type of disability. Hence, they would be attractive to defense attorneys in cases where such injuries were claimed. Their form of advocacy also amounts to an issue bias. Alternatively, some experts may deliberately develop data, research, or other information supporting a position or issue that they champion that will make them attractive to attorneys who are litigating particular issues.

*Advocacy Begets Advocacy.* If the defense has an expert who is a side-oriented or issue-oriented advocate for them and the plaintiff has only an expert who is unbiased, intellectually painstakingly "honest," or taking great effort to not act as an advocate in any way, then the plaintiff may be at a serious disadvantage. Disadvantage occurs because the position of advocacy is often intended to create a compromise most likely resolved with nonpatient advantage. That is, if one advocating expert claims that the person is 50% disabled and the other claims the person is only 10% disabled, then a trier of fact that has no reason to believe one expert versus the other would be expected to give a compromising judgment of 30% disability. Yet, if the "10% expert" is an advocate who might have otherwise judged the person to be 50% disabled if providing their most objective and independent opinion, then the disability rating would actually have be judged to be 50%, a significant difference for the plaintiff. Hence, the advocacy system as such could be seen consistently to benefit the side that hires an expert to be an advocate for their position.

The exception to this rule would of course be that too much of an extreme difference between expert opinions could backfire, particularly for the defense, against whom large damages could be potentially justified and awarded. That is, if the person is obviously 100% disabled for work purposes and the defense doctor opines that there is 0% disability and the defense rests their case upon this position, an overwhelming verdict might well be awarded to the plaintiff in a civil case. On the other hand, if the defense expert simply asserts that, yes, the person is quite disabled, perhaps even 75%, but makes a convincing argument that the disability is overreaching, exaggerated, or misrepresented, then the trier of fact may well award a verdict based on the apparent "honesty" of the defense's position.   In this situation the verdict is much more friendly to the nonpatient even if the actual level of disability (if it could be discovered) was truly 100%.

In effect, one could reason that the advocacy system tends to benefit the side that can obtain the most sophisticated advocacy from an expert. Yet, if the defense gets a painstakingly "honest" or nonadvocating expert and the plaintiff has an advocate, then the plaintiff has an advantage, thus motivating the defense to find an advocate. This reasoning makes it fairly clear that in the arena of litigation advocacy creates advocacy. Hence, one way to bring more honesty to the dueling of experts is to have some way to expose or measure the advocacy of an expert because advocacy is generally successful to the degree that it is not recognized as advocacy.

There may be some benefit seen to the attorney who has an expert having both favorable issue biases and favorable collaborative biases that are unobtrusive. Such a combination can be most effective when the expert has published an authoritative article or research describing an issue salient to a case in ways that are supportive of the attorney's client. The attorney may very ably disguise this subtle form of bias.

## PROBLEMS CAUSED BY FAILURE OF ADVOCACY

Looking at both sides of the advocacy issue can also be helpful. In fact, in many cases a plaintiff's injuries or simulations are not sufficiently represented or conceptualized by the evaluation. Professionals sometimes try so strongly to avoid advocacy that they can do a disservice to the plaintiff or the defense by failing to formulate a clear opinion or present that opinion and its basis with the full degree of confidence that it deserves. What then occurs could be termed a failure on the part of the expert to advocate their own opinion.

**Probabilistic Fallacy**

One reason for the expert's failure to make a proper presentation of his or her opinion can be due to what might be termed "the probabilistic fallacy." A probabilistic fallacy occurrs when a professional adopts a position grounded in the assumption that all opinions concerning human behavior are based on statistical reasoning about probabilistic events and that therefore nothing can or should be opined with certainty.

It is true that the results and conclusions provided by psychologists from their research are generally based on statistical probabilities. However, it does not follow that all psychological opinion should be properly categorized as merely a guess based on statistics. Weiner (1995) provided wise advice for practitioners who are likely to face legal scrutiny of their assessments by observing that, because all test batteries produce some frequency of false negative results, "assessors will be well advised to avoid ruling out the possibility of disorder or handicap, no matter how free from indices of disorder or handicap the test findings appear to be " (p. 100). Weiner's advice appears founded on his belief that any absolute statement about a probabilistic event can expose a psychologist to embarrassment and criticisms. The psychologist could be viewed as reckless in his or her judgments or as having made unwarranted overstatements. Weiner's statement underscores the fact that psychological assessments are more than the reporting and probabilistic interpreting of test results alone. A probabilistic analysis can be applied to any diagnosis or assessment whereby some attempt will be made to classify the accuracy of those diagnoses and assessments, but that does not make the diagnoses or assessments probabilistic.

A simple example is given by the comparison of a Minnesota Multiphasic Personality Inventory-2 (MMPI–2) profile being used in the diagnosis of depression. The MMPI–2 provides probabilistic evidence of depression or its absence. On the other hand, a clinical diagnosis can be made quite independently of statistical probabilities. For instance, depression can be diagnosed from clinical observations and reports that a patient has attempted suicide, feels great sadness after a break-up of a marital relationship, lost 20 pounds, and increased sleep from 7 to 12 hours per day. In the absence of other signs of illnesses, a diagnosis of depression must be made. Though one could apply statistical reasoning to the diagnosis and find the probability that such a diagnosis would be correct, this does not change the nature of the assessment from its being a clinical diagnosis based on awareness of the body of knowledge about depression and other illnesses as distinct from one based on probability alone. In fact, in the case of a blind MMPI–2 assessment an expert would rightly conclude that the diagnosis from the MMPI–2 is only a probable one, whereas the diagnosis from clinical examination would be a clinical diagnosis based on the presence of the signs and symptoms of depression, a diagnosis of reasonable medical or psychological certainty. In fact, the very validation of the MMPI depression scale is based on a clinical identification of persons suffering from clinical depression. The purpose of obtaining MMPI scores is to provide additional important data that will contribute to the diagnosis. Nonetheless, the criterion used to evaluate the validity of a probabilistic indicator is ultimately a clinical diagnosis. In short, the clinical diagnosis is the *sine qua non* for a diagnosis and not just one more probabilistic event. In this regard it is also true that psychological testing often provides data that add to the patient's history and manifest behavior.

The probabilistic fallacy leads some to believe that there can be no certain or absolute conclusion rendered on virtually any issue addressed. However, in clinical sciences absolute statements and conclusions are often made, conditional upon clinical exigencies. For instance, given a certain score on a psychological test index, a psychologist might well opine that there is a high probability that the individual suffered a brain injury, yet not be able on the basis of that score alone to conclude that brain injury is more than highly probable. However, if psychologists were limited to such statistical assessments, then this would put the psychologist at considerable and unnecessary disadvantage compared to the neuropsychiatrist. The neuropsychiatrist simply opines that the patient suffered brain damage on the basis of a thorough clinical examination and history taking, given the fact that in his or her assessment the presence of brain damage is determined by certain clinical signs according to defined criteria set up by the Mild Traumatic Brain Injury Committee of the Head Injury Interdisciplinary Special Interest Group of the American Congress of Rehabilitation Medicine (1993) as presented in Table 2.1.

The neuropsychiatrist might simply identify that the patient suffered an on-site loss of consciousness witnessed by multiple observers at the time of an auto accident. The only subsequent issue then to be addressed would be to determine the severity of the brain injury and its temporary and/or lasting effects on the individual. Yet the psychologist or neuropsychologist caught by the probabilistic fallacy might be unable to diagnose brain injury if he or she relied solely on conditional statistical probabilities represented by psychological test scores. In order to provide the diagnosis of brain injury, the psychologist or neuropsychologist must make a clinical diagnosis that goes beyond the probabilistic use of test scores. A clinical diagnosis can be based on knowledge of psychological, neuropsychological, neurological, biological, or other structures and functions in the same way that the diagnosis of a broken arm bone can be made upon knowledge of what the structure and function of an arm should be like in comparison with the structure and function of the identified patient's arm.    In fact, as neuropsychology has progressed in its development it appears to be moving away from statistical assessment toward clinical assessment of structure and function.

TABLE 2.1
Criteria for Mild Traumatic Head Injury

---

1. Any period of loss of consciousness.
2. Any loss of memory for events immediately before or after the accident.
3. Any alteration in mental state at the time of the accident (e.g., feeling dazed, disoriented, or confused).
4. Focal neurological deficit(s) that may or may not be transient; but where the severity of the injury does not exceed the following:

   - Loss of consciousness of approximately 30 minutes or less.
   - After 30 minutes, an initialGCS of 13–15.
   - Posttraumatic amnesia (PTA) not greater than 24 hours.

---

**Functional Versus Organic Fallacy**

There are many areas that can be examined in order to elucidate some of the practical implications of the conflicting roles of the expert. One interesting dichotomy is that between assigning pathology to that which is neuropathologically based and assigning it which is psychopathologically based, a distinction that can be referred to as the *functional versus organic dichotomy.* This is almost always a very difficult distinction with large areas in the middle that could be judged to be in either category depending on one's perspective. Whereas it is often argued that it makes no difference whether the disability is organically or functionally based, financial judgments are usually greater when the disability is judged to be organically based.  And although the basic issue for the court is often that of determining the actual level of ecologically relevant disability (cf. Sbordone, 1998), the degree to which the disability is perceived as fundamentally beyond the ability of the person to mitigate appears to be the underlying critical issue influencing the trier of fact. In the case of disabilities that are seen as permanent and organically based, the ability of the person to mitigate their disability is generally perceived to be virtually nonexistent. However, disabilities that are seen as functionally based, the ability of the person to mitigate that disability is generally raised as an issue of significance. Hence, some experts can undermine an injury claim by simply referring to it as a psychological injury, as though it was not real, permanent, or truly disabling. The nonpatient attorney may imply, or the trier of fact may infer, that the injured party actually bears responsibility for their own injuries!

**Emotional versus Cognitive Fallacy**

One issue that is often confused with the functional/organic dichotomy is the distinction between emotional and cognitive damage following brain injury cases. All too often one encounters the implicit assumption in experts, attorneys, and the trier of fact that not emotional disorders, only cognitive disorders, can be the direct result of brain injury. This is a confusion that appears to date back to primitive times when emotions were thought to be in the body whereas the intellect was in head. The fallacy could also involve the belief that people are responsible for emotions, but cognitive abilities are God-given and cannot be modified. The assumption is consistent with the reasoning that if a person is brain damaged, it is not their own fault, but if they have an emotional disorder it is indeed their own fault. In fact, the research literature is replete with studies showing that the brain is the seat of the emotions and that certain types of brain injury cause certain types of emotional disorder directly (Heilman & Satz, 1983; Lichter & Cummings, 2001; McAllister & Flashman, 1999). There is also strong research support for the finding that people suffering from "functionally" based emotional disturbance can have diminished cognitive performances as a result of that emotional disturbance (Bremner, Krystal, Southwick, Krystal, & Charney, 1995; Markowitsch, Kessler, Van der Ven, Weber-Luxenburger, Albers, & Wolf-Dieter, 1998; Veiel, 1997). Awareness of the emotional/cognitive fallacy is extremely important because it is easy for the trier of fact to be misled when circumstances of the case contradict popular, although fallacious, assumptions.

**Base-Rate Fallacy**

The base-rate fallacy is the belief that one needs to know the base rate for a phenomenon in order to be able to confidently opine that it is present. In most clinical situations, statistics rarely predict an individual's behavior.

Beliefs about the accuracy of base rates or assumptions regarding the appropriateness of discrete statistical analysis are usually inaccurate. Predicting individual behaviors from the sampled group data is always risky. Finn and Kamphuis (1995) reviewed the uses of base rates by clinicians and provided suggestions on how base rates can be used to assist the clinician in decision making. However, even Finn and Kamphuis in their championing of base-rate usage pointed out the difficulties involved in using base rates and how base rates can mislead clinicians in their judgments. The base rates of most neuropsychological disorders are generally unavailable. However, the psychology of an individual and the history of an individual almost certainly contain the "historical rates" for certain types of behavior for that individual. The person's work history may show that the patient had only 5 days of absence from work over 5 years prior to injury, but the individual had 205 days of missed work in 3 years post injury.

It is a misunderstanding of assessment to conclude that the clinician's principal responsibility is to beat the base rates. Base rates are simply additional information that a clinician can learn to use when making an assessment or formulating an opinion. Otherwise, rare conditions would never be diagnosed because it would be safest to diagnose everyone with the most common mental disorder, depression.

An example of the meaninglessness of base rates was evident to me one evening in Las Vegas. I walked by a craps table that was very lively with excitement. I stopped and asked someone what was going on. An observer replied that the man shooting the dice had just thrown seven sevens in a row. Being aware of the rarity of this run I stopped to watch as the man then threw his eighth seven in a row. This seemed impossible so I bet against him, increasing my bets progressively as I lost because he continued throwing sevens. I quit betting after losing about $600 but watched him throw sevens right up to the 17th in a row. The base rate for the occurrence of that sequence of 17 sevens is astronomical despite the fact that throwing a seven is a one in six probability each time. In fact, in the real world highly improbable events happen all the time.

Gouvier (1999) correctly pointed out that reliance upon test signs in ignorance of base rates can lead even a well-meaning expert to false conclusions. However, two issues that are inadequately addressed by base-rate analyses should be considered. First, many psychological and neuropsychological assessments are not grounded solely in statistical probability. Second, base rates can be misleading in many circumstances. For instance, I once administered the Thematic Apperception Test (TAT) to a person in the pretrial phase of a legal proceeding. One of the patient's responses to the TAT provided words and concepts that could have come only from a person who witnessed the crime scene of a murder. The prosecutor's office shared the information with me, but it had not yet been provided to the defense. Only a person who had access to the crime scene could have known the details. The client denied being at the crime scene, knowing anyone who was at the crime scene, or having any knowledge of the crime. The TAT had functioned as it was supposed to by allowing the person to project their underlying thoughts and motives into the stories so they could be detected and assessed by the examiner. The same TAT cards could be administered to a thousand inmates with none of the protocols revealing a direct incontrovertible link to one of their specific crimes, yet this would not in the least diminish the confidence of the conclusion in the aforementioned case in which the test clearly provided unequivocal psychological evidence that the individual had direct knowledge of the crime scene. No proper comparison of clinical versus statistical prediction as described by Meehl (1954) could be made on such issues as the previous example because it is a rare event that required knowledge of specific situational facts.

Psychological tests of malingering also provide examples of the base-rate fallacy. First it must be recognized that without an actual confession on the part of an individual that they in fact were malingering, there is no absolute criteria to verify that malingering has occurred, so the base rate of malingering is likely to remain unknowable. Most psychological tests of malingering were developed in controlled situations where an individual is required to respond in ways that allow one to judge if the person is exaggerating symptoms and dysfunction. Statistical comparisons between experimental groups establish cut-off scores suggestive of malingering respondents. For many situations, clinical observations provide adequate evidence of malingering. Consider the following examples.

A person presented for assessment with a translator claiming brain injury from an accident. In the initial session I asked the patient if he knew the English alphabet. Knowledge was demonstrated by his quickly rattling off the first half of the alphabet in about 2 seconds. A week later the patient was administered the Wechsler Memory Scale–Revised (WMS–R). When asked to recite the alphabet as quickly as possible, he responded in a halting fashion, "A & B & C & E & G," and so on, with many omissions. Also, he did not complete the sequence within the generous time allowed by the test publisher. This was strong evidence of malingering conditional upon earlier performance. Interestingly, the same patient was unobtrusively observed getting into his car, at which time he threw his arm sling into the back seat, briskly hopped into the front seat, and whipped his bright and shiny new car very quickly and adeptly out of the parking lot in a manner that clearly was the antithesis of the disabled and faltering behavior presented in the consult room.

Even if this patient performed with no signs of malingering on the standardized tests of malingering, one might have to reasonably conclude that he was malingering and sophisticated enough to avoid detection on the standardized tests. Another clinical example comes from a man who a defense attorney described as suffering a "concussive closed head injury." The man had been initially diagnosed by a neuropsychologist as suffering from brain injury, but when the patient was retested months later the neuropsychologist changed his opinion, and concluded that the patient was malingering. When examined for a second opinion by the present author, the patient asserted that staff at the rehabilitation center had treated him poorly and were retaliating against him by saying he was malingering because he had complained about them. When asked to write his name on top of a blank page as part of a testing procedure, the patient demonstrated an inability to spell his first name correctly (and it was a name of four letters), leaving one letter out of the sequence and showing great awkwardness in forming all the letters. He presented as if he were a young child writing his name for the first time. Later in the session, the patient provided a further different and incorrect variant to the spelling of his first name. Examination of the patient's extensive medical records revealed some 30 examples of his signature and name written by himself at various times after the accident, the most recent dated a few days prior to the examination described earlier. When the patient was first admitted to the hospital after head injury, his signature was without flaw; when the patient signed a lien agreement with his attorney, his signature was excellent, and so fourth. The determination of malingering appeared evident from a knowledge of the patient's history and the neuropsychological functions involved supporting such behavior. Furthermore, neither prior neuropsychological testing at the rehabilitation center nor my neuropsychological testing revealed any meaningful pattern of disabilities consistent with this patient's apparent name dysgraphia. A diagnosis by clinical reasoning could be made with a great degree of psychological and professional certainty in this exemplary case based primarily on behavioral observations, tangible evidence of the patient's behavior, and knowledge of psychological and neuropsychological structure and function, rather than on base rates or statistical data.

**Objectivity and Balance**

Diamond (1973) reported that a "scrupulously honest" expert can seldom testify in a way that will have significance to the trier of fact (also see Diamond, 1959, 1983). Ziskin (1995a, 1995b, 1995c), on the other hand, asserted that the expert should "present a balanced picture that does not go

## Minimization of Confidence in the Opinion

Finally, consider the situation where the expert fails to understand that the court is asking for a medical or professional opinion held with medical or professional certainty, not an absolute conclusion beyond any reasonable doubt. The professional recognizes the shortcomings of psychological assessment techniques and, not wanting to overstate the certainty of these methods, he or she yields an opinion that would actually meet the standard of medical or professional certainty required by the court, but then proceeds to present the opinion as though it did not meet the criteria of medical or professional certainty. This can be seen in the many admonitions in the literature that no one can opine that a person is actually malingering or is a malingerer. In fact, there are many instances where such opinions are completely justified and appropriate. Ellard (1993–1994) discussed this problem in some detail. Nash (1982) in fact recommended the use of psychologists for the defense because their arguments are statistical and support reasonable-doubt arguments.

## Reasonable Medical Certainty Standard

Expert medical opinion is allowed when a person qualifies to have special knowledge in an area and can offer such information. However, an expert's opinion may be excluded if it has been rendered with the use of such qualifiers as possible or maybe (Beresford, 1992). The expectation within the legal arena is that the psychological expert will hold an opinion with reasonable medical certainty or reasonable medical probability. Diamond (1985) discussed the meaning of the term reasonable medical certainty and suggested that it should be defined by the scientific, not the legal community. One operational definition of reasonable medical certainty is that a doctor offers an opinion with the same level of certainty that he or she offers any diagnosis that the doctor gives, that is, that there is no special level of confidence required in the legal arena. The doctor does not have to be 51% or 80% confident, but needs simply to meet the criteria for the diagnosis that the doctor would normally use outside of court in general or specialty practice.

## Appropriate Advocacy

A good argument can be made for independent *advocacy of an expert's own opinion* and of the underlying clinical condition it represents. This is quite different from being an advocate for the plaintiff or the defense irrespective of the underlying clinical condition. It is entirely ethical for an expert to make a forceful presentation of data and reasoning for an opinion that the expert holds. Heilbronner and Karavidas (1997) gave voice to this approach in recommending that the expert neuropsychologist be "an advocate of the facts." Singer and Nievod (1987) provided the following advice that embodies the spirit of appropriate advocacy of opinion:

> To function well in the courtroom, the expert must be an articulate, interesting, and believable teacher. Most clinicians and professors live a protected life in which they talk of personality, behavior, and social interactions in abstractions and jargon that others (mostly students) are forced to adapt to by learning to decipher sphinxlike riddles. The forensic psychologist, on the other hand, must be able to explain technical and theoretical concepts in a manner that interests the juror in what is being said, in a style of language free from jargon, and with a demeanor that gives no hint of condescension. The elegance of well-reasoned, jargon-free explanations of behavior can be appreciated by judge and jury. The effective giving of expert testimony demands the expert maintain a quiet warmth and poised dignity, while keeping his or her emotions under control. The expert's attitude should imply knowledge and a willingness to be informative.
>
> It is the jury who literally decide how believable the testimony appears; the jury will base their decision on the total content, conduct, and person of the witness. The skills that enable one to be a credible and persuasive witness—speaking clearly in ordinary language, being adept at explaining ideas, having conviction in the knowledge one has and flexibility in admitting what one doesn't know—combined with an ability to relate in a warm, professional way are the same skills needed for effective consultation with attorneys. Truly forensic work is for psychologists well beyond their first years in the field for it appears to take some time to know one's field well enough to explain its workings in simple yet elegant terms. (p. 540)

Recently, Sweet and Moulthrop (1999) proposed a series of self-examination questions that neuropsychologists can ask themselves to determine how adversarial they might be in their practice (see Table 2.2).

Table 2.2
Self-Examination Questions
Recommended by Sweet and Moulthrop (1999)

---

1. Do I receive referrals from only plaintiff attorneys or only defense attorneys?
2. Do I almost always reach conclusions favorable to the side that has retained me?
3. Have I moved away from being an expert witness to being an advocate?
4. Do I form opinions of plaintiff or defense positions prematurely, without having enough facts for a solid opinion?
5. Have I taken a position, in very similar cases, when retained by an attorney from one side that I did not take when retained by the opposite side?
6. Do I routinely apply the same decision-rules for establishing brain dysfunction no matter which side retains me?
7. Have I been reaching the same diagnostic conclusion at a much higher base rate than my colleagues or at a higher rate than described in the literature?
8. Has my initial written opinion been altered by the time of deposition or trial testimony?

---

Self-examination may produce greater self-awareness when experts believe themselves to be objective, although secondary gain provided by success and financial reward may bias them. Questions about secondary gain are customarily addressed in the cross-examination of opposing experts. Exigencies suggest that in the short-run the expert is likely to be shaped toward greater advocacy by his or her participation in the adversarial system.

There is an increasing trend by the courts to examine and demand scientific validity and not just "general acceptance in the relevant professional community," which has come to be known as the Frye Test of the admissibility of expert evidence *(Frye v. U.S.,* 1923; Goodman-Delahunty, 1997; and Greenberg & Shuman, 1997). The U. S. Supreme Court ruling on *Daubert v. Merrell Dow Pharmaceuticals, Inc.* (113S.Ct. 2786, 1993) has raised the stakes in this matter. The court ruled that expert opinions should be supported by scientifically valid evidence and set the standard for making a "preliminary assessment of whether the reasoning or methodology underlying the testimony is scientifically valid and whether that reasoning properly can be applied to the facts in issue" (U.S. Supreme Court, 113S.Ct. 2786, 1993, p. 592). Hence, greater pressure is being placed upon experts to support their advocacy. Publications in peer review journals represent one method for establishing expert advocacy. However, it is unlikely that a neuropsychologist can consistently publish positions regarding current case work given the amount of work involved and the delays inherent to review and publication practices. A second and more accessible process is to incorporate scientifically and empirically sound statistical methods into the evaluation process. When properly constructed, hypothesis testing can be conducted at a clinical level by the examiner using all data available, including statistical methods, to develop clinical reasoning. Inclusion of a wide variety of evaluation techniques helps develop opinions held with reasonable medical or professional certainty that are most likely to reduce or or identify evaluator bias, the magnitude of injury effects, establishing loss effects, and differentially select between multiple putative etiologies and diagnoses.

## ACKNOWLEDGMENTS

Appreciation is expressed to Dr. Ronald D. Franklin, Dr. Jeffrey T. Barth, and law professor Mark Oring for their review and comments on the present article.

## REFERENCES

American Congress of Rehabilitation Medicine (The Mild Traumatic Brain Injury Committee of the Head Injury Interdisciplinary Special Interest Group). (1993). Definition of mild traumatic brain injury. *Journal of Head Trauma Rehabilitation, 8,* 86–87.

Beresford, H. R. (1992). Neurologist as expert witness. *Neurological Clinics: The Neurology of Trauma, 10,* (4), 1059–1071.

Bremner, J. D., Krystal, J. H., Southwick, S. M., Krystal, J. H., & Charney, D. S. (1995). Functional neuroanatomical correlates of the effects of stress on memory. *Journal of Traumatic Stress, 8,* 527–553.

Bronstein, D. A. (1999). *Law for the expert witness* (2nd ed.)., Boca Raton, FL: CRC Press.

*Daubert v. Merrell Dow Pharmaceuticals, Inc.,* 113 S. Ct. 2786 (1993).

Diamond, B. L. (1959). The fallacy of the impartial expert. In J. M. Quen (Ed.), *The psychiatrist in the courtroom: Selected papers of Bernard L. Diamond, M.D.* (pp. 221–232). Hillsdale, NJ: Analytic Press.

Diamond, B. L. (1973). The psychiatrist as advocate. *The Journal of Psychiatry and Law, 1,* 5–21.

Diamond, B. L. (1983). The psychiatrist as expert witness. In J. M. Quen (Ed.), *The psychiatrist in the courtroom: Selected papers of Bernard L. Diamond, M.D.* (pp. 233–248). Hillsdale, NJ: Analytic Press.

Diamond, B. L. (1985). Reasonable medical certainty, diagnostic thresholds, and definitions of mental illness in the legal context. *Bulletin of the American Academy of Psychiatry & the Law, 13,* 121–128.

Ellard, J. (1993–1994). Why the psychiatrist is an unsatisfactory witness and should remain one. *International Journal of Mental Health, 22,* 81–89.

Finn, S. E., & Kamphuis, J. H. (1995). What a clinician needs to know about base rates. In J. N. Butcher (Ed.), *Clinical personality assessment: Practical approaches* ( pp. 224–235). New York: Oxford University Press.

Foster, K. R., & Huber, P. W. (1997). *Judging science: Scientific knowledge and the federal courts.* Cambridge, MA: MIT Press.

*Frye v. U.S.,* 293 F. 1013 (D.C. Cir., 1923).

Goodman-Delahunty, J. (1997). Forensic psychological expertise in the wake of Daubert. *Law and Human Behavior, 21,* 121–140.

Gouvier, W. D. (1999). Base rates and clinical decision making in neuropsychology. In J. J. Sweet (Ed.), *Forensic neuropsychology: Fundamentals and practice* (pp. 25–37). Lisse, Netherlands: Swets & Zeitlinger.

Greenberg, S. A., & Shuman, D. W. (1997). Irreconcilable conflict between therapeutic and forensic roles. *Professional Psychology: Research and Practice, 28,* 50–57.

Hagen, M. A. (1997). *Whores of the court: The fraud of psychiatric testimony and the rape of American justice.* New York: HarperCollins.

Heilbronner, R. L., & Karavidas, T. (1997). Presenting neuropsychological evidence in traumatic brain injury litigation. *The Clinical Neuropsychologist, 11,* 445–453.

Heilman, K. M., & Satz, P. (Eds.). (1983). *Neuropsychology of emotion.* New York: Guilford.

Huber, P. W. (1991). *Galileo's revenge: Junk science in the courtroom.* New York: Basic Books.

Jones, S. E. (2001). Ethics code draft published for comment. *Monitor on Psychology, 32*(2).

Kuvin, S. F. (1986). Psychiatric disability evaluations: Malingering, advocacy, bias. *American Journal of Forensic Psychiatry, 7* (10), 23.

Lichter, D. G., & Cummings, J. L. (Eds.). (2001). *Frontal-subcortical circuits in psychiatric and neurological disorders.* New York: Guilford.

Marcus, E. H. (1983). Reality and psychiatric reality in litigation. *American Journal of Forensic Psychiatry, 4,* 167–168.

Marcus, E. H. (1985). Unbiased medical testimony: Reality or myth? *American Journal of Forensic Psychiatry, 6,* 3–5.

Marcus, E. H. (1986a). Psychiatric disability evaluations: Plaintiff and defense perspectives. *American Journal of Forensic Psychiatry, 7,* 11–19.

Marcus, E. H. (1986b). Response to Dr. Kuvin's letter "Call for common sense." *American Journal of Forensic Psychiatry, 7* (24), 40, 58.

Markowitsch, H. J., Kessler, J., Van der Ven, C., Weber-Luxenburger, G., Albers, M., & Wolf-Dieter, H. (1998). Psychic trauma causing grossly reduced brain metabolism and cognitive deterioration. *Neuropsychologia, 36,* 77–82.

McAllister, T. W., & Flashman, L. A. (1999). Mild brain injury and mood disorders: Casual connections, assessment, and treatment. In N. R. Varney, & R. J. Roberts (Eds.), *The evaluation and treatment of mild traumatic brain injury* (pp. 347–373). Mahwah, NJ: Lawrence Erlbaum Associates.

Meehl, P. E. (1954). *Clinical versus statistical prediction: A theoretical analysis and a review of the evidence.* Minneapolis: University of Minnesota Press.

Moser, R. S., & Barbrack, C. R. (2000). An urgent call: Treating psychologists are not expert witnesses. *The Independent Practitioner, 20,* 279–281.

Nash, B. (1982). The psychologist as expert witness: A solicitor's view. *Issues in Criminological & Legal Psychology, 3,* 32–38.

Sbordone, R. J. (1998). The ecological validity of neuropsychological testing. In A. M. Horton, D. Wedding, & J. Webster (Eds.), *The neuropsychology handbook: Behavioral and clinical perspectives* (pp. 1–51). New York: Springer.

Simkins, C. N. (1997). Analysis and evaluation of traumatic brain injury from the perspective of a trial lawyer. *Seminars in Clinical Neuropsychiatry, 2,* 216–221.

Singer, M. T., & Nievod, A. (1987). Consulting and testifying in court. In I. B. Weiner & A. K. Hess (Eds.), *Handbook of Forensic Psychology* (pp. 529–554). New York: Wiley.

Sweet, J. J., & Moulthrop, M. A. (1999). Self-examination questions as a means of identifying bias in adversarial assessments. *Journal of Forensic Neuropsychology, 1,* 73–88.

Veiel, H. O. F. (1997). A preliminary profile of neuropsychological deficits associated with major depression. *Journal of Clinical and Experimental Neuropsychology, 19,* 587–603.

Weiner, I. B. (1995). How to anticipate ethical and legal challenges in personality assessments. In J. N. Butcher (Ed.), *Clinical personality assessment: Practical approaches* (pp. 95-103). New York: Oxford University Press.

Ziskin, J. (1995a). *Coping with psychiatric and psychological testimony: Vol. 1. Basic information* (5th ed.). Los Angeles: Law and Psychology Press.

Ziskin, J. (1995b). *Coping with psychiatric and psychological testimony: Vol. 2. Special topics* (5th ed.). Los Angeles: Law and Psychology Press.

Ziskin, J. (1995c). *Coping with psychiatric and psychological testimony: Vol. 3. Practical guidelines, cross-examination, and case illustrations* (5th ed.). Los Angeles: Law and Psychology Press.

Ziskin, J., & Faust, D. (1988). *Coping with psychiatric and psychological testimony* (Vols. 1–3, 4th ed.). Marina Del Rey, CA: Law and Psychology Press.

# Neuropsychological Hypothesis Testing

**Ronald D. Franklin, Ph.D.** [1]
*St. Mary's Hospital, and Florida Atlantic University*

> *The rationale for conservatism in statistical testing for sample differences is strikingly similar to the one that guides the proceedings in a U.S. court of law. The rule in a criminal trial is that the defendant is to be presumed innocent and can be judged guilty only if the prosecution proves guilt beyond a reasonable doubt. Furthermore, the trial can yield one of only two possible verdicts: guilty or not guilty. Not guilty, in this context, is not synonymous with innocent; it means only that guilt was not demonstrated with a high degree of certainty. Proof of innocence is not a requirement for this verdict; innocence is a presumption, and like the null hypothesis, it is to be rejected only on the basis of compelling evidence that it is false. (Nickerson, 2000 p. 243).*

This chapter addresses many issues that, in their own right, have been the topics of books. Consequently, treatment of each is limited, focusing upon those appearing with some frequency in the neuropsychology literature as well as in my personal experience in the teaching and practice of clinical neuropsychology. Many clinicians enter practice having received instruction in introductory statistics, test and measurement, and perhaps one additional course in nonparametric or parametric modeling [2]. The present

---

[1] Please address correspondence to PO Box 246, Candor, NC 27229 or rdfphd@yahoo.com.

[2] Readers with less preparation, or those who may be a bit "rusty" are encouraged to review one of the recent texts on these topics cited in this

chapter is written with this reader in mind. My interns often view probability statements as a form or evidence of "proof." Discussions between practitioners at national and international meetings provide me with little basis for thinking that the views of interns change after graduation. Because psychology is so prone to confirmation bias (see Faust, Ziskin, & Hiers; 1991 Nickerson, 1998), a clear understanding of statistical modeling is particularly important in clinical applications. The purpose of this chapter is to provide readers with the requisite tools for using formal hypothesis testing as a method for reducing the confirmation bias that might otherwise occur in their clinical work.

The clinical literature rarely discusses hypothesis testing in the practice of psychological assessment, and less often for the sub-specialty of neuropsychology. Informal reviews of the workshop titles I have received during the preceding year suggests the range of hypothetical questions presented in clinical practice focuses on permutations of eight issues. These issues all relate to predicting diagnosis, prior function, or outcome. There are three principal goals to this chapter. First I discuss restating hypotheses in forms that are suitable for statistical testing. Consumers of the neuropsychological literature often read about the importance of *alpha*, base rate and effect size. Inconsistent use of these terms in the literature has produced considerable confusion among clinical practitioners. A second goal of this chapter is clarification of those terms that are important to the objective evaluation of clinical hypotheses. The third goal addresses use of computer programs such as spreadsheets, which have become so "user friendly" that clinicians may be tempted to apply *t*-tests indiscriminately to each measure they administer, even though most neuropsychological tests violate the data assumptions for which parametric models are appropriate. Also I identify psychological tests that are most appropriate for parametric analysis and those most appropriate for analysis using nonparametric tests. The overuse of parametric test statistics in neuropsychology could lead readers to believe that parametric models are superior to nonparametric models. This is not the case. Superior evaluation occurs when the neuropsychologist applies the statistical test that is most appropriate to the available data. In keeping with the three principal goals of the chapter, it is organized into three sections.

---

work.

The first section discusses hypothesis formulation addressing prediction of prior, future, and current neuropsychological function. The second section describes technical components of hypothesis testing. Included in this section are descriptions of independent and dependent variables as well as error, power, and specificity. Two probability models are described, Frequentist and Bayesian. The third section reviews statistical tests appropriate for evaluating significance and association of psychological and neuropsychological test data.

## HYPOTHETICAL QUESTIONS

When a neuropsychologist first meets a patient and asks "How may I help you?" the evaluation begins. On occasion the evaluation opens with reviews of medical or other historical information. This first encounter often produces an "initial impression" that forms the basis of subsequent hypothesis testing. Further assessment serves to either support or modify this primacy effect. Social psychology research addressing the primacy effect demonstrates its potential for producing considerable bias. Critics of neuropsychological methods, such as Faust, et al. (1991) claim that bias is pervasive within neuropsychology. One way to control for this type of bias is to carefully identify diagnostic and treatment hypotheses and test them using statistical models. Three types of questions must be addressed during each evaluation: questions regarding the patient's current status, prior status, and future status.

### Questions Regarding Current Patient Status

Many questions arise during and following neuropsychological assessment. The following examples represent variations of the themes presented previously.

*Are findings abnormal?* Do the patient's signs and symptoms correspond with normal variations or do they reflect a pathological process? Is malingering a concern? What sorts of secondary gain might symptoms provide the patient or family members? If a history of injury or disease is reported, do the complaints correspond to the disorder? Faust et al. (1991) presented evidence that neuropsychologists grossly over diagnose pathology. Neuropsychologists tend to overly rely on historical information, in particular the diagnoses of medical professionals, and attribute infrequency (i.e., in this context, low scores on tests or unusual response patterns) to pathology.

*Are Findings Characteristic of a Pathological Process?*
Researchers experienced in model systems recognize that individual differences occurring within simple species (ie., rats) are huge! Normal variations in humans have even larger ranges. Consequently, carefully constructed psychological tests are often the best tool for identifying behavior patterns in humans that deviate from normal in subtle ways. They can also prove helpful in classifying the degree of abnormality. Classification of intellectual abilities, as well as some learning disorders, using standardized testing has been codified by government agencies. Though controversy remains in these classifications, the superiority of psychological test measures over other mechanisms of stratification has been established for some time.

*Which Pathological Process is Suggested?* Typically they are developed independently of medical nosology. Tests and measures evaluate constructs not diseases. For decades neuropsychologists have "mined" test data and developed new tests in hopes of finding response patterns that can serve as markers for specific disorders. Few markers of disease have emerged. Yet, test findings are often helpful in establishing both differential diagnosis and identifying treatment strategies.

*Are Multiple Pathological Processes Implicated?* Because neuropsychological tests evaluate brain function rather than pathology, multiple disorders can produce similar neuropsychological findings. Statistical adjuncts to hypothesis testing can identify differences in data structures unapparent on visual inspection.

*Of All Possible Pathological Processes Suggested, Which Is Most Likely?* Statistical hypothesis testing provides an important tool for identifying which of two diagnoses is more likely. When multiple diagnostic options exist, sequential comparisons are helpful in decision making as well.

### Questions Regarding Prior or Future Status

*Do Findings Represent a Change From Prior Function?* For traumatic injuries, the most important question in litigation often addresses cognitive and affective changes attributable to a specific injury. Few patients can provide data representing prior function. Statistical methods are sometimes the only practical option for estimating preinjury abilities.

***Do Findings Represent a Change Since Initial Diagnosis?***
Progressive conditions, such as dementia of the Alzheimer's type, produce decline in cognitive function over time. Other forms of dementia present frank clinical signs but show stability over time. The use of statistical adjuncts to data interpretation allows neuropsychologists to identify trends earlier and more precisely than does visual inspection alone.

***Do Findings Indicate Additional Improvement Is Likely?*** For patients who have sustained head injuries, a determination regarding when maximal medical improvement (MMI) is reached is necessary for the settlement of compensation claims. It is also an important issue in litigation following traumatic injury. Well-planned integration of statistical methods with hypothesis testing clarifies change analysis.

***If Additional Improvement Is Likely, Do Findings Suggest Which Interventions May Benefit the Patient?*** On occasions where assessment indicates that additional interventions will be helpful, statistical analysis may be useful in establishing the type of treatment that will offer greatest benefit. Analysis may also indicate which order of treatment will provide most improvement in the least time.

## HYPOTHESIS MODELING

### General Considerations

In science, hypotheses are stated in terms that are observable, replicable and objective. Formal (or *classical*) hypothesis testing involves comparisons of objective observations, referred to as data samples. Statistical evaluation compares one sample with another or with a hypothetical distribution. Table 3.1 presents the possible outcomes associated with hypothesis testing.

***Type I Error ($\alpha$, False Alarm).*** Two possibilities exist for the null hypothesis. It is either rejected or it is not. When a hypothesis is rejected but is in fact true, researchers commit a Type I error. Establishment of a maximum acceptable Type I error rate is fixed in advance when a null hypothesis is used (typically as .01 or .05 by convention), and referred to as $\alpha$. Error rate, when used in connection with $\alpha$, is often misinterpreted to be the actual rate of the commission of Type I error, when it really is the rate only under certain assumptions, one of which is that the null is true. Type I errors are possible only when the hypothesis is true.

TABLE 3.1
Probabilities associated with hypothesis testing

| Actual Effect | Concluded Effect | |
|---|---|---|
| | (Reject H$_o$)<br>*Accept* | (Do not Reject H$_o$)<br>*Reject* |
| *Accept*<br>(H$_o$ False) | Sensitivity<br>1 minus β<br>Power | Miss<br>β<br>Type II Error |
| *Reject*<br>(H$_o$ True) | Type I Error<br>α<br>False Alarm | True Negative<br>1 minus α<br>Specificity |

***Type II error ( β, Miss ).*** A Type II error occurs when an evaluator fails to reject the null hypothesis when the hypothesis is actually false, and its probability is represented by β. Note, α can be fixed by the evaluator in advance but β can be fixed in advance only when a specific alternative hypothesis is stated or assumed. Type II errors are possible only when the hypothesis is false.

***Power (sensitivity).*** Power (1- β) is often interpreted as having two meanings. Most often it represents the probability of detecting an effect. Alternatively, power represents the probability of accepting the alternative hypothesis conditional on its being true. Following Cohen's (1988) recommendations many investigators consider .80 an "acceptable" power and .90 as "desirable." Establishment of acceptable levels of α and β is a *subjective* process set by each neuropsychologist, based on their personal values and the knowledge available to them about the evaluation conditions. Factors influencing the establishment of α and β levels in neuropsychology would include: a. cost of evaluation or treatment relative to each error rate; b. availability of similar less expensive evaluations or treatments; c. seriousness of disorder and d. potential for misdiagnosis or iatrogenic reactions.

*Specificity.* In diagnostic testing, the term *specificity* is used to denote the probability that an individual who does *not* have the disorder under study will test negative for the disorder (i.e., the probability of true negative).

## Probability Models

Two types of probability models are common to hypothesis testing, *Frequentist* and *Bayesian*. The Frequentist models evaluate data error and recognize three major divisions:  estimation , hypothesis testing, and confidence intervals. Bayesian statistical methods are distinctive at every level, most notably by the inclusion of subjective or prior (posterior) knowledge parameters. They differ from frequentist methods with respect to the formal probability models that are used, the meaning associated with the probabilities in the models, how the variables within the models are manipulated in analyses and the results. Two Frequentist models have been developed, Neyman-Pearson and Fisherian. The Neyman-Pearson is the older model.

### *Frequentist Models*

*Neyman-Pearson.* The Neyman-Pearson approach tests which of two hypotheses is more probable. Statistical test procedures are evaluated in terms of error probabilities. The probabilistic properties of the Neyman-Pearson model apply to a decision-making procedures of a statistical test, thereby representing properties of the test procedures, not of results. These properties measure the expected, or long-run average, performance of the procedures.

*Fisherian.* Fisher began comparing data observations to a preselected critical region of an expected distribution.  In doing so he became the first to mention a "null" hypothesis ($H_o$) as opposed to two hypotheses as used in Neyman-Pearson. $H_o$ states that no difference exists between two or more data sets with respect to some parameter (usually the mean).  Implied is an *alternative hypothesis* ($H_A$ ) stating that some difference is present.  Statistical tests used in the evaluation of this hypothesis are referred to as Null Hypothesis Statistical Tests (NHST). Probabilities can represent either absolute or relative relationships, but

NHSTs *always* test *relative* relationships. Fisher's modification appears today in two types of assessment, known as *p*-value procedures (or Acceptance Support Null Hypothesis Testing, AS-NHST) and rejection trials (or Rejection Support Null Hypothesis Testing, RS-NHST) (Meehl, 1997 ).

Statistical significance is not equivalent to importance. Rather, in null hypothesis testing, Snow (1977, cited in Pedhazur & Schmelking, 1991) stated "it is the probability that specific evidence appears if the null hypothesis were true" (p. 201). Nickerson (2000) noted: To say that a result is statistically significant is to say that the probability of obtaining that result if there were no factors operating but chance is small. Application of NHST to the difference between two means yields a value of $p$, the theoretical probability that if two samples of the size of those used had been drawn at random from the same population, the statistical test would have yielded a statistic (e.g., $t$ ) as large or larger than the one obtained. (p. 263) Misconceptions regarding null hypothesis testing are common and a summary adapted from Nickerson appears in Table 3.2. Much of this chapter is based on Nickerson's eloquent review of hypothesis testing appearing in Volume five of *Psychological Methods*.

*AS-NHST (p-Values procedures).* Acceptance of the null hypothesis supports the view of the evaluator. AS-NHST is often considered as representative of the "strength of evidence." But, inherent in the $p$ value is the probability of both what was observed *and* what was not observed. So AS-NHST as a measure of strength of evidence is weak. Because $p$ values vary with sample size, a given $p$ value does not have a fixed meaning. The meanings of Type I and Type II errors become transposed from those presented in Table 3.3 during AS-NHST.

In psychological assessment, differences between test scores are termed "significant" when the relative frequency of the observed score in the standardization sample is low. Jerome Sattler (1988) provided tables for comparing many test score differences at .05 and .01 significance levels. This practice has been adopted by test publishers as well, the Psychological Corporation (1997) for example.

*RS-NHST (Rejection-Support).* This is another term used for the more common and stronger model of null hypothesis testing. In this view, $H_o$ represents what the evaluator *does not* believe. Rejection of $H_o$ implies that it is false, thereby supporting the beliefs of the evaluator. *Rejection trials* represent the hypothesis whose nullification, by statistical means,

TABLE 3.2
Common Misconceptions Associated With NHST

---

- $p$ is the probability that $H_o$ is true and $1-p$ is the probability that $H_A$ is true.
- Rejection of $H_o$ establishes the truth of a theory that predicts it to be false.
- A small $p$ is evidence that results are replicable.
- A small value of $p$ means a treatment effect of large magnitude.
- Statistical significance means theoretical or practical significance.
- $\alpha$ is the probability that if one has rejected $H_o$ one has made a Type I error.
- The value at which $\alpha$ is set for a given experiment is the probability that a Type I error will be made in interpreting the results of that experiment.
- The value at which $\alpha$ is set is the probability of Type I error across a large set of experiments which $\alpha$ is set at that value.
- Failing to reject $H_o$ is equivalent to demonstrating it to be true.
- Failure to reject $H_o$ is evidence of a failed experiment.
- $\beta$ is the probability that $H_o$ is false, conditional on having failed to reject it.
- $\beta$ is the absolute probability of committing a Type II error.

---

*Note.* From Nickerson (2000), Copyright 2000 by the American Psychological Association, adapted by Ronald D. Franklin.


would be taken as evidence in support of a specified alternative hypothesis ($H_A$). However, the alternative hypothesis is not the opposite of the null (e.g., $H_A \cong 1- H_o$ rather than $H_A = 1- H_o$). A RS-NHST can be disproved but not proved, rejected but not accepted. If $H_o$ is tested and fails, it is rejected; if not, it may be replicated under similar or different circumstances. Rejection trials are viewed as challenges to the single nullhypothesis. If the observation is in the rejection region, then the hypothesis fails the challenge and is rejected; otherwise the result is "Do not reject $H_o$."

### Bayes as Evidence

Two approaches to Bayesian analysis appear in the psychological literature; *estimation of posterior probabilities* and *likelihood ratios*. For a more complete discussion of estimation see Chapter 4. The Bayesian method offers several advantages in hypothesis testing. First, it permits evidence to strengthen either $H_o$ or $H_A$. Second, Bayes' methods allow inferences regarding the population effect (see Rouanet, 1996, 1998). Third, Bayes relates prior knowledge from base rates (i.e., $br_p$) to outcome. Fourth, Bayes' methods provide procedures for cumulating the effects of evidence across studies over time.

***Estimation of Posterior Probabilities.*** Posterior probabilities consider the likelihood of the null hypothesis given the data ($p(H_o|D)$) where $p$ represents probability, $H_o$ the hypothesis, and D the data.

$$p(Ho|D) = \frac{p(H)o * p(D|Ho)}{p(D)} \quad (3.1)$$

***Likelihood Ratios.*** Likelihood ratios ($\lambda$), also known as *Bayes factors*, are discussed in chapter 5. They represent the ratio of probabilities associated with two hypotheses. The ratio is based on the law of likelihood and compares the relative abilities of measures to identify one distribution as more likely to contain a particular observation than another distribution.
See chapter 4, this volume, for additional discussion.

$$\lambda = \frac{p(H)o}{p(H)_A} \quad (3.2)$$

## STATISTICAL METHODS FOR HYPOTHESIS TESTING

As hypotheses are developed, factors influencing the evaluation of each hypothesis should be considered. These factors should minimally include identification of independent and dependent variables, data characteristics of dependent variables, and the assumptions necessary for statistical testing.

**Type of Hypothesis Being Tested (Independent Variables).**

The questions presented earlier form the basis of independent variables. Table 3.3 presents each statement and then re-forms each statement as an hypothesis.

**Type of Data Available (Dependent Variables)**

*Observations*

Qualitative aspects of a patient's presentation are often incorporated into the evaluation. Many behavior patterns have been identified as indicative of "pathological" states (Goldberg, 1987; Golden, Purisch, & Hammeke, 1991). When present, qualitative information can be evaluated as occurring or not occurring. Interrater and intrarater reliability measures may be helpful for demonstrating both reliability of measurement and symptom presentation (see Franklin, Allison, & Gorman, 1997). Observations such as these may be evaluated using nonparametric statistical tests as can other measures having pass/fail criteria. Likewise, completion of certification programs such as high school, general equivalent diploma, trade school, or college can be included in statistical testing.

Some tests for which no adult populations are reported in the standardization samples (i.e., the *Motor Free Visual Perception Test* or the *Vineland Adaptive Behavior Scales*) can be evaluated similarly because adults would be expected to master all of the items.

*Performance Ratings*

Nonparametric testing is also recommended for comparison of ranked data. The following categories of measures rank data, but are unable to demonstrate the assumption of equal intervals between score points as is appropriate for parametric testing.

*Equivalent Scores.* Tests of academic abilities often provide age or grade equivalents for raw score values. Both equivalent measures represent rankings. Adults with brain damage may not perform at a level appropriate to their age, but their performance on ranked tests may be helpful in measuring treatment progress. Also, scores from ranked tests may be available from school records and serve as a basis for establishing a preinjury performance level against which current function can be evaluated.

TABLE 3.3
Restatement of Referral Questions as Testable Hypotheses
Suitable for Independent Variables

| Question | Hypothesis |
| --- | --- |
| *Are findings abnormal?* | Test scores presented by the patient are no different from the average score presented by the "normal" standardization group. |
| *Which pathological process is suggested?* | Test scores presented by the patient are no different than average scores observed in groups of patients known to have a given disorder. |
| *Are multiple pathological processes implicated?* | Test scores presented by the patient are no different than average test scores of individuals having more than one known pathological process. |
| *Of the possible pathological processes suggested, which is most likely?* | Data are more like findings from Diagnosis Group A than from Diagnosis Group B. |
| *Do findings represent a change from prior function?* | There is no difference between test scores at Time 1, preinjury, and Time 2, postinjury (now). |
| *Do findings represent a change since initial diagnosis?* | There is no difference between test scores at Time 1, prediagnosis, and Time 2, postdiagnosis (now). |
| *Do findings indicate additional improvement is likely?* | Changes in scores observed between testings at Time 1 and Time 2 are no different than changes observed in patients who improve further. |
| *If additional improvement is likely, do findings suggest which interventions may benefit the patient?* | Scores are more like patients who improve when receiving Treatment A than like patients who improve when receiving Treatment B. |

*Impairment Ratings.* Ratings of impairment (see chap. 9, this volume) such as the Glasgow Coma Scale, Halstead Impairment Index, and the Disability Rating Scale provide interval comparisons. Many have been correlated with other measures such as outcome.

## Tests From Neuropsychological Laboratories

Nonparametric statistical tests should be used with specialty tests developed in neuropsychology laboratories. At the time of this writing, none of the laboratory- developed tests reviewed by Spreen and Strauss (1998) or Miturshina, Boone, and D'Elia (1999) provided adequately stratified standardized samples to demonstrate properties appropriate to analysis using parametric statistical tests. Many of the instruments report "norms," but their reliance on subjects of convenience and small sample sizes for both experimental and control groups makes nonparametric statistical analysis more appropriate for hypothesis testing. Dependent variables reported for this group of instruments include means, standard deviations, and occasionally standard scores.

*SS (Including Percentile Scores).* Care must be taken in interpreting standard scores for many neuropsychological tests. Data distributions for experimental groups termed "brain damaged" likely contain considerable skew and kurtosis. Inferences from parametric tests, particularly the Pearson product-moment correlation, is misleading under these conditions.

*Effect Size.* Evaluation of effect size using Sign, $\phi$, and $\chi^2$ provide the most appropriate comparisons when the evaluation produces as few as 4-7 data points. Computer programs such as Quattro-Pro and Excel provide $\chi^2$ analysis as do statistical software packages. The sign test and $\phi$ are available in software packages also. *Statistica* (Statsoft, 1994) provides all three as well as providing the user with excellent data management and graphics capabilities.

*Correlational Studies.* Excellent nonparametric measures of association are available as well. Spearman's $R$, like the parametric Pearson, is based upon proportion of variability and has similar interpretation. The Kendall *tau* provides the probability that two variables are in the *same order* in the data set. Tied observations are not uncommon in neuropsychological evaluation using nonparametric data. On occasions when visual inspection of compared scores indicates many ties, the Gamma statistic is preferred. Like the *tau,* the Gamma statistic evaluates the probability of comparable ranks.

## *Census-Stratified, Randomly Sampled Standardization Groups*

Psychological tests having standardization groups that were randomly selected from stratified samples matching census data are appropriate for analysis using parametric statistical tests. Conormed tests are preferred. The difficulty in comparing two census-matched samples that have not been conormed arises from two principal areas: differences in the standardization groups and differences in age cohorts within each standardization group (see Table 3.4).

TABLE 3.4
Age groupings from six neuropsychological tests

| Std. Prog. Matrix | Color Prog. Matrix | Advance Prog. Matrix | Design Fluency Test | Modified Stroop Test | PASAT |
|---|---|---|---|---|---|
| 18-22 | 55-65 | 18-22 | 14-55 | 17-29 | 16-29 |
| 23-27 | 65-74 | 23-27 | 58-72 | 30-39 | 30-49 |
| 28-32 | 75-85 | 28-32 | | 40-49 | 50-69 |
| 33-37 | | 33-37 | | | 60-69 |
| 38-42 | | 38-42 | | | 70-79 |
| 43-47 | | 43-47 | | | 80+ |
| 48-52 | | 48-52 | | | |
| 53-57 | | 53-57 | | | |
| 58-62 | | 58-62 | | | |
| 63-67 | | 63-67 | | | |
| 68+ | | 68+ | | | |

When test authors provide descriptions for their standardization groups, direct comparisons with other tests are quite difficult. Test publishers rarely provide adequate statistical descriptions of their samples. Consequently, direct comparisons of test scores are often misleading. Poorly organized presentations of standardization samples are also problematic.     The *Wechsler Adult Intelligence Scale-v. 3(WAIS-III)/Wechsler Memory Scale-v.3 (WMS-III)* provides so many tables that determining the percentages of each gender in the standardization sample is a labor-intensive process, especially because the tables are cross-referenced with many other bits of information, such as age and education level. Consequently, psychologists often ignore these important differences in their evaluations, instead relying on comparisons of correlated scores between the tests while ignoring standardization concerns. Correlations all to often rely on small sample sizes. For example, *Technical Manual* comparisons between the WAIS-III and Stanford Binet, v. 4 (SB-IV) are based on only 26 subjects. The procedures described by Chluney in chapter 6, this volume, are appropriate for comparing tests with census-matched samples. However, the effects of regression to the mean are unknown for many tests and standard error likely underestimates true error to a statistically significant degree.

*Standard Scores (Including Percentile Scores)*. Standard scores are preferred by many as the dependent variable of choice. I prefer standardized *z* scores for discussions with patients because they provide the easiest conversions to effect size and more clearly communicate strengths and weaknesses. The standardized *z* score converts all "problem" scores to minus values so the sign of the score is indicative of performance direction. Differences between scores are more clearly communicated when they are presented as absolute values. For statistical calculations *directionally adjusted standard scores* are preferred. Again, directionally adjusted refers to converting all deficits to below the mean. This sounds difficult but is easily accomplished on a spread sheet by first converting to standardized *z* scores and then converting back to a standard score. The procedure results in a conversion of all scores to the same mean and standard deviation (see internet site at http://www.geocities.com/rdfphd/index.html).

$$d = \frac{S_1 - S_2}{\sigma} \qquad (3.3)$$

*Effect Size*. Pearson's R can be used to measure effect size directly or Cohen's *d* can be calculated from scores standardized to the same mean and standard deviation as shown in Equation 3. However, interpretations of the size of effect for the two measures differ (see Table 3.5). A larger *d* than *r* is necessary for an effect size to be considered "large" (.80 compared to .50 ).

TABLE 3.5
Effect Size Equivalents of $r$ and $r^2$

| $d$ | $r$ | $r^2$ |
| --- | --- | --- |
| 0.50 | .243 | .059 |
| 1. | .447 | .200 |
| 1.50 | .600 | .360 |
| 2.00 | .707 | .500 |
| 3.00 | .832 | .692 |
| 4.00 | .894 | .800 |

*Correlational Studies.*  Pearson's product moment correlation is used to compare *Population Samples* (note population here refers to census-matched standardization groups rather than the universal population associated with statistical theory).  Correlations measure the degree of association between two samples and the square of Pearson's correlation ($r^2$ - *coefficient of determination*) measures the degree to which Variable A predicts Variable B.  Therefore, from a Pearson correlation ®) of .80 between Test A and Test B (or Test A at Time 1 vs. Time 2), the predicted score is correct 64% of the time, incorrect 36% of the time.

**Statistical Assumptions Appropriate to the Dependent Variables**

Measurements taken in evaluation of the independent variables must be reliable and valid for the testing purpose.  Volumes have been written on these topics by others (Faust, et al. 1991; Lezak, 1995; Thorndike, 1997; and Sattler, 1988 to name a few).  Still, the following points can not be over emphasized.  Because many psychological and most neuropsychological disorders are of low incidence, base rates and effect size estimates are of particular relevance.

*Reliability*

Reliability refers to the degree that a test is free of both systematic and unsystematic error.  Each test item should produce the same response from a subject each time it is presented unless there has been some change in either the respondent or the testing condition.  Likewise, persons administering tests should do so in the same way each time, under similar circumstances each time.  Control of item administration can be preserved as is reflected in excellent reliability correlations for many test items.  Yet, test environments often vary significantly and environmental effects may be unknown. Differences in test scores taken in hospital may produce very different responses than might be obtained in a quiet and comfortable office setting postdischarge. Score differences between inpatient and outpatient settings may have nothing to do with the patient's abilities but reflect the stress and uncertainty of hospitalization. Does, for example, a Child Orientation and Amnesia Test (COAT) score of two standard deviations below age mean constitute adequate criteria for initiating neuropsychological assessment of acute care patients following head trauma as proposed by Taylor, Wade, Yeates, Drotar, and Klein (1999)? This, and similar practices, must be questioned because rating scales such as the COAT have weak psychometric properties and scores can reflect a wide variety of conditions in awareness. Reliability problems can originate from two principal sources, measurement constraints and behavior constraints. (For a discussion see Pedhazer & Schmelkin, 1991.)

The level of acceptable reliability as measured by correlation has been the subject of debate. Nunnally has recommended both .50 and .70 (cited in Pedhazur et. al, 1991). Cohen (1988) recommended .80. Because the degree of shared variance represented by the square of the correlation coefficient of .80 provides 64% predictive power, Cohen's position is more acceptable when the use of data can have lifelong consequences for a patient. A maximum predictive power that is no better than chance, as occurs when $r$ falls below .71, is clearly unacceptable.

*Validity*

Validity refers to an overall *evaluative judgment* regarding the meaning of test scores, rather than some property of the test (Messick, 1995). In Cronbach's view (1971) validity includes implications for action associated with these evaluative judgments: "As such, validation combines scientific inquiry with rational argument to justify (or nullify) score interpretation and use" (p.443). In clinical practice, one often hears the question "validity for what?" Yet, Hagen (1988) argued that validity does not represent a criterion against which any form of inference should be measured. Ultimately, then, the validity of neuropsychological findings relies on the training and judgment of the clinician, rather than on findings from a series of neuropsychological tests. The true meaning of validity is how well data generalize to real life. In recent years, metaanalysis techniques have demonstrated the ability to produce reasonably robust predictors by combining several weak predictors (Rosenthal, 1984).

*Types of Validity.* Classical measurement theory describes three validity functions: *predictive, assessment,* and *trait measurement* (Nunnally, 1972). Predictive validity is based on the statistical correlation between a measure and the behavior that measure is intended to predict (it is more commonly referred to as *criterion validity,* and is referenced as such hereafter). Assessment validity refers to measuring the "effectiveness of performance" at a given point in time, also termed *content validity.* Trait measurement validity, or *construct validity* in this chapter, refers to evaluation of a psychological term, such as *brain damaged.*

TABLE 3.6
Validity for Forensic Issues

---

- It is the basis for determining what a *fact* means.
- A test may be a satisfactory method of determining current performance in some other realm but may be of minimal usefulness for predicting future performance.
- One wishes to know how scores on the test relate to pragmatic aspects of current, future, or past status, such as whether an individual is intellectually capable of resuming work, now or in the future.

---

Gresham (1997) discussed two approaches for validity in psychometric tests, classical test theory and generalizability theory. For a complete review of generalizability theory, see Cook and D. T. Campbell (1976, 1979). The theory describes *statistical conclusion validity,* construct validity, internal validity, and external validity. Statistical conclusion validity refers to the appropriate use of conclusions and inferences drawn from statistical tests. *Internal validity* addresses the effects of the independent variable on the dependent variable. *External validity* measures generalizability of findings across different populations or to representative target populations.

*Validity Constraints.* Diagnosis may be the most important clinical activity for neuropsychologists because it forms the core of their financial support. *The Diagnostic and Statistical Manual of Mental Disorders* 4th ed. – Text Revision_ (DSM-IV-TR; American Psychiatric Association, 2000) serves as the standard for diagnosis in psychology; however, it poorly represents neurocognitive syndromes. What is more, few neuropsychological tests were designed to represent diagnostic constructs from either *DSM* or *International Classification of Disease (ICD)*. Neuropsychological findings are more often "consistent with" than "markers for" a given diagnosis. For these and other reasons Faust et al. (1991) criticized the validity of neuropsychological tests as it relates to forensic issues. Table 3.6 summarizes their concerns, all of which address external validity.

*External Validity.* The validity of neuropsychological tests has also been criticized because test measures poorly predict outcome (see chap. 9, this volume). Test patterns that are predictive in clinical settings but not others lack external validity. This problem is often termed "limited ecological validity" in neuropsychology.

## Data Distributions

Data are the dependent variable measures. In hypothesis testing, data are often classified and compared based on the distribution of scores. Two types of data groupings, nonparametric and parametric, are made based largely on the way data are distributed. Hopefully, readers are familiar with nonparametric data types (nominal and ordinal) as well as parametric types (interval and ratio). Readers unfamiliar with these data distinctions should review an elementary statistics text.

*Nonparametric.* No assumptions are made about distributional properties of scales; therefore, these tests are appropriate for all levels of measurement. The relatively less frequent use of nonparametric models and tests in neuropsychology may reflect an inaccurate belief in the superiority of parametric models. As Cliff (1996) observed:

> Ordinal statistics can increase the scientific value of much of our research. Certain ordinal methods and approaches are emphasized over others because I feel that they are the most likely to enhance that scientific value. First, if we make ordinal conclusions, it should be based on ordinal characteristics of the data. Second, ordinal analysis avoids the criticism that a different although equally defensible version of the variable might lead to different conclusions, or latent variables might be different from that on their monotonically related observed version. Third, an inferential conclusion is always with respect to some parameter of the distributions, typically means or other

measures of location or some measure of correlation. Such conclusions are conditional on assumptions regarding the characteristics of underlying data distributions. ( p. 27)

Many, if not most, conclusions drawn from psychological and neuropsychological data are ordinal. For example, if the patient is or is not demented, has or has not attained MMI, did or did not sustain functional life changes are all ordinal-level conclusions. Ordinal conclusions are best drawn from ordinal-level analysis of data.

***Parametric.*** Parametric measures are appropriate when dependent variables are measured on *approximately* an interval level and distances between scores can be presumed as equal. Assumptions regarding the distribution of scores within the population of interest are also assumed to have interval qualities. Cliff (1996) observed that assumptions for parametric tests, correlations in particular, require linearity and homoskedasticity. When data are linear, a straight line (regression line – or mean) is the best predictor of unknown scores. Homoskedasticity assumes that residuals (differences between observed and predicted scores – an error measure) have constant variance.

## Bayes

Bayes' Rule may be applied to probability problems. According to this rule, samples of data are viewed as unions of mutually exclusive events. Box and Tiao (1992) described methods for applying Bayesian inference to small samples for which no sufficient statistics exist (e.g., norms for low-incidence neuropsychological populations), thereby improving sensitivity in the presence of departures from central theorem assumptions. No assumption is made within the Bayes model that data are linear, independent, or normally distributed (see Florens, Mouchart, & Rolin, 1990; Gammerman & Thatcher, 1990; Mendenhal, Scheaffer, & Wackerly, 1981).

## Base-Rate Effects

Matarazzo and Herman (1984) defined base rate as the "clinical meaningfulness" of the data by documenting how frequently differences between test scores occurred in the WAIS-R standardization sample. Base-rate (*br*) data have demonstrated greater efficacy in diagnostic predictions than in actuarial studies (Willis, 1984). Two meanings of base rate are reported by Gouvier, Hayes, and Smiroldo (1998): symptom sequella and test performance. In either situation, it is a prior probability ratio (e.g., suitable for Bayesian analysis) reflecting the number of cases with a condition as a proportion of the number of cases in the population (see Equation 4). If data for the population are known, then probability equals the relative frequency of an event's occurrence. A "population," therefore, is composed of base rates for all etiologies and diagnoses if it accurately reflects "normality."

$$br = \frac{\text{Number of cases with the condition}}{\text{Number of cases in the population}} \quad\quad (3.4)$$

For clinical purposes $br$ for a disorder can be considered comparable to either incidence or lifetime prevalence statistics (whichever is available, use prevalence if both are available). Yet, Gouvier et al. (1998) cited Bar-Hillel and Gordon's view that $br$ reflects current population prevalence. This seems to be an academic distinction, because current prevalence cannot be known as it changes minute-by-minute. I distinguish prevalence and incidence base rates as $br_p$ and $br_i$, respectively.

***Prevalence.*** The percentage of a population that is affected with a particular disease at a given time (Merriam-Webster, 1996) or the absolute number of cases presently existing and active in a given population at any particular time (R.J. Campbell, 1981) refers to prevalence base rate $(br_p)$. Prevalence data are compiled from cross-sectional population samples rather than from reported numbers of cases presenting for treatment. Consequently, prevalence includes both new and established cases, reflecting the relative distribution of the disorder within the population. The World Health Organization (*http://www.who.int/whosis/*) and the Centers for Disease Control (*http:// www.cdc.gov/nchs/fastats*) provide occurrence data for disorders classified under the ICD system. The most direct access to $br_p$ is Dialog's proprietary Incidence and Prevalence Database (*http://www.dialog.com*). At the time of writing the search price per diagnosis was $19.25 for account holders and around $25 for everyone else through Dialog's open-access account.

***Incidence.*** Merriam-Webster (1996) defined incidence ( $br_i$ ) as the rate of occurrence or influence. R. J. Campbell (1981) used the epidemiology definition of the number of new cases of any disorder that develops in a given population in a given period of time. Incidence rates are usually expressed per year, per 100,000 population. The exposed population may be the entire population, or particularly when the illness in question begins during only a limited period of years or is confined to one gender, it may be specifically limited to an age group or gender within the total population. Hence, parameters of time or specificity are usually placed on measures referenced as incidence. Incidents rates are compiled from reports of disorders submitted to the Centers for Disease Control, the World Health Organization, or similar epidemiological agency by physicians, hospitals, or other health care organizations. Incidence is of particular importance in the evaluation of brain-damaged subjects because of the limited window of opportunity within which rehabilitation shows maximal effectiveness.

***Score Concordant.*** Base rates derived from test scores or test score differences can be distinguished from other definitions as $br_s$. In organizational psychology, $br$ is described as the proportion of people whose performance is "satisfactory" on employment measures regardless of their status on predictor measures. Pedhazur and Schmelkin (1991) described base rate as "the *proportion* of people from a given pool of applicants [who are] expected to succeed when no selection, or random selection, is used"(p. 40). Therefore, the proportion of people expected not to succeed equals $1 - br$. Sattler (1988) referred to $br_s$ as "objective measures obtained from the observed cumulative frequencies of particular differences between scores" (p. 40). For example, differences between verbal and performance intelligence scores of 16 points occur in 15.3% of the normative sample for individuals whose Full-Scale IQ falls between 90 and 109 (The Psychological Corporation, 1997). For special populations, such as adults with brain lesions, dementia, or psychiatric disorders, $br_s$ are not widely available (McLean, Kaufman, & Reynolds, 1989). Also, the revision practices of test publishers result in $br_s$ data that are *always* obsolete. Base rates may be used in conjunction with effect size to support both confidence in diagnosis and degree of impairment.

***Effect Size ($\delta$).*** Ambiguity surrounds the meaning of effect size because the term is used interchangeably to refer to magnitude of effects, the importance of effects, or the meaningfulness of effects (Pedhauzer & Schmelking, 1991). Effect size also changes as sample size, $\alpha$, and power change. Power probabilities are conditional, given a particular relationship between abilities and test scores. With a constant sample size and $\alpha$, power increases and $\beta$ decreases as the strength of the relationship between the ability (independent variable – IV) and test score ( dependent variable – DV) increases. Effect size is generically referenced by the symbol $\delta$, but notation often differs to reflect various measures of $\delta$ associated with different statistical significance tests (see Table 3.7). In neuropsychology, δ is best considered a statistical measure of the size of the effect produced by the independent variable. Because effect size is associated with strength, importance, and meaningfulness of findings rather than purely statistical considerations, the use of effect size is often presented in an attempt to separate statistical and clinical significance. If it is true that one person's noise is another person's music, then it is also true that one person's importance and meaningfulness is another person's irrelevance and uselessness. Pedhazur et al. argued that the meaning of effect size in socio-behavioral research may be meaningless, especially when data lack equal intervals between scores. Consequently, well-respected statisticians such as Cohen (1988) recommended using *ordinal* terms such as *small, average,* and *large* when discussing the magnitude of an observed effect. Values associated with size of effect vary with different statistical tests as illustrated in Table 3.7. The use of effect size has been popularized by meta-analysis, where comparisons of effect size allow researchers to circumvent problems in comparing studies derived from different scales of measurement or evaluation using esoteric statistical tests into a single, seemingly simple, metric.

Table 3.7 presents comparisons of the size of nominal effect associated with differing effect size measures. Effect size, power and α vary with sample size. The smallest sample sizes reported by Cohen (1988) are identified in the table. Sample size refers to numbers of observations, not numbers of individuals. Therefore, for a neuropsychological evaluation it refers to data points or discrete test scores. It is possible, for example, to use each test item as a data point, although this practice is not recommended. Bear in mind that within each data set (test battery) each data point must be an independent observation, rather than a replication of a prior observation.

## SELECTING STATISTICAL TESTS

Many books have been written addressing the selection of statistical tests. This section considers tests of significance and association that are readily available in spreadsheet statistical functions and inexpensive statistical packages. Many of the significance tests can be obtained at no charge from university computing centers or public-domain software. I present examples of nonparametric and parametric models.

### Tests of Significance

Significance refers to the likelihood of making *error* when predicting an outcome. Significance testing is a method for quantifying the differences between observations and predictions that might occur as a result of measurement error.  In psychological testing, the $p$ level is sometimes inappropriately interpreted as the likelihood of error involved in accepting the prediction that a test score or observation is a valid representation of someone with a specific brain-related disorder, injury, or disability. Methods discussed next  represent models that are appropriate for the individual practitioner.  No attempt has been made to provide exhaustive listings of tests or their descriptions.

TABLE 3.7
Effect Size ($\delta$) Characteristics With Power = .25[a]

| | Parametric | | | Nonparametric | | |
|---|---|---|---|---|---|---|
| **Test** | $t$ | $r$ | $r_1 - r_2$ | **Sign** | $\phi$ | $\chi^2$ |
| $\delta$ symbol | $d$ | $r$ | $q$ | $g$ | $h$ | $w$ |
| Nominal $\delta$ | | | | | | |
| Small | .20 | .10 | .10 | .05 | .20 | .10 |
| Medium | .50 | .30 | .30 | .15 | .50 | .30 |
| Large | .80 | .50 | .50 | .25 | .80 | .50 |
| $p$ | $\alpha{=}.01/$ $d$ | $\alpha{=}.01$ $/r$ | $\alpha{=}.01$ $/r_1{-}r_2$ | $\alpha{=}.01$ $/g$ | $\alpha{=}.01$ $/\phi$ | $\alpha{=}.01$ $/\chi^2$ |
| *smallest n* | 4 | 4 | 6 | 7 | 4 | 4 |

[a] *Note.* Adapted from Cohen (1988)

### Nonparametric

**Chi-Square ($\chi^2$).**  The $\chi^2$ is used for making inferences about a population proportion. It considers the relative frequencies of observations either compared with expected frequencies or with frequencies occurring in a different condition.   Cohen (1988) specified two applications for $\chi^2$, contingence testing and goodness of fit.

*Contingency testing ( $\chi^2_i$ )* evaluates observed frequencies of two different variables using a two-way table for the purpose of testing their joint frequencies against $H_o$. For example, Table 3.8 presents symptoms obtained from a patient during intake where screening suggests the presence of memory loss, problems with executive function, questions of intellectual capacity, complaints of word-finding problems, inattention, and anxiety. The patient denied social or work problems and presented no evidence of unusual activity levels, hallucinations, delusions, or depression. The patient brings a hospital discharge summary indicating that a motor vehicle accident several months earlier produced an abnormal CT and MRI. The patient's presentation and history suggested vascular dementia following a closed head injury. The example presents observed and expected symptoms of vascular dementia as defined in *DSM-IV-TR*. Criteria include four groups of symptoms: (a) memory impairment, (b) either aphasia, apraxia, agnosia, or executive function impairment, (c) impairment in social or occupational function and, (d) focal neurological symptoms or laboratory evidence of focal neurological symptoms. Preferring to think that the patient is well error. except for dementia, I hypothesize that there will be no difference between the patient's symptoms and those characteristic of demented patients (RS-NHST). I establish a significance level ($\alpha$) of .05 as acceptable error before applying $\chi^2_1$. Following testing, the *p* value of $\geq$.4076 is much greater than .05. Therefore, I fail to reject the hypothesis that our patient's presentation is no different from a demented individual because the likelihood of making a Type I error if I rejected the null would be large. I am unable to say the patient is demented, but cannot say the patient is normal. Alternatively, I could use an AS-NHST. Here I would assume the patient is demented and $\alpha$ means "reject when false." With the same $\alpha$ (.05) I would fail to reject the hypothesis that the patient is demented.

Information recorded as "observations" in the 2x2 table come from patient report, especially items identified as social or occupational problems. Additional screening allows analysis using a goodness-of-fit model.

*The goodness-of-fit test.* ( $\chi^2_0$ ) evaluates categories of sample frequencies or proportions against a separate set of expected frequencies or proportions that comprise $H_o$. Neuropsychologists often subsume several constructs within a major category such as "memory." They may speak of short-term, remote, working, delayed components and differentiate between sensory modalities such as vision, memory, and touch. Suppose in the vascular dementia example the evaluator screens six memory components in Category I, five neuro-behavioral functions for Category II, two adaptive

TABLE 3.8
$\chi^2_1$ Analysis of Initial Interview Information
Comparing Patient Signs and Symptoms
With Diagnostic Criteria for Vascular Dementia

| Observed | | Expected | |
|---|---|---|---|
| | | Yes | No |
| | Yes | Memory loss Exec Function CT/MRI | Intelligence Language Attention Anxiety |
| | No | Work Problems or Social Problems | Activity Hallucinations Delusions Depression |

*Statistical Contingency Table Analysis*

| | Column 1 | Column 2 | Row Totals |
|---|---|---|---|
| Frequencies, row 1 | 3 | 4 | 7 |
| Percent of total | 25.0% 33.3% | 58.3% | |
| Frequencies, row 2 | 1 | 4 | 5 |
| Percent of total | 8.3% 33.3% | 41.6% | |
| Column totals | 4 | 8 | 12 |
| Percent of total | 33.3% 66.6% | | |

| | | |
|---|---|---|
| Chi-square (df=1) | .69 | p = .4076 |
| V-square (df=1) | .63 | p = .4279 |
| Yates corrected Chi-square | .04 | p = .8360 |
| Phi-square | .06 | |
| Fisher exact p, one-tailed | | p = .4242 |
| two-tailed | | p = .5758 |
| McNemar Chi-square (A/D) | .00 | p =1.0000 |
| Chi-square (B/C) | .80 | p = .3711 |

behaviors for Category III, and grouped signs and symptoms into two domains for Category IV.    The patient meets criteria for one screening item in each category so the diagnosis of vascular dementia is confirmed using DSM-IV-TR criteria.  However, there is no indication of degree of impairment.  From the goodness-of-fit data presented in Table 3.9 we can calculate likely effect size ($w$) as shown in Table 3.10.  Based on Cohen's (1998) classification, the difference observed constitutes a "large" effect size (see Table 3.7).  Calculation of $\chi^2_1$  from nominal data using spread sheets is not recommended even though many spreadsheets include the function.

TABLE 3.9
$\chi^2_0$ for goodness of fit.

| Category | Expected | Observed |
|---|---|---|
| I Memory | $1/6 = .17$ | $4/6 = .67$ |
| II Other | $1/5 = .20$ | $1/5 = .20$ |
| III Social or Occupational | $\frac{1}{2} = .50$ | $2/2 =$   1.00 |
| IV Signs or Symptoms | $\frac{1}{2} = .50$ | $\frac{1}{2} = .50$ |

*Note.* Chi-square $= 1.970588$; df $= 3$; $p < .57840$

TABLE 3.10.
Effect Size of $\chi^2_0$

| $E$ | $O$ | $E\text{-}O$ | $E\text{-}O^2$ |
|---|---|---|---|
| 0.17 | 0.67 | 0.5- | 0.25 |
| 0.20 | 0.20 | 0.0 | 0.00 |
| 0.50 | 1.00 | 0.5- | 0.25 |
| 0.50 | 0.50 | 0.0 | 0.00 |
| | | Sum | 0.50 |
| | | w | 0.70 |

***Sign Test.*** Cohen (1988, p. 145) described the sign test as "H$_o$ : $p$ = .50," testing the null hypothesis that the proportion of the population is .50. This question is of particular interest in forensics where "beyond a reasonable degree of medical certainty" literally means "there is more than a 50% probability" (Brigham, Babitsky & Mangraviti, 1996). Three situations arise in the neuropsychological evaluation where "beyond a reasonable degree of medical certainty" has particular value: estimating causation, comparing preinjury with postinjury function, and establishing MMI. In each of these situations, evaluation using the sign test is similar. Table 3.11 presents three sets of data gleaned from medical records. The first comes from reports of signs and symptoms before the patient was diagnosed with and treated for communicating hydrocephalus (pre shunt).

TABLE 3.11
Sign Test Supporting Causal Inference

| *Dependent Variable* | *Pre shunt* | *Post shunt* | *Post MVA* |
|---|---|---|---|
| abnormal EEG | NO | NO | YES |
| MR > L ventricle | YES | NO | NO |
| memory complaints | YES | NO | YES |
| urinary incontinence | YES | NO | NO |
| complaints of confusion | YES | NO | YES |
| gait disturbance | YES | NO | NO |
| decorticate posturing | NO | NO | YES |
| MR with hematoma | NO | NO | YES |
| aphasia noted | NO | NO | YES |
| seizures observed | NO | NO | YES |

| *Comparison* | *No. of Non ties* | *Percent* $v < V$ | Z | p |
|---|---|---|---|---|
| Pre shunt vs. Post shunt | 05 | 100.0 | 1.78 | .073 |
| Pre shunt vs. Post-MVA | 08 | 037.5 | 0.35 | .723 |
| Post hunt vs. Post-MVA | 07 | 000.0 | 2.26 | .023 |

*Note.* MVA = motor vehicle accident.

The second column presents observations reported following treatment (post shunt). The last column compares observations following a motor vehicle accident (post-MVA). The patient's neuropsychological status is significant for dementia and the legal issue centers on when the dementia began. The plaintiff's family claims there was no dementia predating the motor vehicle accident from which the patient sustained significant and well-documented brain damage. The defendant claims that the patient was demented before the accident, citing as evidence information presented in the first column as taken from medical records. Plaintiff's attorney alleges that the clearing of symptoms following shunt placement strongly suggests that current symptoms are attributable to the vehicular accident. Data are presented in temporal order. Using RS-NHST, I hypothesize that it is unlikely differences between the plaintiff's presentations before and after MVA, with post shunt placement serving as the prior measure, exceed .50. I establish .05 as an acceptable $\alpha$, recognizing that this level includes strong bias for failing to reject the null. Because the observed $p$ level is .023, I fail to accept the null hypothesis. Data support the opinion that beyond a reasonable degree of medical certainty, it is likely that damage sustained in the MVA accounts for observed vascular dementia.

***Wilcoxin Matched Pairs.*** When comparing two distributions of rank-ordered data for the differences between variables the Wilcoxin Matched Pairs Test is recommended. This test allows comparison of samples of convenience with other samples of convenience or with samples obtained using random selection. Table 3.12 shows findings from scores compared to the expected average score of 100. The Wilcoxin is useful for evaluating a neuropsychological construct for which multiple tests provide overlapping scores, but none of the tests adequately assesses the construct individually. In the example presented, tests relying heavily on "visual processing" present ranges of scores suggestive of problems in this area. Using a RS-NHST model, with $\alpha$ set at .05, I reject the hypothesis of no difference between obtained scores and average scores. This finding suggests that the overall below average performance on tasks involving visual processing is unlikely the result of measurement error. It implies that on some tasks (viz., Trails A, Block Design, and Picture Arrangement) factors other than visual processing could account for observed average performance.

TABLE 3.12
Evaluation of Tests Requiring Visual Processing[a]

| Test | Obtained Score |
|------|----------------|
| Trails A | 100 |
| Trails B | 095 |
| Block Design | 100 |
| Rey Complex figure | 065 |
| WRAT-III Arithmetic | 075 |
| Picture Completion | 090 |
| Picture Arrangement | 100 |
| Dynamic Visual Retention Test | 085 |
| Progressive Matrices | 070 |
| Wisconsin Card Sorting Test | 050 |
| Category Test | 075 |
| Visual Memory | 082 |

*Wilcoxin Matched Pairs Test*

| N | T | Z | p Level |
|---|---|---|---------|
| 12 | 0.00 | 2.66 | .0077 |

[a] *Note. Obtained Scores* are compared to the average score of 100 (not shown).

### Parametric

**Student's-t.** For most clinical purposes, the parametric test of choice for comparing differences between or within conormed tests is student's $t$. The test is robust and readily available. Figure 3.1 presents probability testing using *Quattro Pro*, a spread sheet included in *Word Perfect Office*. Similar capabilities exist in most spreadsheets. Note that column A represents the average score, and all scores are converted to a $\bar{x}$

of 10 and σ of 3. Patient data are compared to other patient data in lines 15 - 24. The cell formula for calculating the *t* test [@TTEST(C3 ..C9,J3..J9,1,2)] includes parameters describing the cells compared (C3..C9,J3..J9); number of tails (1 or 2); and, if the data are paired or repeated (1), two samples of equal variance (2), or two samples of unequal variance (3). Aggregate comparisons such as this are more helpful in evaluating the overall level of disability rather than identifying specific deficits. Differences between individual tests and the average scores appear under the effect size (ES) column, calculated as described in Table 3.8. Pair-wise calculations of effect size differences are also possible and may provide benefit during the evaluation. Spreadsheet functions for this purpose are available at *http://www.geocities.com/rdfphd/index.html*.

**Tests of Association**

Many neuropsychologists equate tests of association with prediction. Predictors of premorbid abilities rely heavily on regression equations as do predictors of recovery. Cohen (1988) observed:   $P_s$ (comparison of proportions) shares with the product moment $r_s$ the difficulty that the standard deviation of the sampling distributions depend upon their population parameters, which are unknown. A consequence of this is that one's ability to detect a difference in magnitude between either population $P_s$ or $r_s$ is not a simple function of the difference as with the case of $r$, a nonlinear transformation of $P$ provides a solution to the problem. (p. 180)

This transformation is provided by the Phi coefficient:

$$\phi = 2 \arcsin \sqrt{P_s} \qquad\qquad (3.5)$$

When testing hypotheses regarding associations, it is tempting to equate $H_o$ with a correlation of zero. Although accepting the $H_o$ implies low correlation, it is not equivalent to no correlation. Meehl (1997) stated that "failing to reject $H_o$ implies high correlation" (p. 391). The conclusion that the correlation between two sets of scores is statistically significant implies that the observed correlation is unlikely if two samples were drawn at random from the same sample. However, this view is not universally accepted (see Abelson, 1995).

*Nonparametric.*    Comparisons between samples can be made using $\phi$, $\phi'$, $r_s$, $\tau$, or $\gamma$. Phi ($\phi$) is used for comparing nominal data using a 2 x 2 table, and $\phi'$ is used if the table is larger. Ordinal data can be compared using Kendall's tau ($\tau$), gamma ($\gamma$), or Spearman's rank-order correlation ($r_s$). Kendall's $\tau$ represents a probability that the order of the variables is the same and the interpretation is not equivalent to Pearson's $r$ as is $r_s$. When your data contain many ties, the $\gamma$ statistic should be used. Again, $\gamma$ is a measure of order similar to $\tau$. I recommend using $\phi$ whenever possible because the relationship between $\phi$ and effect size is known. To my knowledge, none of the popular spreadsheets include nonparametric measures of association in predefined functions. Cohen (1988) provided effect size and power tables for sample sizes (i.e., data points) as few as 10.

*Parametric.* Pearson's product-moment ®) may be the most often used statistic in psychology. With sample sizes as small as 8, it is possible to determine power and effect size. The statistic is an index of the *linear* relationship between two variables. It provides a "best fit" for a straight line (regression line) constructed between variables *standardized to the same variability.* Confusion arises in the use of $r$ because it has different meanings when used descriptively versus inferentially. In descriptive statistics, no assumptions about the shape of the distribution, equal variability of data sets, or homoskedasticity are necessary. In the inferential use of $r$ (as in hypothesis testing) Cohen (1988) stated that "assumptions of normality and homoskedasticity are formally invoked" (p. 75). Exception is granted only when $n$ is large. Although a large $n$ remains undefined, Cohen's power tables suggest a number greater than 500 or 1,000.[3] Because $r$ serves as a measure of effect size and is easily calculated from spreadsheets, it is of particular interest to neuropsychologists when data allow its use. Also, for clinical purposes $r$ is functionally equivalent to $z$ when $r \leq .50$. Multiple $r$ s can be compared directly when their sample sizes are equal. When sample sizes are unequal, the effect size measure $q$ (see Table 3.8) must be used.

Figure 3.1 includes calculations for both $r$ and $r^2$. Sometimes it is necessary to "trick" spreadsheets into calculating an answer. In this example, an error message is returned when all of the "average" scores presented in column A are 10. By changing one score (the first) to 9.99999, the sheet displays 10, but calculates correlations and coefficients of determination for those columns compared to A.

---

[3]The type of sample will determine how large $n$ should be. When observations from a patient suspected of having a disorder prevalent in only .1% of the population are compared to those from a group of "normal" subjects, the standardization sample size must contain at least 1,000 subjects .

## SUMMARY

In this chapter I have attempted to provide readers with an understanding of how clinical questions can be stated as hypotheses that are suitable for statistical analysis. I have provided review of important constructs central to hypothesis testing, pointing out inconsistencies in usage where appropriate. I have reviewed several statistical models useful in the parametric and nonparametric analysis of neuropsychological test data.

| | | MQ | SSE | ES | | SS | ES | | SS | ES |
|---|---|---|---|---|---|---|---|---|---|---|
| | WMS=III | | | | Performance WAIS-III | | | Verbal WAIS-III | | |
| SS | | MQ | SSE | ES | | SS | ES | | SS | ES |
| 10 | Auditory Immediate | 70 | 4 | -2 | Picture Completion | 6 | -1 | Vocabulary | 6 | -1 |
| 10 | Visual Immediate | 65 | 3 | -2 | Digit Symbol | 6 | -1 | Similarities | 7 | -1 |
| 10 | Immediate Memory | 51 | 0.2 | -3 | Block Design | 7 | -1 | Arithmetic | 7 | -1 |
| 10 | Auditory Delayed | 58 | 1.6 | -3 | Matrix Reasoning | 11 | 0 | Digit Span | 13 | 1 |
| 10 | Visual Delayed | 72 | 4.4 | -2 | Picture Arrangement | 10 | 0 | Information | 8 | -1 |
| 10 | Auditory Recognition Delayed | 65 | 3 | -2 | Symbol Search | 4 | -2 | Comprehension | 9 | -0 |
| 10 | General Memory | 59 | 1.8 | -3 | Object Assembly | 5 | -2 | Letter-Numbering | 10 | 0 |
| | | p A:E | | | | p E:J | | | p J:M | |
| t | | 0.00000536 | | | | 0.00378833 | | | 0.08295716 | |
| r | | -0.429378366607954 | | | | 2.34469456256E-16 | | | 0.435695430863 | |
| r² | | -0.858758733215908 | | | | 4.68938912512E-16 | | | 0.871390861725 | |
| | | p A:M | | | | P E:M | | | p A:J | |
| t | | 0.06840631 | | | | 0.00005000 | | | 0.00482167 | |
| r | | 0.478344603107461 | | | | -0.329994591135205 | | | 0.170782512766 | |
| r² | | 0.228813559322034 | | | | 0.108896430178491 | | | 0.029166666667 | |

FIG. 3.1.  Quattro Pro calculations of $t$ and $r$.

Different approaches to testing hypotheses are necessary for tests standardized using random and stratified samples versus those tests standardized in the neuropsychological laboratory or rehabilitation setting. Unfortunately, the outcome of null hypothesis testing is often uninformative. It is more likely to provide information regarding "what a score does not represent" than "what a score represents." For the purposes of clinical decision making, the replacement of null hypothesis testing with Bayesian analysis would be more helpful.

**REFERENCES**

Abelson, R. P. (1995). *Statistics as principled argument.* Hillsdale, NJ: Lawrence Erlbaum Associates.

American Psychiatric Association. (2000). *Diagnostic and Stastical Manual of Mental Disorders* (4th ed., Text Revision). Washington, DC: Author.

Box, G. E. P., & Tiao, G. C. (1992). *Bayesian inference in statistical analysis.* New York: Wiley.

Brigham, C. R., Babitsky, S., & Mangraviti, J. J. (1996). *The independent medical evaluation report.* Falmouth, MA: SEAK, Inc.

Campbell, R. J. (1981). *Psychiatric dictionary* (5th ed.). New York: Oxford University Press.

Cliff, N. (1996). *Ordinal methods for behavioral data analysis.* Mahwah, NJ: Lawrence Erlbaum Associates.

Cohen, J. (1988) . *Statistical Power Analysis for the Behavioral Sciences.* (2nd ed.). Hillsdale, NJ: Lawrence Erlbaum Associates.

Cook, T. D., & Campbell, D. T. (1976). The design and conduct of quasiexperiments and true experiments in field settings. In M. D. Dunnette (Ed.), *Handbook of industrial and organizational psychology* (pp. 223-325). Chicago: Rand McNally.

Cook, T. D., & Campbell, D. T. (1979). *Quasi-experimentation: Design & analysis issues for field settings.* Chicago: Rand McNally.

Cronbach, L. J. (1971). Test validation. In R. L. Thorndike (Ed.), *Educational measurement* (2nd ed., p. 443 - 507). Washington, DC: American Council on Education.

Faust, D., Ziskin, J., & Hiers, J. B. (1991). *Brain damage claims: Coping with neuropsychological evidence* (Vol. 1). Los Angeles: Law and Psychology Press.

Florens, J. P., Mouchart, M., & Rolin, J. M. (1990). *Elements of Bayesian statistics.* New York: Marcel Dekker.

Franklin, R. D., Allison, D. B., & Gorman, B. S. (1997). *Design and analysis of single-case research.* Mahwah, NJ: Lawrence Erlbaum Associates.

Gammerman, A., & Thatcher, A. R. (1990). Bayesian inference in an expert system without assuming independence. In M. C. Golumbic (Ed.) *Advances in artificial intelligence* (pp. 232-265). New York: Springer-Verlag.

Goldberg, S. (1987). *The four-minute neurological exam.* Miami, FL: MedMaster, Inc.

Golden, C. J., Purisch, A. D., & Hammeke, T. A. (1991). *Luria-Nebraska Neuropsychological Battery: Forms I and II.* Los Angeles: Western Psychological Services.

Gouvier, W. D., Hayes, J. S., & Smiroldo, B. B. (1998). The significance of base rates, test sensitivity test specificity, and subjects' knowledge of symptoms in assessing TBI sequelae and malingering. In C. R. Reynolds (Ed.), *Detection of malingering during head injury litigation* (pp. 55-80). New York: Plenum.

Gresham, F. M. (1997). Treatment integrity in single-subject research. In R.D. Franklin, D.B. Allison, & B.S. Gorman, B. S. (Eds.), *Design and analysis in single-case research* (pp. 93-118). Mahwah, NJ: Lawrence Erlbaum Associates.

Hagen, R. L. (1998). Comment: A further look at wrong reasons to abandon statistical testing. *American Psychologist, 53*(7), 797-798.

Lezak, M. D. (1995), *Neuropsychological assessment* (3rd ed.). New York: Oxford University Press.

Matarazzo, J. D., & Herman, D. O. (1984). Base rate data for the WAIS-R: Test-retest stability and VIQ-PIQ differences. *Journal of Clinical Neuropsychology, 6*(4), 351-366.

McLean, J. E., Kaufman, A. S., & Reynolds, C. J. (1989). Base rates of WAIS-R subtest scatter as a guide for clinical and neuropsychological assessment. *Journal of Clinical Psychology, 45*(6), 919-925.

Meehl, P. E. (1997). The problem is epistemology, not statistics: Replace significance tests by confidence intervals and quantify accuracy of risky numerical predictions. In L. L. Harlow, S. A. Maulaik, & J. H. Steiger (Eds.), *What if there were no significance tests?* (pp. 391-423). Mawah, NJ: Lawrence Erlbaum Associates.

Mendenhal, W., Scheaffer, R. L., & Wackerly, D. D. (1981). *Mathematical statistics with pplications.* Boston: Duxbury Press.

Merriam-Webster, Inc. (1996). *Merriam-Webster's collegiate dictionary* (10th ed.). Springfield, MA: Author.

Messick, S. (1995). Validity of psychological assessments. *American Psychologist, 50*(9), 741-749.

Miturshina, M. N., Boone, K. B. & D'Elia, L. F. (1999). *Handbook of normative data for neuropsychological assessment.* New York: Oxford University Press.

Nickerson, R. S. (1998). Confirmation bias: A ubiquitous phenomenon in many cases. *Review of General Psychology, 2*(2), 175-220.

Nickerson, R. S. (2000). Null hypothesis significance testing: A review of an old and continuing controversy. *Psychological Methods, 5*(2), 241-301.

Nunnally, J. C. (1972). *Educational measurement and evaluation* (2nd ed.). New York: McGraw-Hill.

The Psychological Corporation. (1997). *WAIS-III/WMS-III Technical Manual*. San Antonio: Author.

Pedhazur, E. J., & Schmelkin, L. P. (1991). *Measurement, design, and analysis: An integrated approach*. Hillsdale, NJ: Lawrence Erlbaum Associates.

Rosenthal, R. (1984). *Meta-analytic procedures for social research*. Beverly Hills, CA: Sage.

Rouanet, H. (1996). Bayesian methods for assessing importance of effects. *Psychological Bulletin, 119*, 149-158.

Rouanet, H. (1998). Significance testing in a Bayesian framework: Assessing direction of effects. *Behavioral and Brain Sciences, 21*, 217-218.

Sattler, J. M. (1988). *Assessment of children* (3rd ed.). San Diego: Author.

Spreen, O., & Strauss, E. (1998). *A compendium of neuropsychological tests: Administration, norms, and commentary*. (2nd ed.) New York: Oxford University Press.

Statsoft, Inc. (1994). *Statistica*. Tulsa, OK: Author.

Taylor, H. G., Wade, S. L., Yeates, K. O., Drotar, D., & Klein, S. K. (1999). Influences on first year recovery from traumatic brain injury in children. *Neuropsychology, 13*(1), 76-89.

Thorndike, R. M. (1997). *Measurement and evaluation in psychology and education*. (6th ed.). Upper Saddle River, NJ: Merrill.

Willis, W. (1984). Re-analysis of an actuarial approach to neuropsychological diagnosis in consideration of base rates. *Journal of Consulting and Clinical Psychology, 52*(4), 567-569.

# Bayesian Inference and Belief Networks

**Ronald D. Franklin**[1]
*St. Mary's Hospital and Florida Atlantic University*

**Joachim Krueger**
*Brown University*

Clinicians routinely draw inferences from test results to the test taker's latent condition. After all, "a large part of medicine is practiced on people who do not have obvious illnesses, but rather have signs, symptoms, or findings that may or may not represent an illness that should be treated" (Eddy, 1984, p. 75). In the simplest case, both test results and latent conditions are dichotomous variables. Tests turn out either positive or negative, and test takers either do or do not have the disease in question. The inference of interest is a predictive judgment of whether a client with a positive test result has the disease. This judgment depends on several cues. Some of these cues are external, such as the information contained in the client's file (including test scores), whereas other cues are internal, such as the prevalence of the disease in the population or the clinician's experience and memory of related cases. In this chapter, we address the integration of external and internal cues in simple Bayesian inference and in more extended belief networks.

Published posthumously, Bayes' (1763) essay on the doctrine of chances became the cornerstone of a theory of probability that accounts for the interplay of internal, or subjective, and external, or objective, cues. The theory provides methods of principled inductive reasoning and it permits probabilistic predictions about individual cases. The centerpiece of this approach is a theorem stating how beliefs are to be revised in light of evidence. A practicing psychologist is interested in the probability that a person has a certain disease given the presence of a positive result on a test designed to detect this disease. To estimate this

---

[1]Please address correspondence to PO Box 268, Candor, NC 27229 or rdfphd@yahoo.com.

probability (i.e., $p(D_o|P_o)$),[2] which is also referred to as the *positive predictive value* of the test, the psychologist needs to consult the following probabilities. The first probability, which is externally provided by test developers, is the *sensitivity* of the test. Sensitivity is the probability that a person obtains a positive test result given that the person is known—by whatever other independent and valid method—to have the disease (i.e., $p(P_o|D_o)$). The second probability, which is also externally provided, is the *specificity* of the test. Specificity is the probability that a person obtains a negative result given that the person is known *not* to have the disease (i.e., $p(P_n|D_n)$). Together, sensitivity and specificity capture the overall accuracy or "efficiency" of the test. The third probability, which is internal, refers to the psychologist's prior estimate that the person has the disease (i.e., $p(D_o)$). If random sampling can be assumed, the prior probability of the disease corresponds to the base rate of the disease in the population. If random sampling cannot be assumed, prior estimates may vary depending to the availability of other cues (e.g., symptoms) and the psychologist's experience with interpreting these cues. The partial subjectivity of prior estimates leaves room for divergent diagnostic inferences drawn from the same test results.

$$P(Do|Po) = \frac{P(Do) * p(Po|Do)}{p(Do) * (p(Po|Do) + (p(dn) * p(Do|Dn)}  \tag{4.1}$$

Bayes' rule shows how internal prior estimates of the disease combine with the external efficiency information to yield the desired positive predictive value. The probability that a person who tested positive is sick is the product of the prior probability of a person to be sick and the so-called diagnostic ratio. The diagnostic ratio is the sensitivity of the test divided by the overall probability of a test result to be positive. The denominator of the diagnostic ratio is the sum of the probability that a person tests positive *and* is sick, and the probability that a person tests positive *and* is healthy. The first of these joint probabilities is the product of the prior probability of being sick, $p(D_o)$, and the test's sensitivity, $p(P_o|D_o)$; the second joint probability is the

---

[2]In this notation, the subscript 'o' stands for 'occurrence' (of a disease or a positive test result), whereas the subscript 'n' stands for 'nonoccurrence.'

product of the prior probability of being healthy, $p(D_n)$, and the complement of the test's specificity, $p(P_o|D_n)$. In other words, $p(P_o)$ is itself a combination of internal and external information. The formula reads

**Diagnosis and Uncertainty**

Consider a hypothetical psychiatric scenario (Cohen, 1994). The base rate of schizophrenia is assumed to be low ($p(D_o) = .021$), and a test designed to diagnose schizophrenia is assumed to have excellent sensitivity ($p(P_o|D_o) = .952$) and specificity ($p(P_n|D_n) = .969$). Then, the probability of schizophrenia in a randomly tested person with a positive result is .40, namely

$$P(Do|Po) = \frac{.021 * .952}{.021 * .952 + .979 * .031} \qquad (4.2)$$

The increase in the estimated probability of schizophrenia from .021 to .4 reflects the degree to which the psychologist has become less certain that this individual is healthy. Because a categorical decision concerning the person's health status has become more, rather than less certain, further testing is indicated. Such testing is most efficient if it is conditionally independent of the initial testing, that is, if the results of the two tests are unrelated within the population of sick people and within the population of healthy people. If such independence can be assumed, the posterior probability of the disease obtained after the first test (i.e., .40) can serve as the prior probability for the second test (Winkler, 1993). In Cohen's (1994) example, confidence in the presence of the disease would rise to .95 if a positive result were obtained again and if the second test were as sensitive and as specific as the first one. If, however, the follow-up tests are not independent, confidence levels will rise more slowly. Still, sequential testing is a powerful strategy because it overcomes the psychometric limitations of single tests. In the present example, a test would have to have extraordinary sensitivity and specificity (with both $p = .999$) so that a single positive result would yield a positive predictive value of .95.

Sequential testing rapidly dilutes initial differences in clinical opinion, an effect that is often overlooked by critics of Bayesian subjectivism. Potentially divergent prior estimates enter the chain of inferences only once, whereas test results accumulate over time (Lindley, 1993; Thorndike, 1986b). For illustration's sake, suppose a more liberal psychologist approaches the diagnosis of schizophrenia with a prior estimate of .2. This belief would result in a posterior probability of .89 after the first test and a posterior of .996 after the second test, at which point the liberal's judgment hardly differs from the conservative's (i.e., by .04).

Bayesian probability estimation is not a recipe for decision making, but it offers a platform on which treatment decisions can be placed. To be able to decide whether to diagnose a suspected disease, diagnosticians must set a confidence threshold (i.e., a minimum predictive value for a positive diagnosis). The location of this threshold depends on the costs and benefits to the patient (Satz, Fennell, & Reilly, 1970). The lower the threshold, the greater the number of patients who receive a false positive diagnosis with the attendant undesirable consequences. The conservative and the liberal diagnosticians in the example would respectively expect 5% and .4% of their treatments to be wasted. For the former, the expected false positive rate would be greater than the rate indicated by the complement of the test's specificity (here: 3%); for the latter, it would be lower.

## Dealing With Base-Rates

As base-rates become more extreme, their effects on diagnostic decisions become larger. This base-rate effect is crucially important because most tests are designed to detect conditions that are rare in the population. A test is most valuable if it allows the diagnosis of a specific case in a way that contravenes base-rate expectation. Critics of clinical decision making often note that people—novices and experts alike—grossly overdiagnose rare diseases (Dawes, 1994; Faust & Ziskin, 1988). Some clinicians hesitate to think probabilistically about individual cases, believing that group statistics are "of no use for the individual case" (Gigerenzer, Hoffrage, & Ebert, 1998, p. 204), or that sensitivity and specificity "predict test scores, not disorders" (Elwood, 1993, p. 230). If taken too seriously, however, this line of reasoning would also keep one from having a preference between a gun containing one bullet and a gun containing 5 bullets in a game of Russian roulette (Dawes, Faust, & Meehl, 1989). Other clinicians may try to think Bayesian but inadvertently confuse predictive accuracy with retrospective accuracy. It is indeed tempting to believe that high test sensitivity directly implies the presence of the disease given a positive result. Yielding to this temptation, many clinicians equate the posterior probability of the disease, $p(D_o|P_o)$, with the sensitivity of the test, $p(P_o|D_o)$, without proper regard for the base-rate of the disease, $p(D_o)$. This error has been variously characterized as overconfidence, base-rate neglect, or the confusion of the inverse, and it has been attributed to fallible judgmental heuristics such as representativeness, availability, or anchoring with insufficient adjustment (see Dawes, 1988, for a review).   In a classic survey, 95% of the participating physicians did not distinguish between the probability of a positive X-ray given cancer and the probability of cancer given a positive X ray (Casscells, Schoenberger, & Grayboys, 1978).   In a conceptual replication study, most AIDS counselors were certain that a positive test indicated that a low-risk testee was infected (Gigerenzer et al., 1998).  To be consistent, anyone who ignores the prior probability of the disease would also have to ignore its posterior probability after the first test when interpreting the results of sequential tests—hardly a desirable prospect.

The over prediction bias may arise not only from the fallibility of statistical intuitions among practitioners, but also from the way in which they acquire medical knowledge.   Students "learn the signs and symptoms that occur with each disease, and most medical knowledge is organized according to disease" (Eddy & Clanton, 1982, p. 1263). Many textbooks offer the mistaken advice that positive test results indicate the presence of the condition in the tested individual regardless of the base-rate of that condition in the population (Eddy, 1982).   Defenders of clinical (and other intuitive) judgment argue that practitioners reason rather well even when their judgmental task is far more complex than the judgment required in the present single-test, single-disease scenario (Eddy & Clanton, 1982).  Base-rates are hardly ever completely ignored (Koehler, 1996), and judgments appear to be more rational when decision utilities are considered in addition to Bayesian probabilities (Birnbaum, 1983).   Others suggest that judgments improve when clinicians are vividly reminded of the relevance of base-rates (Garb & Schramke, 1996) or when the input data are presented as frequencies (Gigerenzer & Hoffrage, 1995).

The latter recommendation is intriguing because it appears to obviate the entire Bayesian enterprise of integrating prior belief (i.e., base-rate information) with empirical evidence (i.e., test results).  Cohen (1994) himself presented his numerical example in a frequency format so that "the situation may be made clearer" (p. 999).  Table 4.1 shows the data.  The marginal frequencies refer to the individuals with each latent status (sick vs. healthy) and each test result (positive vs. negative), and the cell frequencies refer to the four joint occurrences.  Given these frequencies, the probability of the disease given a positive test is easily obtained by dividing the frequency of co-occurrence of the disease and a positive test result (here: 20) by the marginal frequency of a positive result (here: 50). No base-rate probability of the disease appears to be necessary. It is also evident that the predictive probability is much smaller than the sensitivity of the test (i.e., 20/21).

TABLE 4.1

Joint Frequencies of the Occurrence of the Disease ($D_o$) versus Its Nonoccurrence ($D_n$) and Positive ($P_o$) versus Negative ($P_n$) Test Predictions

|       | $D_o$ | $D_n$ | Total |
|-------|-------|-------|-------|
| $P_o$ | 20    | 30    | 50    |
| $P_n$ | 1     | 949   | 950   |
| Total | 21    | 979   | 1000  |

But where do frequency tables originate? If clinicians were able to classify each incoming case correctly into one of the four cells of the table, test information would be superfluous. The clinician would already know if the person was really sick! Alas, such knowledge is not available in the real world, and diagnosticians cannot count on "natural sampling" of signs and diseases. Instead, they require probabilities to derive frequencies. The frequency of joint occurrence of a positive result and the disease, for example, is the sensitivity of the test times the base-rate of the disease times the total number of cases (i.e., $f(P_o$ and $D_o) = p(P_o|D_o) * p(D_o) * N) = .969 * .021 * 1,000 = 20$). The computation of frequencies is easily computerized (Sedlmeier, 1997). Once obtained, the visual display of frequencies is an effective aid to clinical inference and to the communication of these inferences to clients (Hoffrage, Lindsey, Hertwig & Gigerenzer, 2000). Nevertheless, because probability information remains essential for the construction of frequency tables, clinicians might as well compute their predictive estimates directly (Dawes, 2000; Jones, 1989).

Because knowledge of base-rates remains vital, we return to the question of what the relevant base-rates are. Although Cohen's (1994) example illustrates the mutual dependencies among conditional and unconditional probabilities, it assumes that testing occurs in a random sample of the general population. In clinical settings, however, patients are rarely sampled randomly. Clinical sampling bias is likely to increase the *available* base-rate. Many clients present themselves or are referred for assessment because other probabilistic cues (e.g., symptoms) suggesting the presence of a condition have already been observed. If, for example, the available base-rate is .5, the posterior probability of the disease lies between the values of test sensitivity and specificity. The need to compile local base-rates for local use highlights a difference between test development and test application (Meehl & Rosen, 1955). Test development can yield excellent levels of sensitivity and specificity because it operates on contrast groups of roughly equal size. The challenge of test construction is to find independent and valid criteria (i.e., a "gold standard", Elwood, 1993) for whether patients have the condition to be detected. In contrast, test application and judgments about individuals must incorporate the counterfactual idea of what the judgment would have been if no test results were in evidence. In other words, sampling bias must be assessed independently of the test results at hand.[3]

**Decomposing Accuracy**

Both test sensitivity and specificity must be known (along with the base-rate of the disease) for a predictive estimate to be reached. In Cohen's (1994) example, both types of accuracy are high, so their differential effects are easily overlooked. A test could be perfectly sensitive and yet diagnostically useless. Such a situation could arise if the test had no specificity so that every test taker would receive a positive result. The overall accuracy of a test is captured by the diagnostic ratio of sensitivity, $p(P_o|D_o)$, over the complement of specificity, $p(P_o|D_n)$.[4] If

---

[3]This requirement highlights the need for multiple assessment methods. Without circularity, results from the focal test cannot simultaneously generate a diagnosis for individuals and base-rate estimates for the available population. Bayes's Rule requires that the latter affects the estimate of the former.

[4]A drawback of this measure is that it has no upper limit. Measures of association (i.e., between clients' actual health status and their test results) that do not depend on variations in the base-rates of $D_o$ and $P_o$ offer useful alternatives (e.g., coefficient g, Goodman & Kruskal, 1954, or coefficients of discrimination derived from signal detection theory, Snodgrass & Corwin, 1988).

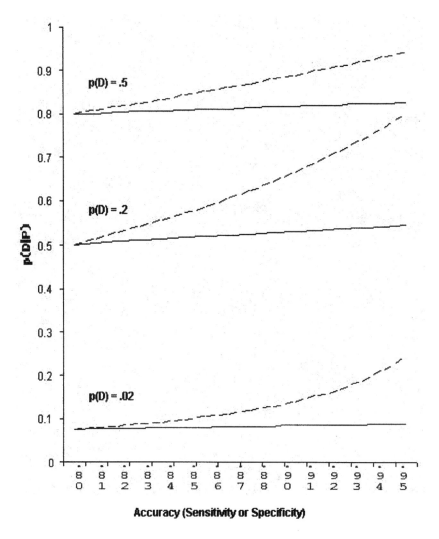

FIG. 4.1. Posterior Probabilities of Disease for Three Base Rates. The solid lines show the effect of variation in test sensitivity for a constant specificity of .8. The dashed lines show the effect of variation in test specificity for a constant sensitivity of .8.

sensitivity and specificity cannot both be maximized, test makers must choose between putting a premium either on  correctly diagnosing the presence of a disease or on correctly diagnosing its absence.   By increasing sensitivity, they risk decreasing specificity, and vice versa. When a test is administered as a screening device for a rare disease, a lack of specificity may seem acceptable because most healthy clients still get a negative result. Often, test constructors' primary goal is to ensure that "if a disease is present, it should be found, even at the risk of getting a high rate of false positive results" (Feinstein, 1978, pp. 111-112).[5]

Contrary to the idea that increases in sensitivity are paramount, Bayes' rule shows that increases in specificity entail the largest increases in positive predictive value. Assuming either a high (.5, top lines), moderate (.2, center lines), or low prior probability of $D_o$ (.02, bottom lines), Fig. 4.1 plots $p(D_o|P_o)$ against test accuracy levels ranging from .8 to .95. When specificity is constant at .8, increases in sensitivity yield hardly discernible increases in diagnostic confidence, as shown by the solid lines. When, however, sensitivity is .8, the same increases in specificity yield dramatic decreases in confidence, as shown by the dashed lines. Bayes' formula reveals why this is so. An increase in sensitivity, $p(P_o|D_o)$, affects both the numerator and the denominator of the diagnostic ratio. In contrast, an increase in test specificity entails a decrease in $p(P_o|D_n)$, which affects only the ratio's denominator. As the denominator becomes smaller, the posterior probability of $D_o$ rises rapidly. When base-rates are low, a tolerance for low specificity reduces predictive accuracy, $p(D_o|P_o)$. Clinicians who overlook this consequence of Bayes's rule may end up making grossly inaccurate judgments.

**Diagnosing Health Without Stating the Obvious**

Even when a test yields a negative result for a low base-rate condition, a revision of belief is in order. In Cohen's (1994) example, a negative test result suggests that the probability of the disease has decreased from .021 to .001. To the client, a negative result may bring the desired peace of mind. This gain is particularly welcome to the extent that prior base rates of being healthy were underestimated. Aside from the disconfirmation of such mistaken expectations, diagnosing health beyond already high base rates can be useful. In genetic testing, for example, prospective parents may wish to assess the risk of having offspring with a recessive disorder. Even if only one prospective parent is tested and obtains a negative result, the probability that offspring will be affected decreases dramatically. Consider again Cohen's hypothetical data and suppose that a genetic defect will be expressed if both parents carry the

---

[5] This preference is not universal. When positive diagnoses lead to risky treatments, the costs of a false positive can be great.

gene. Assuming that mate selection is not affected by the presence of this gene, the probability of a defect is the product of the two base rates (i.e., $p(D_o)^2 = .02^2 = .004$). If, after testing, the probability of one parent to be a carrier can be said to be reduced to .001, the probability of risk falls to .00002 (i.e., .02 * .001). Because people are not sensitive to differences among extreme probabilities (Mellers & McGraw, 1999), test administrators may wish to express the gain as improved odds. In the present example, the negative test result suggests a 20-fold reduction of risk (i.e., from 40 to 2 in 100,000).

One of the authors experienced a counselor's difficulty of communicating the implications of a negative test result. When asked how much the risk of carrying the Tay-Sachs gene had been reduced by a negative test, the counselor insisted that the test produces few false negatives.[6] As Bayes's rule states, however, high specificity (i.e., a low $p(P_o|D_n)$) by itself does not reveal how improbable the condition is given a negative result (i.e., a low $p(D_o|P_n)$). Predictive judgments of health after a negative test result vary more with changes in specificity than with changes in sensitivity. These decreases in $p(D_n|P_n)$ are still small, however, because the posterior probability of health after a negative test result cannot be smaller than the prior probability of health, which is high when sampling is random. In sum, a loss of specificity selectively affects diagnoses of disease if, as is usually the case, the base rate of the disease in the population is below .5.

**A Neuropsychological Example**

Solomon et al. (1998) reported impressive efficiency data for a brief ("7 minute") screening test for Dementia of the Alzheimer Type (DAT). In a cross-validation sample, the test was 92% sensitive and 96% specific. Combined with the base-rate probabilities for DAT among the elderly (Evans et al., 1989), the test's efficiency leads to positive predictive values of .42, .84, and .95 for persons aged 65 – 74, persons aged 75 –

$$\frac{P(Po \mid Do)\, p(Do)}{p(Po \mid Dn)} > \frac{p(Dn)}{p(Do)} \tag{4.3}$$

---

[6]Gigerenzer et al. (1998) reported that "if the client asked for clarification more than twice, the [AIDS counselors] were likely to become upset and angry, experiencing the client's insistence on clarification as a violation of social norms of communication" (p. 202).

84, and persons older than 85, respectively (see Table 4.2, center).   As Cohen's (1994) example already illustrated, a single positive result may lead to the "paradoxical consequence that *deciding on the basis of more information can actually worsen the chances of a correct decision*" (Meehl & Rosen, 1955, p. 202, emphasis in the original).   When, for example, the test result is used for the youngest subgroup of the elderly, 2.76% of diagnoses are correct positives (i.e., $p(D_o)$ * $p(P_o|D_o)$ * 100) = .03 * .92 * 100) and 93.12% of diagnoses are correct negatives (i.e., $p(D_n)$ * $p(P_n|D_n)$ * 100 = .97 * .96 * 100).  The sum of correct diagnoses is 95.88%, which is worse than the 97% accuracy that would be achieved if, following the base rate, everyone were judged to be healthy.   To improve predictive accuracy beyond base rate accuracy, the ratio of the true positive rate (sensitivity) to the false positive rate (1-specificity) must be larger than the ratio of the negative base rate to the positive base rate (Meehl & Rosen, 1955).   That is, For the young old, the diagnostic ratio and the base rate ratio are 23 and 32, respectively, indicating that additional testing remains necessary. Perfect reliability and validity cannot be expected from psychometric tests.   Even if the sensitivity of the 7-minute test were to increase to from .92 to .99, with specificity remaining at .96, the positive predictive value for the young old would still be .42.  Conversely, as our foregoing analysis suggested, huge losses in sensitivity are compensated by small gains in specificity when the base rate of the disease is low.  A drop in sensitivity .46 would be offset by an increase in specificity to .98.

TABLE 4.2
Bayesian Diagnosis of Alzheimer's Disease

|  | Age Group | | |
| --- | --- | --- | --- |
|  | 65-74 | 75-84 | =>85 |
| Prior probability of DAT | .030 | .190 | .470 |
| Prior probability of other dementia | .003 | . 018 | .045 |
| Positive predictive value | .420 | .840 | .950 |
| Revised positive predictive value | .400 | .780 | .870 |
| Spoiling effect | .020 | .060 | .080 |

**The Spoiling Effect**

Solomon et al. (1998) constructed a screening test for DAT by contrasting a group of patients with known DAT with a community control group—of equal size—in which no one showed evidence of neuropsychological impairment. The estimate of specificity was "pure" in the sense that the available sample did not include patients who might have tested positive because of pathologies other than DAT. The drawback of the contrast-group method is that it tends to overestimate the specificity of the test in the general population (Ransohoff & Feinstein, 1978). Evans et al. (1989) estimated that 8.8% of the demented patients "have only a cause of dementia other than Alzheimer's disease" (p. 2554). Because these patients are more likely than normals to test positive, the false positive rate is higher and thus the predictive value of a positive result is lower than the test construction data suggest. Inasmuch as the base rates of different dementias are correlated, the size of the spoiling effect increases with the base rate of DAT. The illustrative values displayed in Table 4.2 show this effect. Values were computed assuming that the false positive rate forthe non-DAT group is the same as the true positive rate for the DAT group.

## BAYESIAN SCORE ESTIMATION

Bayesian models offer a way of thinking through uncertainty by combining expectations with evidence in a disciplined way. The categorical prediction tasks we have considered so far are relatively simple examples from clinical practice. The range of applicability for Bayesian methods is much broader, however. Before they can make clinical diagnoses, for example, neuropsychologists often need to integrate psychometric test data with other cues to infer a person's true performance level. Similarly, they need to integrate test scores to estimate true performance levels and predict future test scores.

Thorndike (1986a) gave an example where a test with a population mean of 100 and a standard deviation of 16 is administered to the same person two years apart (Equation 4.4). The stability correlation for this interval $(r = .85)$ determines the precision with which a score at Time 1 predicts a score at Time 2. The standard error of this prediction is $SE_{pre} = 16 * (1 - .85^2)^{.5} = 8.43$. The reliability coefficient of the test at Time 2 $(r = .94)$ determines that the standard error of measurement at Time 2 is $SE_{meas} = 16 * (1 - .94)^{.5} = 3.92$. If a test taker scored 115 at Time 1 and 125 at Time 2, then we estimate the that the individual's true score lies a bit closer to the second test score than to the first

$$\frac{\dfrac{\text{Score 1}}{SE^2_{pred}} + \dfrac{\text{Score 2}}{SE^2_{meas}}}{\dfrac{1}{SE^2_{pred}} + \dfrac{1}{SE^2_{meas}}} \Rightarrow \frac{\dfrac{115}{8.43^2} + \dfrac{125}{3.92^2}}{\dfrac{1}{8.43^2} + \dfrac{1}{3.92^2}} = 123.5 \quad (4.4)$$

test score because the reliability coefficient at Time 2 (.94) is greater than the stability coefficient for predictions of Time 2 scores from Time 1 scores (.85).   Most important, the standard error of the integrated estimate is smaller than the standard error of the Time 2 score (i.e., 3.92). Taking into account prior information (i.e., the Time 1 score), the test interpreter can revise and sharpen inferences from evidence gathered at Time 2.[7] Using Thorndike's statistical methods, the computer program "The Rev." estimates true scores from multiple test scores (and the means, standard deviations, and reliability coefficients of each test; Franklin & Allison, 1992).

Franklin and Crosby   (2001) presented the application of Bayesian methods to improve the diagnostic accuracy of the neuropsychological assessment by combining data from observational, parametric, and non-parametric analysis.

Diagnostic accuracy is improved in subsequent examinations where the Posterior odds$_1$ replaces base rate of the disorder.   Table 4.3 shows the effect of sequential assessment as described in Equations 4.5 - 4.7.   Posterior$_1$ shows a much poorer effect (.191) than expected from  a .05 significance level when the base rate (.010) is considered.   Posterior$_2$ replaces Posterior$_1$ for base rate in a second testing.   Because AS-NHST (see chap. 2, this volume) is used in Equations 4.5 and 4.6, probability calculations are reversed.   Here, .041 reflects a much improved level of conditional probability.   Equations 4.5 and 4.6 account for AS-NHST by flipping the probability ratios.   Posterior$_3$ reveals after third testing that our probability has fallen to .004, a statistical finding that inspires confidence.

---

[7]Using the same Bayesian approach, Thorndike (1986b) showed how information from different (but correlated) tests can be integrated and how test scores may be used to predict future performance on correlated tests.

$$\text{Posterior}_1 = \frac{(1 - \text{Base Rate})}{\text{Base Rate}} * \frac{(1 - p_1)}{p_1} \qquad (4.5)$$

$$\text{Posterior}_2 = \frac{\text{Posterior Odds}_1}{(1 - \text{Posterior Odds}_1)} * \frac{p_2}{(1 - p_2)} \qquad (4.6)$$

$$\text{Posterior}_3 = \frac{\text{Posterior Odds}_2}{(1 - \text{Posterior Odds}_2)} * \frac{p_3}{(1 - p_3)} \qquad (4.7)$$

Table 4.3
Effects of Sequential Bayesian Testing

| | DV | BR/(1-BR) (1-p)/p RS-H$_o$ or PO/(1-PO) or p/(1-p) AS-H$_o$ | |
|---|---|---|---|
| Symptom Base Rate | 0.010 | | |
| RS-H$_o$  Test p1 | 0.050 | | |
| *Posterior 1* | *0.191* | 0.010 | 19 |
| AS-H$_o$  Test p2 | 0.850 | | |
| *Posterior 2* | *0.041* | 0.237 | 5.6 |
| *AS-H$_o$  Test p3* | 0.910 | | |
| *Posterior 3* | *0.004* | 0.043 | 10 |

## Bayesian Networks

Bayesian networks are statistical models that evaluate relationships between sets of data, combining prior and current knowledge into one belief statement—such as diagnoses—about individual cases (e.g., Shafer, 1996). Thanks to these models "decision problems that, in the past, were hopelessly complex and unmanageable, are made both visually simple and intuitively obvious largely due to assumptions about conditional independence" (Mellers, Schwartz, & Cooke, 1998, p. 464). Networks perform three main functions. First, they represent observed phenomena. Second, they represent phenomena for which action is required without precise knowledge of the requisite data being available. Third, they integrate a priori expectations (e.g., beliefs) and outcome data (e.g., test scores) to generate lawful but fallible (i.e., probabilistic) inferences (Pearl, 1988).

In clinical settings, each new patient represents a  "case" requiring a diagnostic judgment. As we have seen, a Bayesian diagnosis reflects a belief of how signs and symptoms presented by the patient correspond to signs and symptoms associated with a specific disease or disorder. The diagnosis then becomes the basis for outcome prediction, intervention selection, or additional evaluation. In Bayesian networks, clinicians serve as "experts," whose experience is captured as the initial relations between variables (often in the form of conditional probabilities). Once the initial relations are specified, Bayesian networks can be fine-tuned by adding statistical findings from prior and new cases.

## Network Construction

Bayesian networks comprise two or more probabilistic variables, or *nodes*, and relations among the variables, or *links*. Nodes may contain discrete (e.g., true vs. false) or continuous (e.g., test scores) data. Links connect a source, or parent node, with a target, or child node. Parent nodes may have multiple child nodes, and child nodes may have multiple parent nodes. Links are unidirectional so that the represented relations may reflect partial or deterministic causation. Any relation between nodes can be represented in contingency tables.

Once constructed, a Bayesian network is applied to specific cases. For each known variable value, information is entered as a finding. Then, the network calculates a probabilistic inference to establish beliefs for all the other variables in the network. As is customary in Bayesian inference, the final beliefs are posterior probabilities (as opposed to the prior probabilities), which enter the network at the input level. As discussed earlier, the shift from prior to posterior probabilities reflects a revision, or updating, of belief.

The set of beliefs represented at each node reflects probabilistic inferences without changing the knowledge base (vis., original "expert" opinion) of the network. An important feature of Bayesian networks is that new findings representing "true examples" of the diagnosis can be added to the data base, thereby increasing diagnostic accuracy. Addition of new information leads to further belief revisions.    An example network is presented in the Appendix.

## Conclusions

The noted statistician and cognitive psychologist Ward Edwards (1998) predicted that "the 21st century [will be] the Century of Bayes" (p. 416). Several areas of psychological inquiry have been using Bayesian methods to good effect. In cognitive-experimental research, for example, Bayesian methods of hypothesis evaluation are beginning to supplement traditional significance testing (Krueger, 2001; Nickerson, 2000). Similarly, Bayes' theorem has served as a model for inductive reasoning processes that generate these data (Kahneman, Slovic, & Tversky, 1982), a development that Edwards himself pioneered (Edwards, 1961).    Other academic and applied disciplines, such as medical diagnosis, forensic judgment, managerial decision making, econometrics, paternity testing, and engineering control theory, have benefited from the use of Bayesian principles as well (Press, 1989; West & Harrison, 1989).

In    clinical    psychology    and    neuropsychology,    however, applications of automated Bayesian inference and the use of Bayesian belief networks lag behind the technological possibilities. Of the 36 tests marketed by American Guidance Service (AGS, 1999), for example, only 39% provide computer scoring. Slightly more than half provide narrative reports, and only two compare findings of one test with another.    Although AGS is not a developer or publisher of neuropsychological tests, many of their measures are useful for the evaluation of children with neuropsychological disorders and of adults whose function is so impaired that tests standardized for "normal" adults are inappropriate.

If we consider the 53 neuropsychological tests published by the Psychological Corporation (1999), we find that only 17 provide scoring software. Only nine have the capability to produce narrative reports, and five can compare findings from one or two other tests (all of which are published in-house).    Unfortunately, test publishers rarely provide interpretative software that is adequate for comparing findings from multiple sources, even though development of user-friendly applications like *Netica* (Norsys Software, 1997) demonstrate availability and cost-effectiveness of Bayesian techniques. What is more, it is unclear which software interpretation programs, if any, include Bayesian evaluation models in their inference engines.

Edwards (1998) expressed concern that "unless psychologists learn about these new tools, they will not be able to compete in the rapidly growing market concerned with training domain experts to make the judgments they require" (p. 417). We hope that the present chapter contributes to a rising willingness among psychologists and neuropsychologists to consider these methods.

## ACKNOWLEDGMENTS

We are indebted to Hal Arkes, Robyn Dawes, and Roy Poses for their generous feedback on a draft version of this chapter.

## REFERENCES

American Guidance Service. (1999). *Clinical catalog*. Circle Pines, MN: Author.

Arkes, H. R., Wortmann, R. L., Saville, P. D., & Harkness, A. R. (1981). Hindsight bias among physicians weighing the likelihood of diagnoses. *Journal of Applied Psychology, 66*, 252-254.

Dascells, W., Schoenberger, A., & Graybors, T. (1978). Interpretation by physicians of clinical laboratory results. *New England Journal of Medicine, 299*, 999-1001.

Bayes, T. (1763). An essay toward solving a problem in the doctrine of chance. *Philosophical Transactions of the Royal Society, 53*, 370-418.

Birnbaum., M. H. (1983). Base rates in Bayesian inference: Signal detection analysis of the cab problem. *American Journal of Psychology, 96*, 85-94.

Cohen, J. (1994). The earth is round ($p < .05$). *American Psychologist, 49*, 997-1003.

Dawes, R. M. (1988). *Rational choice in an uncertain world*. San Diego: Harcourt Brace.

Dawes, R. M. (1994). *House of cards: Psychology and psychotherapy built on myth*. New York: The Free Press.

Dawes, R. M. (2000). Proper and improper linear models. In T. Connolly, H. Arkes & K. R. Hammond (Eds.), *Judgment and decision making: An interdisciplinary reader* (2nd ed., pp. 378-394). New York: Cambridge University Press.

Dawes, R. M., Faust, D., & Meehl, P. E. (1989). Clinical versus actuarial judgment. *Science, 243,* 1668-1674.

Eddy, D. M. (1982). Probabilistic reasoning in clinical medicine: Problems and opportunities. In D. Kahneman, P. Slovic, & A. Tversky (Eds.), *Judgment under uncertainty: Heuristics and biases* (pp. 249-267). Cambridge, England: Cambridge University Press.

Eddy, D. M. (1984). Variations in physician practice: The role of uncertainty. *Health Affairs, 3,* 74-89.

Eddy, D. M., & Clanton, C. H. (1982). The art of diagnosis: Solving the clinicopathological exercise. *The New England Journal of Medicine, 306,* 1263-1268.

Edwards, W. (1961). Behavioral decision theory. *Annual Review of Psychology, 12,* 473-498.

Edwards, W. (1998). Hailfinder: Tools for and experiences with Bayesian normative modeling. *American Psychologist, 53,* 416-428.

Elwood, R. W. (1993). Clinical discriminations and neuropsychological tests: An appeal to Bayes' theorem. *The Clinical Neuropsychologist, 7,* 224-233.

Evans, D. A., Funkenstein, H. H., Albert, M. S., Schaer, P. A., Cook, N. R., Chowan, M. J., Hebert, L. E., Hennekens, C. H., & Taylor, J. O. (1989). Prevalence of Alzheimer's disease in a community population of older persons. *Journal of the American Medical Association, 262,* 2551-2556.

Faust, D., & Ziskin, J. (1988). The expert witness in psychology and psychiatry. *Science, 241,* 31-35.

Feinstein, A. R. (1978). On the sensitivity, specificity, and discrimination of diagnostic tests. *Clinical Biostatistics, 17,* 104-116.

Franklin, R. D., & Allison, D. B. (1992). The Rev.: An IBM BASIC program for Bayesian test interpretation. *Behavior Research Methods, Instruments, & Computers, 24,* 491-492.

Franklin, R. D., & Crosby, F. X. (2001). Early stopping rules in forensic neuropsychological evaluations. *Journal of the International Neuropsychological Society, 7*(4), 416.

Garb, H. N., & Schramke, C. J. (1996). Judgment research and neurological assessment: A narrative review and meta-analysis. *Psychological Bulletin, 120,* 140-153.

Gigerenzer, G., & Hoffrage, U. (1995). How to improve Bayesian reasoning without instruction: Frequency formats. *Psychological Review, 102,* 684-704.

Gigerenzer, G., Hoffrage, U., & Ebert, A. (1998). AIDS counselling for low-risk clients. *AIDS Care, 10,* 197-211.

Goodman, L. A., & Kruskal, W. H. (1954). Measures of association for cross classifications. *American Statistical Association Journal, 49,* 732-764.

Hoffrage, U., Lindsey, S., Hertwig, R. & Gigerenzer, G. (2000). Communicating statistical information. *Science, 290,* 2261-2262.

Jones, W. P. (1989). A proposal for the use of Bayesian probabilities in neuropsychological assessement. *Neuropsychology, 3,* 17-22.

Kahneman, D., Slovic, P., & Tversky, A. (1982). *Judgment under uncertainty: Heuristics and biases.* Cambridge, England: Cambridge University Press.

Koehler, J. J. (1996). The base rate fallacy reconsidered: Descriptive, normative, and methodological challenges. *Behavioral and Brain Sciences, 19,* 1-53.

Krueger, J. (2001). Null hypothesis significance testing: On the survival of a flawed method. *American Psychologist, 56,* 16-26.

Lindley, D. V. (1993). The analysis of experimental data: The appreciation of tea and wine. *Teaching Statistics, 15,* 22-25.

Meehl, P. E., & Rosen, A. (1955). Antecedent probability and the efficiency of psychometric signs, patterns, and cutting scores. *Psychological Bulletin, 52,* 194-216.

Mellers, B. A., & McGraw, P. (1999). How to improve Bayesian reasoning: Comment on Gigerenzer and Hoffrage (1995). *Psychological Review, 106,* 417-424.

Mellers, B. A., Schwartz, A., & Cooke, A. D. J. (1998). Judgment and decision making. *Annual Review of Psychology, 49,* 447-477.

Nickerson, R. S (2000). Null hypothesis significance testing: A review of an old and continuing controversy. *Psychological Methods, 5,* 241-301.

Norsys Software Corp. (1997). *Netica manual.* Vancouver,BC, Canada: Author.

Pearl, J. (1988). *Probabilistic reasoning in intelligent systems: Networks of plausible inference.* San Mateo, CA: Morgan Kaufman.

Press, S. J. (1989). *Bayesian statistics: Principles, models, and applications.* New York: Wiley.

The Psychological Corporation (1999). *The catalog for neuropsychological assessment & intervention resources.* San Antonio, TX: Author.

Ransohoff, D. F., & Feinstein, A. R. (1978). Problems of spectrum and bias in evaluation the efficacy of diagnostic tests. *The New England Journal of Medicine, 299,* 926-930.

Satz, P., Fennell, E., & Reilly, C. (1970). Predictive validity of six neuropsychological tests: A decision theory analysis. *Journal of Consulting and Clinical Psychology, 34,* 375-381.

Sedlmeier, P. (1997). BasicBayes: a tutor system for simple Bayesian inference. *Behavior Research Methods, Instrumentats and Computers, 27,* 328-336.

Shafer, G. (1996). *Probabilistic expert systems.* Philadelphia: SIAM.

Snodgrass, J. G., & Corwin, J. (1988). Pragmatics of measuring memory: Applications to dementia and amnesia. *Journal of Experimental Psychology: General, 117,* 34-50.

Solomon, P. R., Hirschoff, A., Kelly, B., Relin, M., Brush, M., DeVeaux, R. D., & Pendlebury, W. W. (1999). A 7 minute neurocognitive screening battery highly sensitive to Alzheimer's Disease. *Archives of Neurology, 55,* 349-355.

Thorndike, R. L. (1986a). Bayesian concepts and test interpretation. *Journal of counseling and Development, 65,* 170-172.

Thorndike, R. L. (1986b). The role of Bayesian concepts in test development and test interpretation. *Journal of Counseling and Development, 65,* 54-56.

West, M., & Harrison, J. (1989). *Bayesian forecasting and dynamic models.* New York, NY: Springer-Verlag.

Winkler, R. L. (1993). Bayesian statistics: An overview. In G. Keren & C. Lewis (Eds.), *A handbook for data analysis in the behavioral sciences: Statistical Issues* (pp. 210-232). Hillsdale, NJ: Lawrence Erlbaum Associates.

APPENDIX

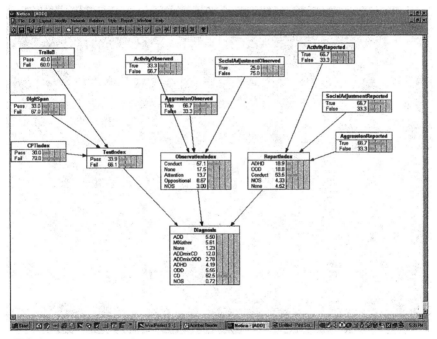

FIG. A.1.  Bayes network for evaluating disorders of conduct.

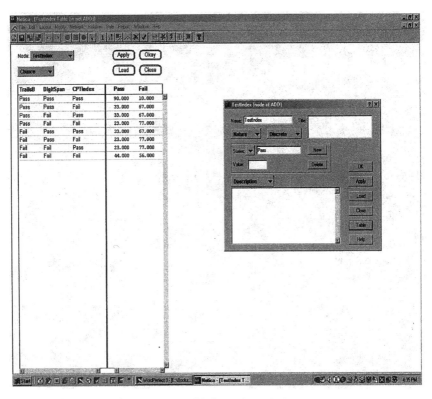

FIG. A.2.  Bayes network contingency table for node TestIndex.

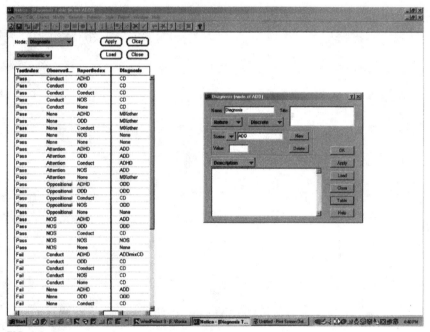

FIG. A.3.  Bayes network contingency table for node Diagnosis.

# Neuropsychological Evaluations
## as Statistical Evidence[1]

**Ronald D. Franklin**
*St. Mary's Hospital and Florida Atlantic University*[2]

**Joachim I. Krueger**
*Brown University*

## EVIDENCE DEFINED

According to Merriam Webster (1996) evidence has different vernacular and legal meanings. In the vernacular it is associated with proof and truth, as well as the observation of events. In law, the term is more precise, referring to "proof of fact(s)" presented at a trial. Evidence is essential in convincing the judge or jury of the facts in a case, thereby enabling the discovery of truth. Legal evidence can include "hard" findings such as photographs, audio recordings, plaster castings, fingerprints, and medical records. More often, however, evidence is provided by a fallible witness who can be questioned and cross-

---

[1]This chapter is prepared with individuals who have received at least one undergraduate and one graduate course in statistics and psychometric theory in mind. Readers lacking this preparation, or those whose exposure to the topics is weak or dated, should review current works such as those prepared by Glenberg (1996) and Thorndike (1997).

[2]Please address correspondence to PO Box 246, Candor, NC 27229 or rdfphd@yahoo.com

examined. In this chapter we consider the evidentiary basis of psychological test data. Psychometric theory, the foundation of psychological test interpretation, evolved from statistical hypothesis testing (see chapter 3, this volume). Recent trends in test interpretation (see Chan, R. C. K, 2001; Martens, Donders, & Millis, 2001; Mitrushina, Boone & D'Elia, 1999; Putzke, Williams, Blutting, Konold, & Boll, 2001; and Rosenfeld, Sands & Van Gorp, 2000) champion interpretation anchored in base rate. Although base rate must be considered as an import component of diagnostic formulation, rarity is not synonymous with disability. For example, it is rare when children are born with extra digits or red eyes, but both are expressions of normal variation and rarely impair growth or development even though they may be associated with other disorders that affect development. In considering psychological findings as evidence it is wise to remember Fisher's (1959) *frequency admonition* "...the infrequency with which, in particular circumstances, decisive evidence is obtained, should not be confused with the force, or cogency, of such evidence" (p. 93).

## THE WITNESS AS EVIDENCE

Courts generally recognize two types of witness, the fact witness and the expert witness.

### The Fact Witness

A witness of fact reports firsthand observations to the court. There is no expectation that the fact witness provide an opinion or personal view. Circumstances may permit statements of views from a fact witness when "(a) [opinions are] rationally based on the perception of the witness, and (b) helpful to a clear understanding of the witness' testimony or the determination of a fact in issue" (Stromberg et al., 1988, p. 646). A fact witness may be compelled to testify with no guarantee of payment. The uncertainty of payment may influence the thoroughness of a fact witness' literature review or examination. In medicine and psychology, a treating clinician is often called upon as a fact witness. When this occurs, the witness can be asked to comment on a variety of topics such as the degree of impairment, or the likely cause of a medical or psychological condition, why specific treatments were recommended (or not recommended), and what prognosis can be made. A psychologist who has evaluated a patient following traumatic brain injury may be asked to witness this fact. Usually fact testimony is limited to when and why a patient is seen. However, "facts" sometimes represent opinions (ie., clinical judgments such as is the patient brain damaged) instead of factual information. What is more, the fact witness may not be allowed to present research findings supporting clinical judgments on the grounds that they are tentative working hypotheses rather than actual facts. Hence there may be rules circumscribing the kinds of information allowable as a fact. What is more, items presented as facts are subject to challenge in cross-examination. When findings provide greater support for one side than the other, an expert may be hired for the purpose of challenging opinions expressed by the fact witness. Challenges of facts typically occur in two forms; cross-examination and testimony by an expert witness. The attorney who cross-examines a fact witness may have a non-testifying expert review reports or notes of the fact witness as well as any depositions taken for the current or prior trials. Reviews of prior trials can include any similar cases for which the fact expert has made public statements, including depositions or trial testimony. When large financial settlements are possible, a consulting expert will likely provide the attorney who cross-examines with information designed to undermine those opinions expressed by the fact witness. There may be no requirement that either attorney inform the fact witness regarding the involvement of either a consulting expert or a testifying expert, although the attorney who calls the fact witness typically provides the fact witness with reports and depositions provided by a testifying expert. Most likely, if an attorney employs a non-testifying expert, neither the fact witness nor the other attorney(s) will have knowledge of the employment. So, a prudent fact witness assumes that every test and test protocol will be scrutinized by a hostile expert who has conducted a thorough literature review and has likely conducted independent research on some aspect of neuropsychology that is relevant to the case.

**The Expert Witness**

The designation of a witness as "expert" by the courts has specific meaning as defined by Federal Rules of Evidence 702 and 703 (http://expertpages.com/federal/federal.htm). These rules allow courts to qualify a witness as expert on the basis of knowledge, skill, experience, training, or education, and to allow admission of scientific data or other information used in the expert testimony. Experts usually enter a case voluntarily and may or may not actually testify. On some occasions, psychologists or other professionals are appointed by the courts to serve as expert witness. Compensation is usually provided for case preparation and testimony. Because the designation as "expert" does not guarantee payment in all jurisdictions, many experts require payment of a retainer before they will meet with either the attorney or the patient. Obtaining a retainer is important because it insures that the neuropsychologist can perform both a thorough literature review and an appropriate examination.

***Psychologists as Expert Witnesses.*** The entry of psychology as experts in the courts dates back to 1962 (Ofloff, Beavers, & DeLeon, 1999). Courts have consistently upheld the right of psychologists to qualify as experts for testimony concerning the presence of brain damage. Courts have historically been less supportive in qualifying psychologists as experts regarding the issue of causality (McCaffrey, Williams, Fisher, & Laing, 1997) but acceptance of psychological testimony for this purpose is growing.

***Neuropsychologists as Expert Witnesses.*** Since its introduction in the legal arena, the use of neuropsychological testimony has been vigorously challenged. In their first edition of *Coping With Psychiatric and Psychological Testimony*, Ziskin and Faust (1998) argued that psychological data were based upon inadequate science. Faust, Ziskin, and Hiers (1991) further described neuropsychological data as inadequate legal evidence. Replies to this claim have been vigorous (see Barth, Ryan, & Hawk, 1992; McCaffrey et al., 1997), many writers noted that Ziskin and Faust's critique targeted the scientific method and its application to psychometric theory. Much of the debate focuses either directly or indirectly on the value of null hypothesis testing (NHST) to diagnosis and outcome prediction (see chapter 3, this volume).

Currently, the role of psychology is being resolved in the courts regarding testimony for both the presence and cause of brain damage. For example, Florida case law recently reversed the disallowance of neuropsychologists testifying with regard to causation:

> Because the practice of psychology has expanded to the point where psychologists who are not [medical] doctors are increasingly becoming involved in areas which were traditionally considered to be purely medical, a blanket prohibition of testimony by psychologists concerning causation of brain injury no longer seems practical. Instead, the more prudent

approach is to allow trial judges, in their discretion, to qualify psychologists and neuropsychologists to testify on causation as any otherexpert would be qualified to testify in his or her area of expertise. (School Board vs. Cruz, 2000)[3]

The Georgia legislature has also defined neuropsychologists as professionals who can diagnose and treat organic brain disorders (T. G. Burns, personal communication 10/15/01).

The view taken in this chapter is that psychology is well suited to litigation because hypothesis testing using psychological test data is consistent with the spirit of the judicial process and because test findings are open to empirical review. Controversy about psychological evidence historically involves two points; variations in the role of hypothesis testing as a basis of neuropsychological evidence and the use of statistical data as evidence of neuropsychological deficit. This chapter reviews salient aspects of these issues, and offers alternatives to currently disputed statistical procedures.

***Statistics in the evidentiary process.***  In contrast to facts, statistics are tools used by experts for the formulation of opinions. While statistical evidence does not directly signify truth, it can be submitted to inferential methods that help estimate the truth of relevant hypotheses. Royall (1997) stated that statistical evidence refers to "which [hypothesis] is better supported. We might reasonably expect that strong evidence cannot be misleading very often" (p. 6). The degree to which statistical evidence constitutes legal evidence is determined by established "rules of evidence." These rules provide judges discretion in allowing or disallowing statistical information as evidence depending upon the circumstances of the case. Rules of evidence permit a judge to limit information provided to juries because jurors "are not totally

---

[3]Jurisdictions are beginning to certify neuropsychologists as psychology sub-specialists. The state of Georgia, for example, (Official Code of Georgia Annotated Section 43-39-1) defines neuropsychology as "concerned with the relationship between the brain and behavior, including the diagnosis of brain pathology through the use of psychological tests and assessment techniques."

rational, they must be shielded from exposure to information which is more likely to be deceptive than illuminating" (Stromberg, et al., 1988, p. 594).

Neuropsychological test scores reflect statistical reasoning at various levels. Statistical modeling is ubiquitous in psychological training, test development, and test interpretation. In best practice, the psychologist interprets statistical information gained from testing in such a way that designated parties in the court (i.e., judges and jurors) can infer "truth." The degree to which neuropsychological testimony aids in the inference of "truth" determines the value of that testimony to the court.

## HYPOTHESIS TESTING
## AS A BASIS OF PSYCHOLOGICAL EVIDENCE

Two statistical models of hypothesis testing are used in psychology, frequentist and Bayesian. The frequentist model is concerned with how frequently certain observations can be expected to occur given a certain hypothetical distribution (such as the number of snake-eye rolls out of 10 tosses of two fair dice). There are two frequentists approaches, often referred to as the Fisherian and Neyman-Pearson schools (see chap. 3, this volume.) In contrast to the frequentist approach, the Bayesian approach (chap. 4, this volume) considers prior probability distributions as well as frequency distributions present at the time of the observation. What is more, the Bayesian approach permits estimates regarding the outcome of single, yet unobserved, events.

### Frequentist Models of Hypothesis Testing

*Fisher's Theory.* According to Fisher, observed data need to be compared with a preselected critical region within a theoretical distribution using Null Hypothesis Significance Testing (NHST). Specifically, NHST yields the probability of finding the observed data—or data more extreme—if the theoretical distribution is assumed to be true. Because the $p$ value can vary considerably depending on the extremity and the number of observations, its interpretation is confounded. A quarter of a century ago, ten of the world's leading applied statisticians, co-authored a paper explaining that trials contain large sample sizes provide stronger evidence than trials containing small sample sizes (Peto et al., 1976, p. 593). Rejection trials (also known as

Rejection Support Null Hypothesis Testing or RS-NHST, see chapter 3, this volume), is a second expression of Fisher's model, that includes an alternative hypothesis with the null. However, the alternative hypothesis associated with the null is simply a statement of what has not occurred.

***Neyman-Pearson Theory.*** In contrast to Fisher's method, the Neyman-Pearson approach to NHST requires setting up a substantive alternative to the null hypothesis. Then, the method permits a choice between two alternative hypotheses given the evidence by evaluating the probability of the data under each of the contesting hypotheses. As in Fisher's method, the data are compared in terms of their abilities to predict long-run averages. Hence, both approaches are less concerned with the meaning or the value of the data than they are with the mathematical relationships between the sets of data.

***The Statistical Relationship Between Test Findings and Diagnosis.*** Frequentist theories evaluate relationships between a distribution of sample data with hypothetical distributions. The typical task of the psychologist, however, is to reach a judgment on individual cases based on actual test findings. Table 5.1 presents the nominal descriptions that are used to indicate relationships between test findings and the presence or absence of a disorder.

TABLE 5.1
Nominal References for 2x2 Hypothesis Decision Matrix.

| test findings +/- | disorder presence+/- | nominal reference |
|:---:|:---:|:---|
| + | + | sensitivity |
| - | - | specificity |
| - | + | 1-sensitivity |
| + | - | 1-specificity |

First defined by Yerushalami (1947), the terms 'sensitivity' and 'specificity' address the same issues of hypothesis testing described in Table 3.1 (chap. 3, this volume). Sensitivity refers to the proportion of the population with the disorder who test positive. Specificity refers to the proportion of the population without the disorder who test negative.

Ideally, psychological tests have both high sensitivity and high specificity. What these indexes have to say about the psychologist's judgment in an individual case also depends on the overall 'prevalence' (i.e., the base rate) of the disorder in the tested population (Meehl & Rosen, 1955).

## The Bayesian Approach to Hypothesis Evaluation

As noted in chap. 4, this volume, Bayesian methods lead to the estimation of likelihood ratios and posterior probabilities of certain hypotheses. This section presents a brief description of both, considering the efficacy of them as evidence.

### *Estimates of Posterior Probabilities.*

Three posterior probability estimates are described in the psychology literature (e.g., Elwood, 1993; Glaros & Kline, 1988).

*Positive Predictive Value.* (PPV) refers to the probability the patient has the disorder given a positive test result $p(D_o|P_o)$. According to Bayes' Theorem, PPV (Equations 5.1 and 5.2) is a posterior probability that depends on the prevalence of the disorder, the sensitivity of the test, and the overall probability of obtaining a positive test result. The latter is the sum of two probabilities: The test score could be positive given the presence (sensitivity) or the absence of the disorder (1-specificity).

$$PPV = \frac{prevalence * sensitivity}{prevalence * sensitivity + (1 - prevalence) * (1\text{-}specificity)} \quad (5.1)$$

or

$$p(D_o|P_o) = \frac{p(D_o) * p(P_o|D_o)}{p(D_o) * (p(P_o|D_o) + (p(D_n) * p(P_o|D_n))} \quad (5.2)$$

**Negative Predictive Value.** (NPV) is the probability the patient does not have the disorder given a negative test result ($p(P_n|D_n)$) as demonstrated in Equation 5.3.

$$NPV = \frac{(1\text{-prevalence}) \times \text{specificity}}{(1\text{-prevalence}) \times \text{specificity} + \text{prevalence} \times (1\text{-sensitivity})} \quad (5.3)$$

**Overall Predictive Value.** (OPV) calculates the probability that a test taker's classification is correct (Equation 5.4) . The probability that a positive diagnosis is correct is the product of PPV and the prevalence of the disorder. The probability that a negative diagnosis is the product of NPV and the complement of the prevalence. OPV is the sum of these two products.

$$OPV = PPV * \text{prevalence} + NPV * (1\text{-prevalence}) \quad (5.4)$$

Clearly, OPV increases as PPV or NPV increase. The role of the prevalence of the disorder is less intuitive, because regardless of PPV and NPV, OPV increases as the prevalence becomes more extreme. If prevalence is .5, the a priori uncertainty regarding the presence of the disorder in the tested individual is at its maximum, which keeps OPV fairly low even if PPV and NPV are high. The question then is whether OPV is high enough to permit the claim that testing has improved the accuracy of the diagnosis beyond what it would be without testing. One way to evaluate such improvement is to ask whether OPV is superior to making a diagnosis randomly, on the basis of prevalence alone (Wiggins, 1973). If, for example, the prevalence of a disorder were .1, one might randomly make a positive diagnosis for every tenth client. The OPV of such a procedure would be .82 (i.e., $.9^2+.1^2$). It is difficult to justify this procedure because it amounts to non-optimal probability matching. If the assessor were to make a negative diagnosis in each case, OPV would be .9. The drawback of this method, of course, is that no positive diagnosis would ever be made, thus precluding any correct identification of the disorder. A good test with high sensitivity and specificity is a necessary tool if psychological assessors are to improve their diagnosis beyond these unsatisfactory alternatives. Such improvement becomes increasingly difficult as prevalence base rates become more extreme (which typically means as disorders become rarer).

To see if testing actually improves diagnosis, the ratio of OPV over the complement of the disorder's prevalence (1-prevalence) may be used (assuming that the disorder is rare; if it is frequent, the ratio is OPV/prevalence). Note that it is possible that both PPV and NPV are greater than their respective base rates (prevalence and 1-prevalence), while OPV is smaller than the accuracy one would achieve making uniformly negative diagnoses (i.e., 1-prevalence if $p(D_o|P_o) < .5$). As an example, consider the case in which the prevalence of the disorder is .2, sensitivity is .6 and specificity is .7. In this case, PPV/prevalence = 1.67, NPV/(1-prevalence) = 1.09, while OPV/(1-prevalence) = .96.

In psychological testing, the term Base Rate has two additional meanings. First, it refers to the frequency distribution of scores within populations – $BR_f$. For example, a standard score of 100 has a frequency distribution of 50% in the normal standardization sample. However the same score of 100 would have a frequency distribution of < 1% in the Huntington's disease sample (The Psychological Corporation, 1997, p. 147). $BR_f$ may help the psychologist understand if a finding is rare, but it conveys no diagnostic information per se. Second, Base Rate is also used to describe the cumulative frequency of the score differences between tests in a given population – $BR_d$. Here, for example, differences of one standard deviation between Verbal and Performance IQ occur at a cumulative frequency of 15.5 % (The Psychological Corporation, 1997, p. 305). Again, $BR_d$ provides no information about diagnosis, unless the rarity of these combined scores exclusively defines a disorder. Confounds occur with each of the three expressions of Base Rate. Prevalence Base Rates ($BR_p$) are problematic because even though estimates of disease prevalence exist they are sometimes disputed, and can vary considerably across cultures and geographic regions. What is more, if $BR_p$ is known psychologists rarely know either the sensitivity or the specificity for most psychological tests associated with a specific diagnosis. $BR_f$ and $BR_d$ are more problematic because they convey no information that is unique, either to the patient or to specific disorders. Score frequencies are largely undefined for specific populations, and where they exist inconsistency is the rule rather than the exception. Remember Fisher's *Infrequency Admonition*.

*Likelihood Ratios.* As noted in chap. 3, this volume, likelihood ratios ($\lambda$) represent the ratio of the probabilities of the data under two hypotheses. When we compare the OPV (see Equation 5.4) of tests measuring two different diagnoses, we can consider ($\lambda$) as a measure of evidence for the first test ($OPV_1$) vis-à-vis the second test ($OPV_2$).

To the degree that two findings measure different diagnoses, the ratio of ($\lambda$) OPV constitutes a likelihood ratio such that:

$$(\lambda) = \frac{OPV_1}{OPV_2} \qquad (5.5)$$

For example, consider the comorbid diagnoses of oppositional defiant disorder (ODD) and attention deficit disorder (ADD). If I have a test for ODD with an $OPV_1$ of .92 given the patient's score on the ODD measure, and a second test for ADD having an $OPV_2$ of .72 given the patient's score on the ADD measure, then by substituting the values for ODD/ADD in Equation 5.5, $(\lambda)$ = .92/.72. We could conclude that evidence supporting the diagnosis of ODD is stronger than the evidence supporting a diagnosis of ADD. Later in this chapter we will consider the strength of this evidence as well as the degree to which this evidence can be weak or misleading. This ratio provides an efficacious measure of statistical evidence for determining which psychological test best characterizes a diagnosis "beyond a reasonable degree of medical certainty" as defined by Brigham, Babitsky & Mangraviti, (1996). See Chapter 3, this volume for further discussion of medical certainty.

Likelihood ratios are problematic when conditional probabilities are equal for both the numerator and the denominator, resulting in the same $\lambda$ when both $OPV_1$ and $OPV_2$ = .9 or when $OPV_1$ and $OPV_2$ = .001. In the first instance, a high degree of confidence is warranted. In the second instance, little confidence is warranted. Also, on those occasions where the denominator is zero, $\lambda$ is undefined.

## THE INADEQUACIES OF STATISTICAL HYPOTHESIS TESTING AS EVIDENCE

Both frequentist models reflect similar views regarding hypothesis testing. Because they are ubiquitously associated with null hypothesis testing in psychology, they both suffer from similar inadequacies as evidence. Royall (1997) argued that both the Neyman-Pearson model (p. 56) and Fisher's model (p. 79) produce invalid outcomes that can "lead to different results in two situations where the evidence is the same." Proofs supporting Royall's statements are beyond the scope of this work and interested persons should review his original text. It is important for readers to understand that his formative arguments represent a Bayesian perspective (see Chapter 3, this volume).

**Null Hypothesis Significance Testing**

Null hypothesis statistical testing (NHST) has become the standard for many scientific publications. Even so, there have been critics of the method since its inception. Tryon (1998) attributed the success of NHST to the ease at which it can be correctly calculated and interpreted. Yet, prominent psychometricians often misinterpret NHST results (Cohen, 1994) and documented misuse of the procedure has occurred for three decades (Dar, Serlin, & Omer, 1994). Most of the introductory psychology textbooks printed between 1965 and 1994 presented NHST inaccurately (McMan, 1995). Critics present three classes of problems associated with NHST: (a) the logical foundations (b) interpretation difficulties and (c) failure to also use supplementary or alternative inference methods (Krueger, 2001).

*Logical Foundation.* The logical foundation of null hypothesis testing was eloquently challenged by Howson and Urbach (1989), who viewed the inductive step of either accepting or rejecting a null hypothesis as capricious. Arbitrary decisions must be taken (i.e., proper statistic derived from "experience" or personal judgment) in order to render a conclusion. A leading advocate of the null hypothesis method proposed by Fisher once stated, "There is no answer to [the question] 'Which significance test should one use  except the subjective one? Personal views intrude always" (Kempthorne, 1966, p. 12).

*Interpretation Difficulties.* Problems interpreting the Neyman-Pearson model lead to the introduction of a distribution having a critical region against which observations could be compared with a test-statistic selected a priori. Rejection criteria were recommended for this critical region and a hypothesis was "rejected" or "failed rejection" dependent on how sample data compared to this critical region. Unfortunately, the meaning of "accept and reject a hypothesis or reject and fail to reject" remain obscure. What is more, it is commonly assumed that acceptance or rejection of a hypothesis may be a function of the size of the sample rather than anything associated with the theory.

Howson and Urbach (1989) described many instances showing how the results of hypothesis testing using either the Fisher or Neyman-Person standard are in conflict with reality. Two well-known examples germane to psychology were reported by Cohen (1994). Meehl and Lykken (cited in Meehl, 1990) cross-tabulated 15 presumably unrelated items taken from 57,000 Minnesota high school students. All of the cross-tabulation were statistically significant, 96% of them at p <

.000001!  Meehl (1990) thus noted that, "the notion that the correlation between arbitrarily paired trait variables will be, while not literally zero, of such minuscule size as to be of no importance, is surely wrong" (p. 212). In the second oft-cited example, Cohen reported a 2% incidence of schizophrenia in adults. One screening for schizophrenia has a sensitivity of 95% and specificity of 97%. Given a positive test for schizophrenia, and a test sensitivity of 95%, one might conclude that the patient with a positive test result has schizophrenia because there is less than a 5% chance the test is in error. However, given the low incidence of schizophrenia, the true probability that the case is normal is about .60 (calculated using the Bayesian model presented in Equation 1; see chap. 4, this volume, for a more detailed description of this problem). As noted by Howson and Urbach (1989): Well supported hypotheses are often rejected by a significance test. Inference by significance test also clashes with entrenched ideas about the nature of evidence, requiring the rejection of hypotheses that seem highly confirmed, allowing (in randomized tests) quite extraneous experiments such as the selection of cards from a pack to influence one's attitude toward hypotheses which have nothing to do with cards. (p. 175)

Psychologists who react to negative beliefs derived from rejection of a null hypothesis as though they are valid, "accept" null hypotheses by behaving as though they were true (Malgady, 1998). Subjective, and possibly unconscious or obscure, value judgment may enter into this inference. Nickerson (2000) cited other criticisms of NHST, which are summarized in Table 5.2

TABLE 5.2
Other Criticisms of Null Hypothesis Statistical Testing

| |
| --- |
| a priori unlikelihood that $H_o$ is true |
| sensitivity of NHST to sample size |
| noninformativeness of test outcomes |
| inappropriateness of all-or-none |
|       decisions regarding significance |
| arbitrariness of the decision criterion test bias |
| possible inflation of Type I errors in the literature |
| presumed frequency of Type II errors |
| ease of violating assumptions of statistical tests |
| influence on experimental designs |

*The Directional Hypothesis.* If a neuropsychologist has reason to suspect that scores from the patient's test protocol will be greater than or less than those obtained from the comparison group, a directional hypothesis is sometimes used. The directional hypothesis is evaluated using a one-tailed statistical test that compares scores with only one half of the theoretical distribution. The one-tailed test effectively doubles the likelihood of finding a "significant" effect (Dietrich & Kearns, 1983). Because the directional hypothesis does not allow inferences in cases where findings are the opposite of those predicted, it should be avoided in clinical practice.

Despite the ongoing criticisms of NHST, the methods have also found its apologists. Hagen (1998), for example, attributes shortcomings to improper use by evaluators. He observed that "the null hypothesis is not a statement about the sample (i.e., the patient), [it] is a statement about the population [e.g., standardization sample] from which the sample is drawn" (p. 801). When investigators and clinicians render conclusions about patients from null hypothesis test results, they make inappropriate attributions. Table 5.3 presents Nickerson's (2000) synopsis of reasons that he believes NHST has withstood the many criticisms (see also Krueger, 2001).

TABLE 5.3
Reasons Null Hypothesis Statistical Testing
Remains Impervious to Criticism

---

lack of understanding of NHST or confusion
    regarding conditional probabilities
the appeal of formalism and the appearance of objectivity
the need to cope with the threat of chance
deep entrenchment of the approach within the field
    [of psychology] as evidenced in the behavior of
    advisers, editors, and researchers
it appears to provide the user with a relatively
    simple and straightforward method for
    separating meaningful and irrelevant data

---

**Standardization Samples in Psychology**

Perhaps because of the ubiquity of NHST in psychology research and test standardization, psychologists often make assumptions about data reported as "norms" for psychological tests. First, they assume that data described by means and standard deviations are measured using equal intervals (i.e., 30 - 35 is the same score difference as 100 - 105). Second, they assume that the distances between scores are equal across tests (i.e., 85 - 95 on Test A: 35 - 45 on Test B). Three, data are assumed to follow a "bell curve" distribution. Spreen and Strauss (1998) published reviews of more than 91 tests and measures that are used by neuropsychologists. Table 5.4 presents an analysis of the standardization samples for tests described therein, clustered into three principle groups. Education refers to tests that were developed for, or whose development has been significantly influenced by, school classification requirements (viz., PL 94-142, PL 99-457; see Sattler, 1988). Specialty tests were developed for special populations, primarily psychiatric inpatients and outpatients. Npsych. addresses those measures that were designed in neuropsychology laboratories (See the web page www.geocities.com/ rdfphd/index.htm).

Of the tests described by Spreen and Strauss (1998), three groups were co-normed (viz.,Woodcock-Johnson Psychoeducational Test Battery; the Wechsler Intelligence Scale for Children - III [WISC-III] and the Wechsler Individual Achievement Test [WIAT]; and, The Wechsler Adult Intelligence Scale III [WAIS-III], The Children's Memory Scale [CMS], and the Wechsler Memory Scale III [WMS-III]). Co-norming refers to administration of multiple tests to the same individuals within the same block of time. Co-norming is described as "linking samples" by the Psychological Corporation. A rather large group of children (N = 1,284) participated in the linking sample for the WIAT with intelligence tests (WISC-III, WPPSI-R, or WAIS-R). No adults participated in the link. The Children's Memory Scale also has "linking samples" with WISC-III and WPPSI-R using 108 children in each of five age groups (Cohen, 1994). · The WAIS-III/WMS-III Technical Manual (the Psychological Corporation, 1997, p. 16) notes that the standardization group for the WMS-III consists of half the WAIS-III standardization group.

TABLE 5.4
Summary of Sample Sizes Reported by Spreen and Strauss (1998)

| Category | Total | Specialty | Education | Npsych. |
|---|---|---|---|---|
| Mean sample size | 2001 | 2519 | 2951 | 548 |
| Standard deviation | 5603 | 2974 | 1061 | 965 |
| Ratio /σ | 2.79 | 1.80 | 0.54 | 1.76 |
| Census match % | 20.8 | 36.0 | 100 | 02.9 |

Several problems arise when parametric statistics are used to evaluate scores taken from tests that were not co-normed. First, age cohorts vary inconsistently and unpredictably across and within samples. Second, cell sizes (typically age cohorts) are often insufficient to generalize information to other populations (cell sizes as small as 2 were reported by Spreen & Strauss, 1998.). Third, standardization samples cannot be generalized due to the persistent use of poorly defined "available" subjects (less than 2% of the samples were large enough to permit meaningful stratification). Fourth, only the Education group provides samples having a standard deviation less than the mean. This suggests that only tests in the Education group can be meaningfully compared using the standard deviation as a measure of effect. These criticisms are particularly germane to the neuropsychology measures. Consequently, direct comparisons of standardized scores across neuropsychological measures is risky. This does not mean that scores from the neuropsychology group are uncomparable, only that direct comparison of average scores or difference scores from a reference mean introduces considerable unknown error. When conditions such as these exist, comparisons using nonparametric statistical tests are recommended. As noted by Cliff (1996):

> The calculations of the power of statistics and the relative power of different statistics must also be done on the basis of assumptions about the characteristics of the data. When the parent distributions have

characteristics different from those assumed, the absolute and relative powers can consequently be different. Since we often have reason to believe that our data do not conform to classical (i.e., parametric) assumptions, working with statistics that have good power under a broad range of situations is preferable to using ones that have optimum power under a narrow range of special ones. (p. 17)

## Bayesian Methods

In considering data as evidence, the classical Bayes model as presented in chap. 4, (this volume) is problematic as well. Different prior probabilities lead to different conclusions. When prevalence data are available, multiple estimates may exist. Bayesian findings are further limited in their evidentiary value because they overly rely on belief, especially when prior probabilities are subjective. A final criticism of the Bayesian model is based on the difficulty of representing complete ignorance by a probability distribution and ignorance represents a form of prior belief. Consider the value calculated for positive predictive power in Equation 1 when the prevalence equals zero (a form of complete ignorance or disbelief in the existence of a disorder).

## Impeachment

Inconsistent testimony can produce impeachment. Opposing attorneys may attempt to discredit a witness's credibility whenever the witness presents strong evidence for or against a client. Videotaped depositions, reviews of prior testimony in deposition for the current or prior trials, discrepancies between published statements and evidentiary statements, and "mousetrap" questioning can result in confusion and a claim of impeachment (Babitsky & Mangraviti, 1999).

The $p$ value has two distinct and conflicting roles in NHST (see chap. 3, this volume). First, it measures the strength of evidence. Second, it represents the probability of obtaining misleading evidence. Because of these conflicting roles, impeachment accompanies all null-hypothesis-based tests of statistical significance. The Bayesian approach (see chap. 4, this volume) has been recommended as a remedy for circumventing this problem (Box & Tiao, 1992; Gouvier, Hayes & Smiroldo, 1998; Harlow, Mulaik, & Steiger, 1997; McCaffrey et al , 1997). One specific form of Bayesian analysis, likelihood ratios, measures evidence in a way that mitigates against impeachment.

## STATISTICAL EVALUATION USING LIKELIHOOD RATIOS AS EVIDENCE OF NEUROPSYCHOLOGICAL DEFICIT

### Theoretical Basis for Using Likelihood Ratios as Evidence

The likelihood ratio ($\lambda$) entails three interrelated notions: the likelihood principle, the likelihood function, and the law of likelihood (Royall, 1997). The *likelihood principle* supposes that when presented with two sets of data, the likelihood of selecting one observation of the same value from either group is equal. The *likelihood function* refers to the likelihood of selecting a single value from a group of values. When the likelihood of observing a specific value is greater in one group than the other, then the likelihood function provides evidence supporting selection from the group having greater likelihood of containing the value of interest; hence, the function provides support for one group vis-à-vis the other. The strength of evidence supporting one group over the other is supported by evidence from the likelihood ratio. The *law of likelihood* applies to two hypotheses and indicates when a given set of observations is evidence for one hypothesis versus the other. It explains how observations should be interpreted as evidence for A vis-à-vis B, but makes no mention of how those observations should be interpreted as evidence in relation to A alone. Neither of the two NHST models (viz., *p* values or rejection trials) provides adequate evidence for hypothesis testing because each is based on the law of improbability or the law of changing probability. The law of likelihood is based on the Bayes model. But, unlike Bayesian probability models, which are useful only when prior probabilities are known, likelihood ratios only evaluate current data. Likelihood ratios remain stable irrespective of prior probabilities. The law of likelihood effectively defines the concept of statistical evidence as it relates to comparison with another set of observations. The question "When do test observations support one conclusion or another" is best answered by the law of likelihood.

Calculation of the likelihood ratio compares two conditional probabilities as expressed in Equation 5.5. Phrased as a question, the ratio asks "Given a score of x, which diagnosis is more likely, A or B?" Royall (1997) equated statistical evidence with this likelihood function: "The evidence in the observations is represented by the likelihood function, and is measured by likelihood ratios. It is not represented and measured by probabilities, either frequentist sample-space probabilities or Bayesian posterior probabilities" (p. 176). Two applications of likelihood are salient to psychology: evaluation of the evidentiary strength of specific neuropsychological measures and evidentiary support of testing specific dependent variables arising out of the individual assessment.

## CALCULATING EVIDENCE

When the psychologist considers test findings as evidence, tests can be grouped into three classes based upon the amount of information available in the research literature. The first group we will call *Diagnostic Tests* because they have known sensitivity and specificity for a disorder with a known prevalence. The second group, *Abilities Tests*, are associated with some and possibly multiple disorders having known prevalence, but the sensitivity and specificity information are either unknown or unassociated. The third group, *Construct Tests,* have theoretical relationships with theoretical disorders that have unknown prevalence and no known sensitivity or specificity. In those situations where it is possible to select tests in advance, the psychologist will use *Diagnostic Tests* if they are available.

*Evidentiary Strength of Diagnostic Tests.* Diagnostic Tests vary in their ability to identify pathological processes. Occasionally inferences about their relative efficacy can be gained form their demonstrated sensitivity and specificity for a given diagnoses. This group of tests is most appropriate for Bayes analysis as described earlier. The psychologist calculates OPV for each test and associated diagnosis, then compares the OPV using ratios as described earlier. See Equation 5.5 and the associated discussion.

*Evidentiary Strength of Abilities Tests.* Perugini, Harvey, Lovejoy, Sandstrom, K., & Webb. (2000) present a method for calculating OPV for tests having known specificity and sensitivity, but unknown prevalence (see Equation 5.6).

$$OPV = \frac{\text{Sensitivity} + (1\text{-Specificity})}{} \qquad (5.6)$$

N

According to E. A. Harvey (personal communication, May 21, 2002) this formula uses sample size to compensate for unknown prevalence. The OPV allows the psychologist to compare these findings with those of other tests for which sensitivity, specificity, and sample sizes are known. When comparing *Abilities Tests* with *Clinical Tests*, this formulation should serve as a lowest common denominator.

*Evidentiary Strength of Construct Tests.* When the psychologist must use a test having unknown sensitivity and specificity, then the standardized percentile rank can be used to compare the patient's relative standings on various tests[4]. When it is necessary to compare Construct Tests with other types of test, the comparison should be made at the percentile rank level. Diagnosis can be made using this process by comparing historical information and psychological test scores to diagnostic criteria listed in the most current version of Diagnostic and Statistical Manual of Mental Disorders (DSM) or the International Classification of Disease (ICD). Neither nosology incorporates psychological test findings in their inclusion or exclusion criteria for most diagnosis. Table 5.5 provides an example for calculating evidentiary strength of construct tests, $\lambda d$ (as defined in Equation 5.6) for the differential diagnosis of Dementia of the Alzheimer's Type (DAT) and Traumatic Brain Injury (TBI) using data presented in the WAIS-III/WMS-III Technical Manual.

The ratio shows a greater likelihood that the patient's observed standard scores (SS) on one measure (Auditory Immediate Memory) are due to DAT rather than TBI (i.e., $\lambda d = 27/2 = 9.04$)[5]. Calculations such

---

[4]The standardized percentile score corrects for direction of deficit, so that all scores compared have either high or low scores reflective of poor performance. For example, in comparing a WAIS-III performance percentile ranking of 75 with theTrails B percentile score of 60, the Trails B score must be subtracted from 100 (i.e., 100 - 60 = 40) in order to standardize the scores because high scores indicate poor performance on Trails B whereas low scores reflect poor performance on the WAIS-III. The resulting comparison of 75/40 produces an Index score (?) of 1.87, a difference that is too small to establish significance "beyond a reasonable degree of medical certainty."

[5]Royall (1997) presented proofs that ratios of 8 and 1/8 are consistent with 5% level of risk. On occasions requiring "quite strong"

as these are easily performed on spreadsheets (the spreadsheet for this table is available from the web page at http: / / www . geocities . com / rdfphd / index . html).

TABLE 5.5.
Likelihood Ratios from WMS-III for Differential Diagnosis[6]

| test | SS | DAT | | | TBI | | | DAT/TBI |
|------|-----|------|------|-----|------|------|-----|---------|
|      |     |      | σ    | %   |      | σ    | %   | $\lambda_d$ |
| AI   | 62  | 68.7 | 11.0 | 27  | 98.3 | 19.3 | 02  | **09.04** |
| VI   | 65  | 70.6 | 10.9 | 30  | 74.9 | 13.9 | 24  | 01.27 |
| IM   | 55  | 62.9 | 11.4 | 24  | 78.9 | 17.7 | 09  | 02.76 |
| AD   | 64  | 66.1 | 09.6 | 41  | 89.6 | 21.8 | 12  | 03.44 |
| VD   | 72  | 67.5 | 08.1 | 71  | 74.3 | 13.9 | 43  | 01.63 |
| ARD  | 65  | 65.6 | 08.6 | 47  | 93.6 | 16.6 | 04  | **11.10** |
| GM   | 62  | 60.4 | 08.6 | 37  | 81.9 | 16.5 | 11  | 05.03 |
| WM   | 74  | 80.4 | 16.6 | 35  | 91.9 | 11.9 | 07  | 05.28 |

***Evidentiary Support for MMI ($\lambda m$).*** Establishing that a patient has attained MMI implies that the patient's condition has become static and no significant additional change is likely. Table 5.6 provides comparisons of the data from Table 5.5 with a second evaluation occurring one year later. Evidence provided by $\lambda m$ indicates the patient has reached MMI ( $\lambda m < 8$ in all categories), conditional upon the

---

evidence, he recommended ratios of 32 and 1/32 where the level of risk is .001. Data are interpreted using the boundries of $\lambda = 8$ or $\lambda = .125$.

[6]For each score above the 50th percentile, you must add $\lambda$ to the $\lambda$ for the cumulative posterior percentilews as demonstrated on the corresponding spreadsheet on the internet web page at HTTP//www. geocities.com/rdfphd/index.htm).

assumption that after one year no further change is expected, where $\lambda$m = Percentile Rank 1/Percentile Rank 2 (i.e., Auditory Immediate $\lambda$m = .271/.302 = 1.114).

TABLE 5.6
Determination of MMI

| | Adm. Standard Scores | | Std. Sample | | Percentile Ranks | | |
|---|---|---|---|---|---|---|---|
| | 1 | 2 | Mean | SD | 1 | 2 | $(\lambda_m)$ |
| Aud. Immediate | 62 | 63 | 68.7 | 11.0 | 0.271 | 0.302 | 1.114 |
| Visual Immediate | 65 | 60 | 70.6 | 10.9 | 0.304 | 0.165 | 0.545 |
| Immediate Memory | 55 | 45 | 62.9 | 11.4 | 0.244 | 0.058 | 0.238 |
| Aud. Delayed | 64 | 74 | 66.1 | 9.6 | 0.413 | 0.795 | 1.922 |
| Visual Delayed | 72 | 82 | 67.5 | 8.1 | 0.711 | 0.963 | 1.355 |
| Aud. Rec. Delayed | 65 | 73 | 65.6 | 8.6 | 0.472 | 0.805 | 1.705 |
| General Memory | 62 | 71 | 60.4 | 8.6 | 0.574 | 0.891 | 1.553 |
| Working Memory | 74 | 81 | 80.4 | 16.6 | 0.350 | 0.514 | 1.470 |

***Evidentiary Support for Posterior Function ($\lambda e$).*** The comparison of posterior with current function has been the subject of many studies[7], yet controversy remains regarding the best way to evaluate this type of change. Table 5.7 provides an example of the equivalent evaluation ratio ($\lambda e$) for this purpose. Here, all tests have the same mean and standard deviation. Rankings are again compared with $\lambda e$ reflecting WISC percentiles/WAIS percentiles. Rather than predict prior abilities, this function evaluates the differences between current and prior scores. The prior scores can originate in academic and other records (preferred) or derivations from predictive equation. In this example, both Digit Span and Block Design reflect boundary differences of sufficient magnitude to opine that abilities were superior during the earlier evaluation.

---

[7]PsycSCAN lists 223 documents between 1990 and 2001 containing the keyword *premorbid*.

TABLE 5.7
Comparison to Posterior Function

| Test | Battery SS | | Percentile Rank | | $\lambda_e$ |
|---|---|---|---|---|---|
| | WISC | WAIS | WISC | WAIS | |
| Vocabulary | 112 | 98 | 0.79 | 0.45 | 1.76 |
| Information | 92 | 87 | 0.30 | 0.19 | 1.54 |
| Similarities | 101 | 83 | 0.53 | 0.13 | 4.10 |
| Comprehension | 98 | 92 | 0.45 | 0.30 | 1.51 |
| **Digit Span** | **105** | **78** | **0.63** | **0.07** | **8.85** |
| Arithmetic | 99 | 82 | 0.47 | 0.12 | 4.11 |
| Picture Completion | 113 | 95 | 0.81 | 0.37 | 2.18 |
| Picture Arrangement | 110 | 101 | 0.75 | 0.53 | 1.42 |
| Object Assembly | 107 | 94 | 0.68 | 0.34 | 1.97 |
| **Block Design** | **114** | **74** | **0.82** | **0.04** | **19.86** |

## DETERMINING IF EVIDENCE IS MISLEADING

The interpretation of likelihood ratios ($\lambda$) requires consideration of the magnitude of the ratio as well as its likelihood of producing weak or misleading evidence. Weak ($w$) evidence refers to low likelihood ratios. Misleading ($m$) evidence refers to data supporting hypothesis A when Hypothesis B is in fact true. Royall (1997) recommended using the bounds of < $\lambda$ 1/8 (.125) or > 8 as evidence of preference for one hypothesis vis-à-vis the other. Table 5.8 presents the probability of obtaining misleading or weak evidence with a $\lambda$ of 8:1/8 and 32:1/32 as adapted from Royall (p 97).

Returning to Table 5.5, we see evidence for every test that the patient' standard scores are more like both DAT and TBI patients than the "normal" standardization sample (based on the "normal" standardization sample mean score of 100 and standard deviation of 15).

From Table 5.7 we can conclude (using Table 5.8) that with eight paired observations (col. 1) the evidence is not likely to be misleading ($m = .01|\lambda = 8:1/8$ or $m = .001| \lambda = 32:1/32$), but it may be weak ($w = .046|\lambda = 8:1/8$ or $w = .202 |\lambda = 32:1/32$). We can also conclude that the test scores alone poorly discriminate between DAT and TBI but they provide good evidence that the patient differs from "normal."

TABLE 5.8
Probabilities of Misleading or Weak Information

| # obs | $\lambda = 8$ or $1/8$ | | $\lambda = 32$ or $1/32$ | |
|-------|------|------|------|------|
|       | $m$  | $w$  | $m$  | $w$  |
| 7     | .005 | .143 | .005 | .143 |
| 8     | .010 | .046 | .001 | .202 |
| 9     | .003 | .083 | .003 | .083 |
| 10    | .006 | .026 | .002 | .120 |
| 11    | .002 | .048 | .001 | .048 |
| 12    | .004 | .016 | .001 | .072 |

**Evaluating Multiple Measures**

*Sequential Bayesian Analysis.* The preceding discussion considered relationships between two data sets or a single score with a reference group. Although many comparisons of test scores employ these models, psychologists also evaluate single abilities or constructs using multiple measures. It is not uncommon to include several measures of attention or memory in a single test battery. Spreen and Strauss (1998) point out that "The process of clinical interpretation takes into account not only the probabilities of individual test results, but also the combination of many test results, the observations during the process of testing, the question posed for the examiner, and the characteristics of a specific disorder"(p. 28). Bayesian models imply that a sequential analysis of data allow each observation or score to serve as an estimation of posterior probabilities for subsequent observations or scores (see Equations 4.5 – 4.7 and accompanying text, this volume). Therein, each new piece of data would increase the positive predictive power of the test battery. However, an empirical study of ADHD appears to contradict this view.

Perugini, et al. (2000) compared permutations of seven tests in their abilities to classify 43 children as either ADHD or control. Table 5.9 presents analysis of the Perugini et al. data using Bayesian definitions of PPV, NPV, OPV, and the ADHD prevalence of .04 (American Psychiatric Association, 2000, p. 90).Using Perugini et al. data, Bayes predictive measures of empirical findings do not support the conventional view that using more tests improves predictive accuracy. This analysis shows best OPV when only 1 test, Trials, is used. Failure in predictive enhancement is likely a consequence of unknown measurement error that may exceed predictive power of the tests. In Bayesian analysis both error and predictive power are magnified. One method for controlling error in Bayesian decision making is to employ a Bayesian network.

***Bayesian Network Analysis.*** Bayes networks evaluate believed relations between sets of variables relevant to some problem. They combine discrete, continuous and propositional (true/false) variables using algorhythms that are capable of incorporating multiple and varied information sources. Figure 5.1 presents a Bayes network for the diagnosis of ADD and related disorders that incorporates the Perugini et al. data with other measures. This analysis is available for download from the web site at http://www.geocities.com/rdfphd/index.html. The network analysis makes no assumptions regarding data distributions. Prior knowledge is included in the decision process. Findings allow inferences about patients rather than data. Findings are simply presented in diagrams. Findings are highly accurate when networks are properly constructed. Networks produce no undefined results. For psychology, the networks are superior to algorithms available for DSM evaluation because they include objective and test data. Also, as new information emerges, networks can "learn" and improve accuracy. This is accomplished by introducing either new cases or research findings. Error is controlled by using multiple data or observation sources .

Currently software for developing and analyzing networks is available. Expert system software, such as *Netica* (www.norsys.com), provides an excellent visual presentation of data that can be understood by most jurors and other consumers of psychological information. At this time Bayes networks provide the most promising method of statistical analysis as evidence in forensic and neuropsychology. There is, however, a pressing need for the construction and validation of Bayes networks for psychological diagnosis.

TABLE 5.9

Bayesian predictive measures for Perugini et al. *

| Tests | Sensitivity | Specificity | PPV | NPV | OPV |
|-------|-------------|-------------|-----|-----|-----|
| 1/7 | .76 | 0.45 | .06 | 0.95 | .94 |
| 2/7 | .62 | 0.91 | .20 | 0.99 | .77 |
| 3/7 | .28 | 1.00 | .25 | 1.00 | .00 |
| 4/7 | .05 | 1.00 | .05 | 1.00 | .00 |
| 1/3 | .76 | 0.59 | .07 | 0.97 | .92 |
| 2/3 | .52 | 1.00 | .52 | 1.00 | .00 |
| 3/3 | .10 | 1.00 | .10 | 1.00 | .00 |
| Trails | .29 | 0.91 | .09 | 0.99 | .88 |
| Digit Span | .38 | 0.95 | .18 | 0.99 | .76 |
| CPT Index | .67 | 0.73 | .09 | 0.98 | .90 |
| Trails | .70 | 0.51 | .05 | 0.96 | .94 |

*Base rate of ADHD = .04 (American Psychiatric Association, 2000,p. 90)

## CONCLUSIONS

The expertise of a psychologist in court is dependent on the evaluator's ability to present statistical evidence as legal evidence that is clear to the trier of fact. Because presentation of complex statistical processes often confuses jurors, psychologist should avoid statistical explanations when possible. However, a thorough understanding of statistical constructs may be necessary during cross examination. Statistical theory is so important in the design, development, and evaluation of psychological tests that psychologists who are unprepared to explain them risk not only professional embarrassment, but could be held liable for malpractice should their client "loose" as a consequence of their poor preparation.

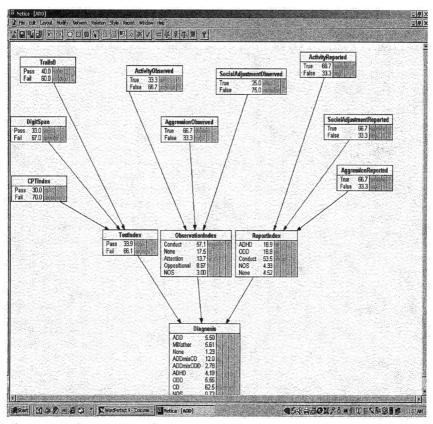

Figure 5.1. Bayes network

Statistical findings constitute evidence when they assist in demonstrating the superiority of one set of data vis-à-vis another. Reliance on NHST as the basis for establishing statistical evidence constitutes impeachment because the measure of significance employed probability model is of value in establishing the efficacy of a test when ($p$) has two different and contradictory meanings. Bayes' posterior prevalence for a neuropsychological disorder is well established, but has questionable value as evidence for the superiority of one set of test results vis-à-vis a second set or when prevalence is unknown. Likelihood ratios provide the best extant model for comparing two sets of data as evidence, but can be challenged because their product can be undefined. Bayes networks offer the most viable analytic alternative for psychological evidence inforensic and neuropsychology but networks need to be constructed and verified.

## CLINICAL IMPLICATIONS

When it is necessary to demonstrate that the difference observed between two test scores is significant *beyond reasonable degree of medical certainty*, the simplest calculation is pair-wise division of standardized percentile scores[8]. The quotient of this division functions as a likelihood ratio ($\lambda$). Table 5.10 presents percentile scores when $\lambda =$ 8 and 32 that are appropriate for pair-wise comparisons. As the table indicates, when the percentile score from Test A = 50 (SS = 100), it would be necessary for the patient to produce a percentile score of 6.25 (SS ~77) on the second test in order to demonstrate a difference that is "beyond a reasonable degree of medical certainty." A percentile score of 0.781 on Test B (SS ~ 62) would be necessary to establish a $\lambda$ of ~32, a difference that is "well beyond a reasonable degree of medical certainty."

Calculation in this way may be less precise than regression-based analysis, but unlike regression models, the analysis allows comparison across data types when correlation coefficients between tests are unknown or when inadequate information exists for calculating Bayesian posterior probabilities. Even qualitative rankings from ordinal data types can be compared in this manner. For example, the classifications of Mild, Moderate, or Severe that are gleaned from hospital, rehabilitation, or other medical records can be assigned percentile values of 10%, 5%, and 1% respectively to indicate their relative relationships. Evaluating findings in this way tends to be more conservative than regression based methods, thereby allowing the clinician to place high confidence in the results.

---

[8]The standardized percentile score corrects for direction of deficit, so that all scores compared have either high or low scores reflective of poor performance. For example, in comparing a WAIS-III performance percentile ranking of 75 with theTrails B percentile score of 60, the Trails B score must be subtracted from 100 (i.e., 100 - 60 = 40) in order to standardize the scores because high scores indicate poor performance on Trails B whereas low scores reflect poor performance on the WAIS-III. The resulting comparison of 75/40 produces an Index score ($\lambda$) of 1.87, a difference that is too small to establish significance "beyond a reasonable degree of medical certainty."

At the time of this chapter's publication, psychologists in clinical settings rely almost exclusively on statistical models that originated in the 19th century. Isn't it time to move on and develop Bayes networks as well as other forms of modern analysis as aids to clinical diagnosis?

TABLE 5.10

Percentile Score Differences Between Value A and Value B
Required for Significance When $\lambda = 8$ and $\lambda = 32$.

| A% | B%@ $\lambda = 8$ | B%@ $\lambda = 32$ |
|----|----|----|
| 1 | 00.125 | 00.016 |
| 5 | 00.625 | 00.078 |
| 10 | 01.250 | 00.156 |
| 15 | 01.875 | 00.234 |
| 20 | 02.500 | 00.313 |
| 25 | 03.125 | 00.391 |
| 30 | 03.750 | 00.469 |
| 35 | 04.375 | 00.547 |
| 40 | 05.000 | 00.625 |
| 45 | 05.625 | 00.703 |
| 50 | 06.250 | 00.781 |
| 55 | 13.125 | 03.128 |
| 60 | 20.625 | 05.156 |
| 65 | 28.750 | 07.118 |
| 70 | 37.500 | 09.375 |
| 75 | 46.875 | 11.719 |
| 80 | 56.857 | 14.219 |
| 85 | 67.500 | 16.857 |
| 90 | 78.750 | 19.688 |
| 95 | 90.625 | 22.656 |

## REFERENCES

American Psychiatric Association. (2000). *Diagnostic and statistical manual of mental disorders.* (4th ed.). Washington DC: Author.

Babitsky, S., & Mangraviti, J. J. (1999). *How to excel during depositions.* Falmouth, MA: SEAK, Inc.

Barth, J. T., Ryan, T. V., & Hawk, G. L. (1992). Forensic neuropsychology: A reply to the method skeptics. *Neuropsychology Review, 2,* 251-266.

Box, G. E. P. & Tiao, G. C. (1992). *Bayesian inference in statistical analysis.* New York: Wiley.

Brigham, C. R., Babitsky, S., & Mangraviti, J. J. (1996). *The independent medical evaluation report.* Falmouth, MA: SEAK, Inc.

Chan, R. C. K. (2001). Base rate of post-concussion symptoms among normal people and its neuropsychological correlates. *Clinical Rehabilitation, 15*(3), 266-273.

Cliff, N. (1996). *Ordinal methods for behavioral data analysis.* Mahwah, NJ: Lawrence Erlbaum Associates.

Cohen, J. (1994). The earth is round (p < .05). *American Psychologist, 49,* 997-1003.

Dar, R., Serlin, R. C., & Omer, H. (1994). Misuse of statistical tests in three decades of psychotherapy research. *Journal of Consulting and Clinical Psychology, 62,* 75-82.

Dietrich, F. H., & Kearns, T. J. (1983). *Basic statistics.* San Francisco: Dellen.

Elwood, R. W. (1993). Clinical discriminations and neuropsychological tests: An appeal to Bayes' Theorem. *The Clinical Psychologist, 7,* 224-233.

Faust, D., Ziskin, J. & Hiers, J. B. (1991). *Brain damage claims: Coping with neuropsychological evidence.* Los Angeles: Law and Psychology Press.

Fisher, R. A. (1959). *Statistical methods and scientific inference.* Edinburgh: Oliver and Boyd.

Glaros, A. G., & Kline, R. B. (1988). Understanding the accuracy of tests with cutting scores: The sensitivity, specificity, and predictive value model. *Journal of Clinical Psychology, 44,* 1013-1023.

Glenberg, A. M. (1996). *Learning from data: An introduction to statistical reasoning.* (2nd ed.). Mahwah, NJ: Lawrence Erlbaum Associates.

Gouvier, W. D., Hayes, J. S., & Smiroldo, B. B. (1998). The significance of base rates, test sensitivity, test specificity, and subjects' knowledge of symptoms in assessing TBI sequelae and malingering. In C. R. Reynolds (Ed.), *Detection of malingering during head injury litigation* (pp. 55-80). New York: Plenum.

Hagen, R. L. (1998). A further look at wrong reasons to abandon statistical testing. *American Psychologist, 53*, 797-798.

Harlow, L. L., Mulaik, S. A., & Steiger, J. H. (1997). *What if there were no significance tests?* Mahwah, NJ: Lawrence Erlbaum Associates.

Howson, C., & Urbach, P. (1989). *Scientific reasoning: The Bayesian approach.* La Salle, Il: Open Court.

Kempthorne, O. (1966). Some aspects of experimental inference. *Journal of the American Statistical Association, 61,* 11-34.

Krueger, J. (2001). Null hypothesis significance testing: On the survival of a flawed method. *American Psychologist, 56,* 16-26.

Malgady, R. G. (1998). In praise of value judgments in null hypothesis testing and of "accepting" the null hypothesis. *American Psychologist, 53,* 797-798.

Martens, M., Donders, J., & Millis, S. R. (2001). Evaluation of invalid response sets after traumatic head injury. *Journal of Forensic Neuorpsychology, 2*(1), 1-8.

McCaffrey, R. J., Williams, A. D., Fisher, J. M., & Laing, W. C. (1997). *The practice of forensic neuropsychology: Meeting challenges in the courtroom.* New York: Plenum.

McMan, J. C. (1995, August). *Statistical significance testing fantasies in introductory psychology textbooks.* Paper presented at the 103rd Annual Convention of the American Psychological Association, New York.

Meehl, P. E. (1990). Appraising and amending theories: The strategy of Lakatosian defense and two principles that warrant it. *Psychological Inquiry, 1,* 108-141.

Meehl, P. E., & Rosen, A. (1955). Antecedent probability and the efficiency of psychometric signs, patterns, or cutting scores. *Psychological Bulletin, 52,* 194-216.

Merriam Webster, Inc. (1996). Merriam Webster's collegiate dictionary (10th ed.). Springfield, MA: Author.

Mitrushina, M. N., Boone, K. B., & D'Elia, L. F. (1999). *Handbook of normative data for neuropsychological assessment.* New York. Oxford University Press.

Nickerson, R. S. (2000). Null hypothesis significance testing: A review of an old and continuing controversy. *Psychological Methods, 5,* 241-301.

Ofloff, J. R. P., Beavers, D. J., & DeLeon, P. H. (1999). Psychology and the law: A shared vision for the 21st century. *Professional Psychology: Research and Practice, 30,* 331-332.

Perugini, E. M., Harvey, E. A., Lovejoy, D. W., Sandstrom, K., & Webb, A. H. (2000). The predictive power of combined neuropsychological measures for Attention-Deficit/Hyperactivity Disorder in children. *Clinical Neuropsychology, 6,* 101-114.

Peto, R., Pike, M. C., Armitage, P., Breslow, N. E., Cox, D. R., Howard, S. V., Mantel, N., McPherson, K., Peto, J., & Smith, P. G. (1976). Design and analysis of randomized clinical trials requiring prononged observation of each patient, I: Introduction and design. *British Medical Journal, 34,* 585-612.

Putzke, J. D., Williams. M. A., Glutting, J. J., Konolid, T. R., & Boll, T. J. (2001). Developmental memory performance: Inter-task consistency and base-rate variability on the WRAMAL. *Journal of Clinical & Experimental Neuropsychology, 23*(3), 253-264.

Rosenfeld, B., Sands, S. A., & Van Gorp, W. G. (2000). Have we forgotten the base rate problem? Methodological issues in the detection of distortion. *Archives of Clinical Neuropsychology, 15*(4), 349-359.

Royall, R. M. (1997). *Statistical evidence: A likelihood paradigm.* London: Chapman & Hall.

Sattler, J. M. (1988). *Assessment of children.* (3rd ed.) San Diego, CA: Author.

School Board vs. Cruz. 25 F.L.W. D1085. (Fla. 5th DCA, 2000).

Spreen, O., & Strauss, E. (1998). *A compendium of neuropsychological tests: Administration, norms, and commentary.* (2nd ed.) NY: Oxford University Press.

Stromberg, C. D., Haggarty, D. J., Mishkin, B., Leibenluft, R. F., Rubin, B. L., McMillian, M. H., & Trilling, H. R. (1988). *The Psychologist's Legal Handbook.* Washington, DC: The Council for the National Register of Health Service Providers in Psychology.

The Psychological Corporation. (1997). *WAIS-III/WMS-III technical manual.* San Antonio, TX: Author.

Thorndike, R. M. (1997). *Measurement and evaluation in psychology and education.* (6th ed.). Upper Saddle River, NJ: Merrill.

Tryon, W. W. (1998). The inscrutable null hypothesis. *American Psychologist, 53*, 796-807.

Wiggins, J. S. (1973). *Personality and prediction.* Reading, MA: Addison-Wesley.

Williams, J. M. (1997). The forensic evaluation of adult traumatic brain injury. In R. J. McCaffrey, A. D. Williams, J. M. Fisher & W. C. Laing, (Eds.). *The practice of forensic neuropsychology: Meeting challenges in the courtroom.* (pp. 37- 70). New York: Plenum.

Yerushalami, J. (1947). Statistical problems in assessing methods of medical diagnosis. *Public Health Reports, 62,* 1432-1449.

Ziskin, J., & Faust, D. (1998). *Coping with psychiatric and psychological testimony.* Los Angeles: Law and Psychology Press.

# Assessing Reliable Neuropsychological Change

**Gordon J. Chelune**[1]
*Cleveland Clinic Foundation*

Neuropsychologists in hospital, clinic, and private-practice settings have long been recognized for their expertise in the measurement and assessment of neurocognitive change associated with known or suspected illnesses or injuries affecting brain functioning. In these settings, issues of reliability and validity have been largely examined within the context of group studies in terms of the diagnostic accuracy of a given neuropsychological assessment compared to some external criterion of brain impairment (i.e., neuroimaging or electrophysiological abnormality). However, as neuropsychologists have begun to increasingly offer their expertise within the courtroom, the emphasis has shifted to diagnostic accuracy in the individual case, and the issues of reliability and validity have come under "public" rather than "scientific" scrutiny (Matarazzo, 1987).

The situation is further complicated within the forensic context by the adversarial nature of legal proceedings, especially in personal injury litigation, where frequently clients are "independently" evaluated by more than one neuropsychologist. In this context, neuropsychologists must not only defend the reliability and validity of their assessment of a client, but also deal with issues of test-retest reliability and practice effects in the individual case (Putman, Adams, & Schneider, 1992). Fortunately, pressures from evidence-based medicine for outcomes accountability have led to a growing body of data concerning methods of assessing reliable change at the level of the individual.

A little over a decade ago the concept of "outcomes management" was introduced by Paul Ellwood, the father of the health maintenance

---

[1] Please address correspondence to: Gordon J. Chelune, PhD, ABPP-CN, Mellen Center (U-10), Department of Neurology, Cleveland Clinic Foundation, 9500 Euclid Avenue, Cleveland, OH 44195, Voice: (216) 444-5984, Fax: (216) 445-6259, E-mail: cheluneg@ccf.org

organization movement (Johnson, 1997). As originally conceived, the costs of health care can be reduced and care improved if reimbursement is provided for only those procedures and treatments that have value and can be objectively demonstrated to positively affect or change a patient's condition in a cost-effective manner. In part, outcomes management was born out of reaction to the fundamental premise that "a substantial portion of health care expenditure in the United States is wasted on unproven or ineffective tests and treatments" (Horwitz, 1996, p. 30). In its place, a value-driven, evidence-based health care system was proposed in which "outcomes accountability and following the outcomes of patients and managing them on the basis of epidemiologic information" (Johnson, 1997, p. 12) is central to the practice of medicine.

Within a value-driven health care system, neuropsychological evaluations for the purpose of diagnosis or description are of value only if they can be shown to enhance the management of a patient's condition. Hence, there is a growing emphasis on clinical outcomes research in which neuropsychological data serve as predictor variables of individual clinical outcomes (e.g., Chelune & Najm, 2001; Chui & Zhang, 1997; Desmond, Moroney, Bagiella, Sano, & Stern, 1998). Alternatively, neuropsychological assessment is also being used as a means of evaluating the neurocognitive outcomes of other procedures such as medications, surgical interventions, medical management, rehabilitation, and so on. In outcomes research, neuropsychological tests are increasingly being given in a serial manner, and neurocognitive change is directly deduced by comparing current test performances against baseline test data.

Whereas the complexities of measuring "change" have been "a persistent puzzle in psychometrics" (Cronbach & Furby, 1970, p. 68), the demands of evidence-based medicine have led to a renewed interest in methods for assessing reliable change. The purpose of this chapter is to examine the nature of neurocognitive "change" within the context of serial assessment. Using a few simple statistical constructs, we review several methods for determining whether observed test-retest changes at the level of the individual are reliable and meaningful.

## Methods for Assessing Change:
## Experimental versus Test-Retest Paradigms

Experimental methods of assessing change generally perform a controlled intervention (e.g., ablation) on a naive subject and then compare its performance with that of a control subject who did not receive the intervention. This paradigm assumes that the experimental case was "normal" prior to the intervention and that the observed difference between the subject and its matched control was due to the intervention. In contrast, the test-retest paradigm uses the subject as his or her own control and attributes changes in the subject's performance to the effects of the intervention. This paradigm assumes reliability and stability of the tests used to evaluate change. Although this is the model most frequently used to assess neurocognitive change in clinical practice, neuropsychological tests do not have perfect reliability nor are they free of bias.

A distinction also needs to be made between a reliable change, or one that is repeatable, versus one that is clinically meaningful. Whether an observed test-retest difference is meaningful depends on how it is evaluated. Common statistical procedures (paired $t$-tests, repeated measures) evaluate whether obtained differences between pairs of related scores are significant in terms of their reliability; that is, at $p < .05$, an obtained difference is likely to occur by chance less than 5 times out of 100. However, as pointed out by Matarazzo and Herman (1984) in their seminal paper examining Wechsler Adult Intelligence Scale–Revised (WAIS-R) IQ scores (Wechsler, 1981), although such differences may be reliable (repeatable), they may be quite common in the normal population, and therefore be of little clinical significance. What is of interest to clinicians is whether an observed difference between two scores is sufficiently rare in the normal population (e.g., occurring less that 5% of the time) that it is more likely to have been drawn from an "abnormal" than "normal" population.

**Factors Affecting Test-Retest Performances:  Bias and Error**

Under ideal test-retest conditions and in the absence of any significant intervening events, one's performance on a test should be the same at retest as it was at the time of original administration. However, in the absence of perfect stability and reliability, one must deal with the residuals of these statistical properties: bias and error. *Bias* represents a systematic change in performance. The most common form of bias on cognitive measures given twice is a positive *practice effect* in which performance is enhanced by previous exposure to the test materials, although negative bias can also occur in the form of proactive interference. Where large positive practice effects are expected, the absence of change may actually reflect a decrement in performance. Another form of bias is aging, with a positive maturational effect in children and a negative bias in the elderly.

Because of increased interest in the serial use of neuropsychological procedures, publishers are beginning to incorporate more extensive information concerning stability in their test manuals. For example, the test-retest sample presented in the manual for the WAIS-R (Wechsler, 1981) consisted of 119 cases, whereas the retest sample for the latest revision, the Wechsler Adult Intelligence Scale—Third Edition (WAIS-III), includes data for 394 cases (The Psychological Corporation, 1997); the Wechsler Memory Scale–Third Edition (WMS-III) included 297 test-retest cases (The Psychological Corporation, 1997). Test-retest stability correlations are generally quite good for the WAIS-III summary IQ scores (range .91 to .96) and for the WMS-III primary Index scores (range .70 to .88). Nonetheless, significant gains are consistently noted on retesting over the 2 to 12-week test-retest interval.

Research over the last decade has demonstrated significant test-retest gains for a wide variety of neuropsychological measures among both neurologically intact and patient groups retested over intervals ranging from 5-7 days to between 1 and 2 years (Basso, Bornstein, & Lang, 1999; Chelune, Naugle, Lüders, Sedlak, & Awad, 1993; Dikmen, Heaton, Grant, & Temkin, 1999; Ferland, Ramsay, Engeland, & O'Hara, 1998; Hermann, et al., 1996; Ivnik, et al., 1999; Kneebone, Andrew, Baker, & Knight, 1998; McCaffrey, Ortega, Orsillo, Nelles, & Haase, 1992; Paolo, Axelrod, & Tröster, 1996; Rapport, Axelrod, Theisen, Brines, & Kalechstein, 1997; Rapport, Brines, Axelrod, & Theisen, 1997; Rawlings & Crewe, 1992; Sawrie, Chelune, Naugle, & Lüders, 1996; Sawrie, Marson, Boothe, & Harrell, 1999; Theisen, Rapport, Axelrod, & Brines, 1998). From these studies, four points can be deduced regarding practice effects. First, significant retest gains are the rule for most neuropsychological measures. Second, retest gains are evident among both patient groups as well as amount neurologically intact samples. Third, retest gains occur across the adult life span, including among the elderly. Fourth, retest gains are not strongly linked to the length of the test-retest interval and they diminish slowly, still being evident after even as much 1 to 2 years.

In addition to the systematic bias introduced by previous experience with the test materials, test measures themselves are imperfect and can introduce an element of random error. For our purposes here, we consider *error* as encompassing two sources of imprecision in measurement, both of which are inversely related to a test's reliability; where $r_{xx}$ is reliability and $(1 - r_{xx})$ represents error. The first source of error pertains to the distribution of random variations in a test score around the true score (see Fig. 6.1). That is, if were possible to administer the same test multiple times without any bias or practice effect, the distribution of these observed scores (X) would fall into a theoretically normal distribution around the true score (T). Thus, any given observed test score (X) is equal to the true test score plus error (X = T + E).

Statistically, the band of error surrounding the observed score is called the *standard error of measurement* ($SE_M$), and it is directly related to the error of the test (1 - $r_{xx}$). The $SE_M$ for a test can be simply calculated with the following formula:

$$SE_M = SD * (1 - r_{xx})^{1/2}$$
(6.1)

where $SD$ = standard deviation of the obtained scores; $r_{xx}$ = test's reliability coefficient; and, $^{1/2}$ = the exponential sign for square root. For a measure such as the WAIS–III Full Scale IQ (FSIQ) score, where the standard deviation is 15 and the average reliability coefficient (using Fisher's $z$ transformation) across ages is .98, the average $SE_M$ is 2.30 (The Psychological Corporation, 1997, p. 50). Thus, 90% of the time a person's true FSIQ score would be expected to fall within $\pm$ 1.64 $SE_M$ of his or her observed score (X): X $\pm$ 3.77 points. If we were to use the stability information for the WAIS-III FSIQ score (The Psychological Corporation, 1997, pgs. 58-61) in which the test-retest reliability coefficient ($r_{12}$) was .95 and the SD of the retest sample was 13.63, the $SE_M$ for this population of retest cases would be: 13.63 * (1 - .95)$^{1/2}$ or 3.05, with a 90% confidence interval of $\pm$ 5.00.

Measures with different test-retest reliabilities and standard deviations will have different $SE_M$s surrounding their true scores. Tests with low reliability have a large $SE_M$ surrounding the true score at both baseline and on retest, and large test-retest differences may occur simply as random fluctuations in measurement. However, even small test-retest differences may be reliable and clinically meaningful for tests with high reliability because they have a small $SE_M$ surrounding the true score. Thus, the clinical significance of change scores must be interpreted in light of their measurement errors.

The second source of error affecting change scores is *regression to the mean*, which pertains to the susceptibility of retest scores to regress to the mean of the scores from the first administration. As baseline scores deviate from the population mean, they are increasingly likely to regress back toward the population mean on retest as a function of the test's reliability. This happens because, on average, an individual's true score (T) is actually closer to the mean (M) of the population than their observed score. On average, one can estimate the predicted true score (T) with regression to the mean having been taken into account by the simple formula proposed by Glutting, McDermott, and Stanley (1987):

$$\text{True score (T)} = M + r_{xx} * (X_1 - M) \tag{6.2}$$

where $M$ = Mean of the population; $X_1$ = Observed score on initial testing; and $r_{xx}$ = reliability coefficient ($r_{12}$ in the case of the test-retest reliability coefficient). The measurement error associated with estimated true scores is described as the *standard error of estimate* ($SE_E$) and is given by the formula proposed by Garrett (1958):

$$\sigma * (r_{xx} - r_{xx}^2)^{\frac{1}{2}} \tag{6.3}$$

where: $\sigma$ = the standard deviation of true scores; and $r_{xx}$ = the reliability coefficient.

Tests with low reliability will produce scores having a greater tendency to regress back toward the mean on retest. Consider the following

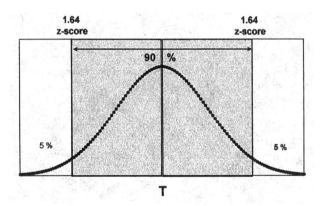

FIG. 6.1 Distribution of measurement error around the true score with a 90% confidence interval.

conditions for observed baseline score X on two tests that both have a population mean of 100, but reliabilities of .90 and .75, respectively. When $M$ = 100 and $r_{12}$ = .90, X = 120, 100 + .90*(120 - 100) the predicted retest score becomes 118, a loss of 2 points. If X = 80, 100 + .90*(80 - 100) = the predicted retest score becomes 82, a gain of 2 points. Or if X = 60; 100 + .90*(60 - 100) the predicted retest score becomes 64, a gain of 4 points. Also if $M$ = 100 and $r_{12}$ = .75, X = 120; 100 + .75*(120 - 100) the predicted retest score becomes 115, a loss of 5 points. If X = 80; 100 + .75*(80 - 100) the predicted retest score is 85, a gain of 5 points, Finally, if X = 60; 100 + .75*(60 - 100) the predicted retest score is 70, a gain of 10 points.

It is apparent from the preceding examples that baseline scores that deviate substantially from the population mean on tests that have low test-retest reliability are more likely to show greater test-retest changes due to regression to the mean, even in the absence of any intervening events, than scores closer to the population mean. Clinically, this can lead to spurious conclusions. Patients in rehabilitation settings who initially perform below the population mean on a measure may appear to get substantially better on retesting (score closer to the population mean) simply due to the effects of regression to the mean. Conversely, patients undergoing open heart surgery who initially perform above the mean on a neuropsychological measure, may appear to deteriorate on post testing as a result of surgery when their change in performance may simply reflect the effects of regression to the mean.

When practice effects are considered together with the effects of regression to the mean, interpretation of change scores becomes more complex.    Low baseline scores may show marked improvements on retesting due to the positive additive effects of both practice and regression to the mean.   Conversely, high baseline scores may show little change because the negative effects of regression to the mean tend to cancel out the positive effects of practice. The effects of bias and error are always present when a test is given twice, and they can confound and obscure the true impact of an intervention or treatment and make the interpretation of meaningful change difficult.   Because of the confounds of practice and regression to the mean, use of alternate test forms  has been offered as a solution. Unfortunately, these procedures do not work well.

**Alternate Forms:  Why They Do Not Work**

Alternative forms have been offered as a means to avoid or minimize the effects of test familiarity.   Considerable effort is needed construct psychometrically sound alternate forms. Typically, construction of such measures requires creation of two scales or tasks of equal content, difficulty, and reliability. There is an underlying assumption that the two forms are independent and can be used interchangeably to obtain comparable scores. Although indeed independent groups may obtain comparable scores on the two alternate forms, this does not mean that a given patient will obtain comparable scores when the forms are administered in a serial fashion. The reason is twofold: a) alternate forms may minimize practice effects due to the carry over of explicit content, but do not control for procedural learning; and b) alternate forms must still contend with issues of measurement error and regression to the mean involved in two scales rather than simply one.

The limitations of the serial use of alternate forms are clearly documented in the research literature. Goldstein et al. (1990) attempted to use alternate forms in a multicenter cooperative study of hypertension in the elderly, and found significant improvements in test performance at follow-up even when alternate forms were employed. Franzen, Paul, & Iverson (1996) looked at the reliability of alternate forms of the Trail Making Test (desRosiers & Kavanaugh, 1987) among three patient groups using a counter balanced design. Patients consistently performed better on the second trial of the test regardless of whether the original form or alternate version was given first. Ruff, Light, and Parker (1996) also noted significant improvements in verbal fluency on alternate forms (C-F-L vs. P-R-W) of the Controlled Oral Word Association Test (Benton, Hamsher, & Sivan, 1994) over a 6-month test-retest interval. Finally, Uchiyama and associates (Uchiyama, et al., 1995) studied the comparability and reliability over 12 months of alternate forms of the Rey Auditory Verbal Learning Test (Rey, 1964) in a large study of 2,059 HIV-seronegative men. Although the two forms of the Rey AVLT were found to be equivalent at initial and follow-up administration, significant practice effects were noted longitudinally, and the authors suggested that appropriate retest normative data are needed. Taken together, alternate forms do not necessarily avoid the problem of practice effects, and the use of two separate instruments with potentially different propensities for regression to the mean only makes interpretation of test-retest change scores more difficult.

## CONTROLLED METHODS OF ASSESSING CHANGE

Bias and error are problems only to the degree that they are unknowns and are not taken into account when interpreting change scores. Two controlled methods for assessing test-retest change scores are advanced here. The first is the *Reliable Change Index* (RCI), a method for deriving cutoff scores that reflect change scores that are clinically rare in the general population. This method is useful for making categorical decisions about whether an individual has shown a meaningful and reliable change, and can generally be derived from information contained in most test manuals. The second approach relies on *Standardized Regression Based Change Scores* (SRB), which are derived from regression-based prediction equations that estimate retest scores based on baseline performance and other demographic considerations.    Both procedures take into account the reliability and stability of the test measure, but only the SRB approach factors in moderating variables. Both procedures are examined in detail in the following subsections, and although they have the appearance of being quite "statistical" in nature, they are merely an elaboration of the concepts of mean, standard deviation, and correlation. However, the reader should note at the outset that difference scores or change scores, while derived from the same test given at two points in time, are independent variables with their own unique statistical properties and, therefore, meaning.

### Reliable Change Index (RCI) Scores

*Observed Distribution of Differences.* Perhaps the most simple and direct way of determining if a reliable and unusual degree of change has occurred between a patient's test and retest score on a given test is to compare it to the distribution of change scores from a comparable group of individuals.    Note, that we are now speaking of the distribution of *difference* scores between baseline and retest and not simply the distribution of scores at time one or at time two. Although in both cases we are interested in the standard deviation (*SD*) as a measure of the distribution of these scores, the *SD* for difference scores is different from that of the scale itself.  That is, just because a test yields standard scores with a mean of 100 and a standard deviation of 15, administration of this test on two occasions will yield a distribution of difference scores with its own unique mean of differences and standard deviation of differences.  For example, Dikmen and colleagues (1999) looked at the test-retest characteristics of an expanded Halstead-Reitan Neuropsychological Battery in a large sample of 384 normal and neurologically stable individuals tested twice over an average of 11 months.  The sample had a mean WAIS FSIQ of 108.8 at baseline with a standard deviation of 12.3. On retest, the group showed a 3-point gain, obtaining a mean retest FSIQ of 111.9 with a standard deviation of 13.1.  However, the standard deviation surrounding the mean test-retest change score of 3 was 4.6. If we wished to set a 90% confidence interval ($\pm$ 1.64 SD) around this expected "practice" score, change scores of 3 $\pm$ 7.54 would be expected to occur in less than 10% (5% above and 5% below the respective cutoff scores) of the population.  To the degree that a patient is similar to the Dikmen et al. normative sample, we can assert

**Distribution of Practice Adjusted Change Scores**

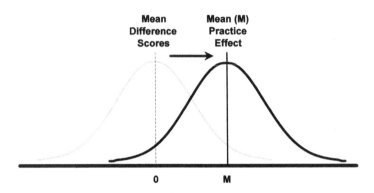

FIG. 6.2. Practice adjusted Reliable Change Index method.

that an increase of 11 or a decrease of 5 FSIQ points on retesting is reliable (probability of .05) and rare in the general population, and most likely represents a real change in performance.

> ***Methods of Estimating Reliable Change.*** Although it is desirable to have direct information concerning the magnitude and distribution of test-retest change scores from samples that are representative of our patients, these data are not always available. In these situations, it is possible to use "reliable change" methods to estimate the distribution of expected change (Jacobson, Follette, & Revenstorf, 1984; Jacobson & Truax, 1991) using basic information (i.e., test-retest means, standard deviations, and reliability) typically contained in any good test manual. In their work looking at   psychotherapy outcomes,   Jacobson and his colleagues (1984, 1991) developed a method of defining reliable change in terms of the *standard error of differences* ($S_{diff}$). The $S_{diff}$ is derived from a measure's $SE_M$, and is given by the formula:

$$S_{diff} = ( 2 (_{SEM})^2 )^{1/2}. \qquad (6.4)$$

The $S_{diff}$ between two test scores describes the spread of the distribution of change scores that would be expected if no actual change had occurred. Because $S_{diff}$ represents area under the normal curve, one can derive

Reliable Change Index (RCI) scores that would be expected to encompass a known percentage of the general population. Similar to the $SE_M$ that describes the distribution of measurement error around an individual's observed score, the $S_{diff}$ describes the distribution of expected test-retest difference scores around a mean of zero (no difference). However, because differences scores imply that a test has been give twice, there is an $SE_m$ both at baseline and at retest. Thus, Jacobson and associates (1984, 1991) simply multiplied the $SE_M$ twice in their calculation of $S_{diff}$. Using $S_{diff}$, a confidence interval or RCI of 90% of the general population can be defined as having observed differences between $\pm$ 1.64 $S_{diff}$ when no real change had occurred, with only 5% of the population expected to show positive changes equal to or greater than +1.64 $S_{diff}$ and only 5% showing negative changes of less than or equal to -1.64 $S_{diff}$.

***Practice Adjusted Reliable Change Index Scores.*** The RCI method developed by Jacobson and Truax (1991) for evaluating reliable psychotherapeutic changes was designed for self-report outcomes measures, and it assumes no systematic bias or practice effect. This is not the case with neurocognitive measures where previous exposure to a test generally enhances performance when the test is administered a second time. Taking this systematic bias into account, our early attempts to use RCI methods to determine reliable changes among patients undergoing surgery for intractable epilepsy led us to a simple modification (Chelune et al., 1993; Sawrie et al., 1996). We derived a $S_{diff}$ from a group of medically refractory epilepsy controls and centered it around their average change (practice) score as depicted in Fig. 6.2 rather than centering the distribution of expected difference scores around a mean of zero. Although this method treats "practice" as a constant and is open to criticism for its failure to consider regression to the mean (Bruggemans, Van de Vijver, & Huysmans, 1997), it does attempt to take into account measurement error and practice.

Several recent studies have employed this methodology and have presented RCI-like data for a number of neuropsychological instruments (Chelune et al., 1993; Hermann et al., 1996; Paolo et al.,1996; Sawrie et al., 1996). For example, in a study of test-retest performance among patients with intractable seizure disorders, Sawrie and colleagues found a mean FSIQ score of their sample to be 90.90 at baseline and 93.31 at retest 8 months later. The test-retest reliability for FSIQ was .94 and the $S_{diff}$ was 3.9. The simple 90% RCI interval for determining reliable change would be $-7 \leq RC \geq +7$. However, because there was a statistically significant practice effect of 2.41 points (retest score minus baseline score), the RCI distribution was adjusted by 2 points, and the adjusted $RC_{90\%}$ in whole numbers becomes $-5 \leq RC \geq +9$. Chelune et al. (1993) demonstrated the utility of this approach in estimating the number of epilepsy surgery patients who show abnormally large changes in verbal memory function following temporal lobectomy.

***Modified Practice-Adjusted Reliable Change Index (RCI-m) Scores.*** Although use of Jacobson and Truax's (1991) $S_{diff}$ [$S_{diff}$ = [ 2( $SE_M$)$^2$]$^{1/2}$] to calculate RCI values appears useful and is empirically grounded, others have suggested alternative methods ranging from use of the standard error of prediction (Paolo et al., 1996) to much more complicated procedures that call for matching control subjects with patients on the basis of pretest scores (Bruggemans et al., 1997). A relatively simple and conceptually straightforward modification has been suggested by G. L. Iverson (personal communication November 13, 1997). Jacobson and Truax's calculation of $S_{diff}$ assumes that the standard error of measurement ($SE_M$) is the same at both test and retest, and hence is simply multiplied by 2. However, given the effects of practice and other factors on subsequent performance, the standard deviation of retest scores is not apt to be the same as at the time of initial testing. Iverson suggested that separate $SE_m$s be calculated for test and retest scores using their respective SDs and the test-retest reliability coefficient in the calculation of both. The modified formula for computing $S_{diff}$ becomes:

$$[S_{diff} = [(SE_{M1})^2 + (SE_{M2})^2]^{1/2}] \tag{6.5}$$

where $SE_{M1}$ and $SE_{M2}$ are the $SE_M$s at test and retest, respectively.

To evaluate how well this modified RCI (RCI-m) formula compares to the original formula, the test-retest data for the Immediate Memory and General Memory Indexes from the new Wechsler Memory Scale-III were examined (Chelune, Sands, Barrett, Naugle, Ledbetter, & Tulsky, 1999). Table 6.1 presents the means, standard deviations, practice effects, test-retest reliabilities, and $SE_M$s for the WMS-III Immediate and General Memory Indexes.

Table 6.2 presents a comparison of the RCI cutoffs using the practice-adjusted standard and modified formulas for calculating $S_{diff}$. As can be seen, Iverson's modified formula results in somewhat larger RCI intervals, but ones that appear to be a better fit of the data in terms of the expected distribution of scores. Using simply the test-retest means, standard deviations, and reliability coefficient it is possible to estimate the actual distribution of change scores. For the test-retest Immediate Memory and General Memory Index scores reported in the *WAIS–III/WMS–III Technical Manual* (The Psychological Corporation, 1997), we found the actual standard deviations of observed change scores to be 10.24 and 8.41, respectively (Chelune, et al., 1999). These observed standard deviations correspond reasonably well with the estimated $S_{diff}$ calculated by the RCI methods, especially when modified to allow for differences in $SE_M$ at baseline and at retest. However, there is some variance between the observed distributions of change scores (SD) for the Immediate and General Memory Indexes and their estimated distributions ($S_{diff}$), even using the RCI-m method.

TABLE 6.1
Test-Retest Means, Standard Deviations,
and Standard Errors of Measurement ($SE_M$)
for the WMS–III Immediate and General Memory Index Scores.

| | WMS-III Immediate Memory Index | | | | WMS-III General Memory Index | | | |
|---|---|---|---|---|---|---|---|---|
| | Test 1 | Test 2 | Test-Retest | | Test 1 | Test 2 | Test-Retest | |
| M | 100.2 | 113.7 | Pract-ice | 13.4 | 100.7 | 112.8 | Pract-ice | 12.1 |
| SD | 015.9 | 019.2 | SD | 10.2 | 015.2 | 017.5 | SD | 08.4 |
| $SE_M$ | 006.2 | 007.5 | $r_{12}$ | 00.8 | 005.3 | 006.1 | $r_{12}$ | 00.8 |

*Note:* Data are based on the sample presented in the *WAIS-III/WMS-III Technical Manual.*, copyright 2002 by The Psychological Corporation. Reproduced by permission. All rights reserved.

***Reliable Change Using the Standard Error of Prediction.*** Although the RCI methods described previously take into account measurement error and adjust for practice, they do not take into account the tendency of scores to regress toward the mean on retest (Basso et al., 1999; Bruggemans et al., 1997). This can be particularly problematic if a test measure has low reliability. To take this additional source of error into consideration we need to approach the relationship between test and retest scores as a matter of prediction: Given knowledge of the degree of association between baseline and retest scores, what is the most probable value of a retest score given a specific value of the variable at baseline. If a test had perfect test-retest reliability ($r_{12} = 1.00$), we could simply obtain the mean difference between test and retest scores as an estimate of practice, and add this value to each person's baseline performance to obtain his or her retest score. However, tests are less than perfectly reliable as are the people to whom the tests are administered.

To estimate the goodness of our prediction of retest scores from our knowledge of baseline scores, we must calculate the *standard error of prediction* ($SE_P$), also known as the standard error of estimate (Garrett, 1958). Essentially, this statistic represents the standard error of a retest score (Y) predicted from a baseline score (X) in a regression equation, where $r_{12}$ is the standardized beta coefficient of the regression. The $SE_P$ is given by the formula:

$$SE_P = SD_Y * (1 - r_{12}^2)^{\frac{1}{2}}, \tag{6.6}$$

where $SE_P$ = the standard error of retest scores predicted from baseline scores; $r_{12}$ = the test-retest coefficient; and $SD_Y$ = is the standard deviation of the observed retest scores.

We can calculate the $SE_P$ for both the WMS–III Immediate and General Memory Index scores from the data presented in Table 6.2. For the Immediate Memory Index the $r_{12}$ is .847 and the standard deviation of retest scores ($SD_Y$) is 19.24, with the resulting $SE_P$ equal to 10.23. This value is nearly identical to the standard deviation of 10.24 of the observed difference scores for the Immediate Memory Index. Likewise, using the $r_{12}$ of .878 and the $SD_Y$ of 17.58 for the General Memory Index, we can obtain a $SE_P$ of 8.41, which is the same as the standard deviation of the observed difference scores. By multiplying these values by ± 1.64 we can establish a 90% RCI interval around the mean practice effect to represent the boundaries of test-retest change, with scores equal to or exceeding these limits in either direction expected to occur in less that 5% of the general population. Identical to the distribution on scores obtained by using the observed standard deviation of differences, the 90% RCI based on the standard error of prediction method captures 90.9% of the WMS–III test-retest sample, with 4.4% of cases falling below and 4.7% falling above this RCI for the Immediate Memory Index score. Using ±1.64 of the $SE_P$ for the WMS–III General Memory Index, again 4.4% of the test-retest sample of 294 cases fell below the 90% RCI interval and 4.7% fell above the interval. Compared to the classification rates in Table 6.2 obtained by using the standard or modified practice-adjusted $S_{diff}$ to estimate the distribution of test-retest differences for these two WMS-III scores, the RCI method using the $SE_P$ produces a closer approximation to the theoretical distribution of practice-adjusted test-retest difference scores, and more closely mirrors the observed standard deviation of test-retest difference scores.

The reader should once again note that the application of RCI procedures requires relatively simple calculations based on the means and standard deviations of a test measure given on two occasions and the degree of association between the baseline and retest scores reflected by the test-retest reliability coefficient. This information is typically tucked away in a brief chapter often labeled "Statistical Properties" in most test manuals, but rarely read by most clinicians with more than passing interest. However, appropriate calculation of the limits of reliable change can be essential in deciding whether the observed differences in a litigant's performance obtained by two forensic experts are within the range of expected fluctuations or perhaps represent true instability. Within the context of outcomes research or clinical accountability, knowledge of whether a patient's change scores are meaningful and reliable is critical in determining whether an intervention or treatment has had a significant effect on the patient's condition.

TABLE 6.2

Standard errors of difference ($S_{diff}$) and confidence intervals for the standard and modified Reliable Change Index (RCI) cutoffs for the WMS–III Immediate and General Memory Indexes.

| | *WMS-III Immediate Memory Index* | | *WMS-III General Memory Index* | |
|---|---|---|---|---|
| | *Standard Approach* | *Modified Approach* | *Standard Approach* | *Modified Approach* |
| $S_{diff}$ | 8.823 | 9.776 | 7.543 | 8.133 |
| 90% RCI | ± 14.47 | ± 16.033 | ± 12.371 | ± 13.338 |
| Adj. RCI | $(-1 \leq M_2)$ - $(M_1 \geq 28)$ | $(-3 \leq M_2)$ - $(M_1 \geq 30)$ | $(-1 \leq M_2)$ - $(M_1 \geq 25)$ | $(-2 \leq M_2)$ - $(M_1 \geq 26)$ |
| < 5% | 7.1 | 4.4 | 6.4 | 5.4 |
| 90% | 83.8 | 89.2 | 86.1 | 88.2 |
| > 5% | 9.1 | 6.4 | 7.4 | 6.4 |

*Note:* The above data are based on the sample presented in the *WAIS-III/WMS-III Technical Manual*, copyright 2002 by The Psychological Corporation. Reproduced by permission. All rights reserved.

## Standardized Regression Based (SRB) Change Scores

The aforementioned RCI methods use very simple summary statistics ($M$, $SD$, and $r_{12}$) to estimate the distribution of test-retest difference scores that is likely to be obtained in the absence of a meaningful intervening variable. Depending on the measure of dispersion that is selected ($SD$, $S_{diff}$, or $SE_p$), confidence intervals can be constructed around the mean change (practice) score to describe the boundaries of reliable change, taking into account regression to the mean and/or measurement error. However, these methods are limited in that they only consider a person's baseline performance and treat "practice" as a constant source of bias. There is some evidence to suggest that the magnitude of practice effects for some variables may vary as a function of baseline performance (Rapport, Brines et al., 1997). Furthermore, the magnitude of change may be differentially affected by the length of the test-retest interval and other demographic variables such as age, education, and gender. Note that just because age-corrected scores are obtained at baseline and again at retest, this does not exempt age from also differentially affecting the degree to which someone can be expected to benefit from previous exposure to the test material. To address these issues we need a more complex approach to account for these factors.

Although still based on simple measures of dispersion, standardized regression-based (SRB) change scores offer a means for not only taking into account measurement error, regression to the mean, and differential practice effects, but also incorporating other demographic variables that may affect test-retest performance. Based upon simple multiple regression techniques, McSweeny, Chelune, Lüders, and Naugle (1993) demonstrated that it is possible to create standardized norms for change by generating regression equations in which the baseline scores for a group of control subjects are regressed against retest scores using a simple prediction equation:

$$Y_p = b * X_o + C, \tag{6.7}$$

where $Y_p$ = the predicted retest score; $b$ = the unstandardized beta weight of the regression formula; $X_o$ = the observed baseline score; and $C$ = the constant of the regression formula. The accuracy of this prediction equation is given by the *standard error of the estimate of the regression* ($SE_{reg}$). Like the other measures of dispersion we have examined, we can construct a confidence interval around a given predicted score ($Y_p$) by multiplying the $SE_{reg}$ by a z-score value to define a given area under the normal curve. For example, by multiplying the $SE_{reg}$ by $\pm 1.64$ we can define a 90% confidence interval around a $Y_p$. In its simplest form and where practice is relatively constant across the range of baseline scores, the $SE_{reg}$ is virtually identical to the $SE_p$. For example, the $SE_p$ for the WMS–III Immediate Memory Index score was 10.23, whereas the $SE_{reg}$ for the prediction of Immediate Memory Index scores from baseline Immediate Memory Index scores was 10.248.

Because the SRB approach to assessing reliable change also allows us to consider multiple predictors of retest scores, we can examine the potential contributions of other factors that might affect retest performance. For example, the length of the test-retest interval is often thought to be an important consideration, with potential practice effects thought to be attenuated by time.   However, in our evaluation of the test-retest performances of normal individuals taking the WAIS-III and WMS–III over an interval of 19 to 83 days (The Psychological Corporation, 1997), the test-retest interval was not a significant predictor of retest scores (Chelune et al., 1999; Barrett et al., 2000).   Similarly, the test-retest interval was not a significant predictor in a clinical sample of medically intractable epilepsy patients tested twice on a variety of neuropsychological measures from 4 to 23 months (Sawrie et al., 1996), although test-retest interval for a group of normal and neurologically stable subjects tested over 2 to 16 months was a predictor for some Halstead-Reitan measures (Timken, Heaton, Grant, & Dikmen, 1999). In addition to the test-retest interval and a patient's baseline

TABLE 6.3
Standardized Regression Based data for predicting WMS-III retest scores
for the Immediate and General Memory Indexes.

| WMS-III Index | R | $SE_{est}$ | Constant | $\beta_{Baseline}$ | $\beta_{Age}$ | $\beta_{Edu.}$ | $^a\beta_{sex}$ |
|---|---|---|---|---|---|---|---|
| Immediate Memory | .85 | 10.24 | 18.45 | 1.00 | -.097 | --- | --- |
| General Memory | .88 | 08.31 | 15.44 | 1.00 | -.063 | --- | --- |

*Note:* Copyright 2002 by The Psychological Corporation, a Harcourt Assessment Company. Reproduced by permission. All rights reserved.

test performance, other relevant demographic characteristics can be considered (e.g., age, education, and gender) to determine whether they enhance the prediction equation. Table 6.3 presents the results of multiple regression analyses in which the WMS–III Immediate and General Memory Index retest scores were predicted on the basis of baseline scores, test-retest interval, age, education, and gender (Chelune et al., 1999). For these two variables, only the subjects' baseline performance and their age were significant predictors of their retest performances. Age was also a significant predictor of WMS-III Visual Immediate and Visual Delayed Memory Index retest scores, whereas gender entered as a predictor of Visual Immediate Memory retest scores and education entered as a predictor of both Auditory Delayed Memory and Auditory Recognition Delay Memory Index retest scores. In no case did the retest interval enter into any of the prediction equations.

To determine whether an individual's retest performance deviates significantly from normal expectations using the SRB method, one merely needs to compare an individual patient's observed retest score with his or her regression-predicted retest score and divide the difference by the $SE_{reg}$. That is, by dividing the difference between a patient's observed and predicted retest scores by the standard error of the regression line [(Observed - Predicted)/$SE_{reg}$ ], one obtains a standardized $z$ score that reflects the degree of departure from the expected retest score in standard deviation units. If we set the confidence interval to 90% ($\pm 1.64 * SE_{reg}$), we can compare the efficacy of the SRB method with that of the RCI methods. For, the WMS-III Immediate Index data presented in Table 6.3, the combination of a subject's baseline performance and age yielded a multiple R of .855 with a $SE_{reg}$ of 10.248. Setting our confidence interval to 90% ($\pm 1.64 * SE_{reg}$), 89.5% of 296 cases fell within this interval with 5.1% falling below the lower cutoff and 5.4% falling above the upper limit. For the General Memory Index, the combination of baseline performance and age resulted in a multiple R of .882 with a $SE_{reg}$ of 8.312. Setting the confidence interval again to 90%, 89.2% of the cases fell within the confidence interval with 5.7% falling below the lower cutoff and 5.1% falling above the upper limit.

Use of SRB-predicted change scores has several distinct advantages. First, they effectively model the expected effects of practice and regression to the mean. They also allow one to equate subjects for differences in baseline ability because the regression line models the effects of regression to the mean and practice at each point along the continuum of baseline scores. Finally, change scores from different tests can be expressed by a common metric ($z$ scores) that takes into account differences between the tests in terms of their respective reliability and stability. Use of SRB normative data for evaluation of clinical outcomes is rapidly being incorporated into studies evaluating surgical outcome among patients being treated for medically refractory epilepsy (e.g., Chelune & Najm, 2001; Davies, Bell, Bush, & Wyler, 1998; Hermann et al., 1999; Jokeit et al., 1997; Martin et al., 1998; Seidenberg et al., 1998).

**Forensic Case Example**

To bring the use of reliable change methods into a forensic context, let us consider the following case. The patient was a 28-year-old, right-handed man with two years of college education. His past medical history was negative for known or suspected illnesses or injuries affecting the brain. He was involved in a motor vehicle accident and found at the scene in an awake but confused and combative state. He was taken to a local hospital where computed tomography (CT) and electroencephalogram (EEG) studies were normal. Over the course of his hospitalization he became increasingly alert and verbal, but was tangential in thought. However, toward the end of his hospital stay he became mute, but still followed commands appropriately. He was subsequently transferred to a rehabilitation facility where a repeat CT scan was normal, in the presence of an EEG revealing mild diffuse slowing, and he was placed on anticonvulsants prophylactically. Memory was a focus of intervention, although the patient was noted to be able to "grossly recall meaningful events" over the course of a day. He was subsequently discharged and underwent a neuropsychological evaluation 4 weeks after his initial injury. At that time, the patient obtained a FSIQ of 106, a Halstead Impairment Index of .14, and had a WMS-R Verbal Memory Index of 95. For his workers' compensation claim, he was seen by a neurologist who felt that the patient had suffered a significant closed head injury with some memory impairment, although there was thought to be a significant amount of "embellishment and functional overlay." The patient was referred by his attorney for a forensic neuropsychological evaluation 12 months after his first evaluation, and obtained a Full Scale IQ of 113 and a WMS-R Verbal Memory Index of 80. Defense counsel referred the patient to our service for a third evaluation 22 months later (35 months post injury). He earned a FSIQ of 102 and his Verbal Memory Index was 69.

Given the patient's history of mild traumatic brain injury, we felt that his neurologic status should be stable and his cognitive difficulties should resolve or improve over time. However, his data appeared rather erratic, and we applied the RCI data from Sawrie et al. (1996) to determine whether the observed discrepancies between the patient's three evaluations were clinically meaningful. His initial 10-point improvement in FSIQ from immediate post injury evaluation to plaintiff's evaluation exceeded expected practice effects and measurement error relative to our comparison group of patients with refractory epilepsy. Such improvement was expected within the context of a resolving head injury. However, his subsequent 11-point decrement in FSIQ was highly unusual, and is relatively rare ($p <$ .05) even among patients with known neurologic conditions. Furthermore, the patient's deterioration in Verbal Memory from a standard score of 95 to 80 over 12 months would be expected to occur by chance in less that 3% of cases in a neurologic population (see Fig. 6.3). Likewise, the additional decrement of 11 points from plaintiff's exam to defense examination would be expected to occur in only 3.5% of cases retested over a similar time period. The overall test-retest Verbal Memory drop of 26 points from immediate post injury to long-term follow-up would occur only about 5 times in 10,000 on the basis of chance ($p < .0005$). In the absence of any known intervening neurologic variables that would account for such losses and in combination with other indicators of exaggeration, a strong case was made for potential symptom magnification.

## CONCLUSIONS

As "outcomes accountability and following the outcomes of patients and managing them on the basis of epidemiologic information" (Johnson, 1997, p. 12) becomes increasingly central to the practice of medicine, it is likely that neuropsychological assessment will be widely used to evaluate neurocognitive outcomes following other procedures such as medications, surgical interventions, medical management, and rehabilitation. As such, it is important that empirical methods be developed to evaluate whether a given patient's observed test-retest changes are clinically meaningful. The methods presented here should help the clinician determine whether observed change scores exceed chance expectations. They can also facilitate outcomes research by providing investigators with criteria for performing relative risk analyses and for computing treatment effects.

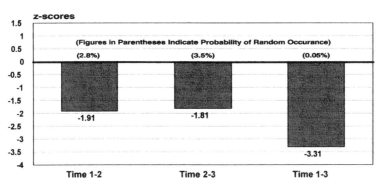

FIG. 6.3. Retest difference scores for Wechsler Memory Scale-Revised (WMS-R) Verbal Memory Index expressed *z* score deviations for expected retest levels in a forensic case.

Methods for assessing whether observed differences between examinations at two points in time are meaningful or simply normal fluctuations in performance due to measurement error and bias are equally important for the forensic practitioner. They provide potentially powerful tools for evaluating the reliability of our assessments and for contrasting our findings with those of opposing experts. Most important, reliability and validity can be considered at the level of the individual and not solely on the basis of group data. Our judgments of reliability and validity can be related to base-rate standards that meet both "public" and "scientific" scrutiny (Matarazzo, 1987).

## REFERENCES

Barrett, J., Chelune, G., Naugle, R., Tulsky, D., & Ledbetter, M. (2000). Test-retest characteristics and measures of meaningful change for the Wechsler Adult Intelligence Scale–III. *Journal of the International Neuropsychological Society, 6,* 147-148.

Basso, M. R., Bornstein, R. A., & Lang, J. M. (1999). Practice effects on commonly used measures of executive function across twelve months. *The Clinical Neuropsychologist, 13,* 283-292.

Benton, A. L., Hamsher, K. de S., & Sivan, A. B. (1994). *Multilingual aphasia examination.* Iowa City, IA: AJA Associates.

Bruggemans, E. F., Van de Vijver, F. J. R., & Huysmans, H. A. (1997). Assessment of cognitive deterioration in individual patients following cardiac surgery: Correcting for measurement error and practice effects. *Journal of Clinical and Experimental Neuropsychology, 19,* 543-559.

Chelune, G. J., & Najm, I. (2001). Risk factors associated with postsurgical decrements in memory. In H. O. Lüders & Y. Comair (Eds.), *Epilepsy Surgery,* (2nd ed., pp. 497-504) Philadelphia: Lippincott-Raven.

Chelune, G. J., Naugle, R. I., Lüders, H., Sedlak, J., & Awad, I. A. (1993). Individual change after epilepsy surgery: Practice effects and base-rate information. *Neuropsychology, 7,* 41-52.

Chelune, G. J., Sands, K., Barrett, J., Naugle, R. I., Ledbetter, M., & Tulsky, D. (1999). Test-retest characteristics and measures of meaningful change for the Wechsler Memory Scale–III. *Journal of the International Neuropsychological Society, 5,* 109.

Chui, H., & Zhang, Q. (1997). Evaluation of dementia: A systematic study of the usefulness of the American Academy of Neurology's practice parameters. *Neurology, 49,* 925-935.

Cronbach L. J., & Furby, L. (1970). How we should measure "change"–or should we? *Psychological Bulletin, 74,* 68-80.

Davies, K. G., Bell, B. D., Bush, A. J., & Wyler, A. R. (1998). Prediction of verbal memory loss in individuals after anterior temporal lobectomy. *Epilepsia, 39,* 820-828.

Desmond, D. W., Moroney, J. T., Bagiella, E., Sano, M., & Stern, Y. (1998). Dementia as a predictor of adverse outcomes following stroke: An evaluation of diagnostic methods. *Stroke, 29,* 69-74.

desRosiers, G., & Kavanaugh, D. (1987). Cognitive assessment in closed head injury: Stability, validity, and parallel forms for two neuropsychological measures of recovery. *Journal of Clinical Neuropsychology, 9,* 162-173.

Dikmen, S. S., Heaton, R. K., Grant, I., & Temkin, N. R. (1999). Test-retest reliability and practice effects of Expanded Halstead-Reitan Neuropsychological Test Battery. *Journal of the International Neuropsychological Society, 5,* 346-356.

Ferland, M. B., Ramsay, J., Engeland, C., & O'Hara, P. O. (1998). Comparison of the performance of normal individuals and survivors of traumatic brain injury on repeat administrations of the Wisconsin Card Sorting Test. *Journal of Clinical and Experimental Neuropsychology, 20,* 473-482.

Franzen, M. D., Paul, D., & Iverson, G. L. (1996). Reliability of alternate forms of the Trail Making Test. *The Clinical Neuropsychologist, 10*, 125-129.

Garrett, H. E. (1958). *Statistics in psychology and education.* New York: Longmans, Green.

Glutting, J. J., McDermott, P. A., & Stanley, J. C. (1987). Resolving differences among methods of establishing confidence limits for test scores. *Educational and Psychological Measurement, 47*, 607-614.

Goldstein, G., Materson, B. J., Cushman, W. C., Reda, D. J., Freis, E. D., & Ramirez, E. A. (1990). Treatment of hypertension in the elderly: II. Cognitive and behavioral function. *Hypertension, 15*, 361-369.

Hermann, B. P., Perrine, K., Chelune, G. J., Barr, W., Loring, D. W., Strauss, E., Trenerry, M.R., & Westerveld, M. (1999). Visual confrontation naming following left anterior temporal lobectomy: A comparison of surgical techniques. *Neuropsychology, 13*, 3-9.

Hermann, B.P., Seidenberg, M., Schoenfeld, J., Peterson, J., Leveroni, C., & Wyler, A. R. (1996). Empirical techniques for determining the reliability, magnitude, and pattern of neuropsychological change following epilepsy surgery. *Epilepsia, 37*, 942-950.

Horwitz, R. I. (1996). The dark side of evidence-based medicine. *Cleveland Clinic Journal of Medicine, 63*, 320-323.

Ivnik, R. J., Smith, G. E., Lucas, J. A., Petersen, R. C., Boeve, R. F., Kokmen, E., & Tangalos, E. G. (1999). Testing normal older people three or four times at 1- to 2-year intervals: Defining normal variance. *Neuropsychology, 13*, 121-127.

Jacobson, N. S., Follette, W. C., & Revenstorf, D. (1984). Psychotherapy outcome research: Methods for reporting variability and evaluating clinical significance. *Behavior Therapy, 15*, 336-352.

Jacobson, N. S., & Truax, P. (1991). Clinical significance: A statistical approach to defining meaningful change in psychotherapy research. *Journal of Consulting and Clinical Psychology, 59*, 12-19.

Johnson, L. A. (1997). Outcomes management a decade out: An interview with Paul Ellwood. *Group Practice Journal, 46*, 12-15.

Jokeit, H., Ebner, A., Holthausen, H., Markowitsch, H. J., Moch, A., Pannek, H., Schulz, R., & Tuxhorn, I. (1997). *Neurology, 49*, 1-7.

Kneebone, A. C., Andrew, M. J., Baker, R. A., & Knight, J. L. (1998). Neuropsychologic changes after coronary artery bypass grafting: Use of reliable change indices. *Annals of Thoracic Surgery, 65*, 1320-1325.

Martin, R. C., Sawrie, S. M., Roth, D. L., Gilliam, F. G., Faught, E., Morawetz, R. B., & Kuzniecky, R. (1998). Individual memory change after anterior temporal lobectomy: A base rate analysis using regression-based outcome methodology. *Epilepsia, 39,* 1075-1082.

Matarazzo, J. D. (1987). Validity of psychological assessment: From the clinic to the courtroom. *The Clinical Neuropsychologist, 1,* 307-314.

Matarazzo, J. D., & Herman D. O. (1984). Base rate data for the WAIS-R: Test-retest stability and VIQ-PIQ differences. *Journal of Clinical Neuropsychology, 6,* 351-366.

McCaffrey, R. J., Ortega, A., Orsillio, S. M., & Nelles, W. B. & Haasen, R. F. (1992). Practice effects in repeated neuropsychological assessments. *The Clinical Neuropsychologist, 6,* 32-42.

McSweeny, A. J., Naugle, R. I., Chelune, G. J., Lüders, H. (1993). "T-scores for change:" An illustration of a regression approach to depicting change in clinical neuropsychology. *The Clinical Neuropsychologist, 7,* 300-312.

Paolo, A. M., Axelrod, B. N., & Tröster, A. I. (1996). Test-retest stability of the Wisconsin Card Sorting Test. *Assessment, 3,* 137-143.

The Psychological Corporation (1997). *WAIS–III/WMS–III technical manual.* San Antonio, TX: Author.

Putman, S. H., Adams, K. M., & Schneider, A. M. (1992). One-day test-retest reliability of neuropsychological tests in a personal injury case. *Psychological Assessment, 4,* 312-316.

Rapport, L. J., Axelrod, B. N., Theisen, M. E., Brines, D. B., & Kalechstein, A. D. (1997). Relationship of IQ to verbal learning and memory: Test and retest. *Journal of Clinical and Experimental Neuropsychology, 19,* 655-666.

Rapport, L. J., Brines, D.B., Axelrod, B. N., & Theisen, M. E. (1997). Full Scale IQ as mediator of practice effects: The rich get richer. *The Clinical Neuropsychologist, 11,* 375-380.

Rawlings, D. B., & Crewe, N. M. (1992). Test-retest practice effects and test scores changes of the WAIS–R in recovering traumatically brain-injured survivors. *The Clinical Neuropsychologist, 6,* 415-430.

Rey, A. (1964). *L'examen clinique en psychologie* [The clinical examination in psychology]. Paris: Presses Universitaires de France.

Ruff, R. M., Light, R. H., & Parker, S. B. (1996). Benton Controlled Oral Word Association Test: Reliability and updated norms. *Archives of Clinical Neuropsychology, 11,* 329-338.

Sawrie, S. M., Chelune, G. J., Naugle, R. I., & Lüders, H. O. (1996). Empirical methods for assessing meaningful neuropsychological change following epilepsy surgery. *Journal of the International Neuropsychological Society, 2*, 556-564.

Sawrie, S. M., Marson, D. C., Boothe, A. L., & Harrell, L. E. (1999). A method for assessing clinically relevant individual cognitive change in older adult populations. *Journal of Gerontology: Psychological Sciences, 54*, 116-124.

Seidenberg, M., Hermann, B., Wyler, A. R., Davies, K., Dohan, F. C., & Laveroni, C. (1998). Neuropsychological outcome following anterior temporal lobectomy in patients with and without the syndrome of mesial temporal lobe epilepsy. *Neuropsychology, 12*, 303-316.

Theisen, M. E., Rapport, L. J., Axelrod, B. N., Brines, D. B. (1998). Effects of practice in repeated administrations of the Wechsler Memory Scale-Revised in normal adults. *Assessment, 5*, 85-92.

Timken, N. R., Heaton, R. K., Grant, I., & Dikmen, S. S. (1999). Detecting significant change in neuropsychological test performance: A comparison of four models. *Journal of the International Neuropsychological Society, 5*, 357-369.

Uchiyama, C. L., D'Elia, L. F., Dellinger, A. M., Becker, J. T., Selnes, D. A., Wescln, J. E., Chen, B. B., Satz, P., van Gorp, W. & Miller, E. N. (1995). Alternate forms of the Rey Auditory-Verbal Learning Test: Issues of test comparability, longitudinal reliability, and moderating demographic variables. *Archives of Clinical Neuropsychology, 10*. 133-145.

Wechsler, D. (1981). *WAIS-R manual.* New York: The Psychological Corporation.

# What Goes Together and What Does Not Go Together – Configural Frequency Analysis in the Practice of Neuropsychology

Alexander von Eye[1]
*Michigan State University*

Christiane Spiel
*University of Li Vienda*

Michael J. Rovine
*The Pennsylvania State University*

This chapter introduces readers to configural frequency analysis (CFA) and its application in clinical neuropsychology. CFA is a method for the detection of types and antitypes in cross-classifications. Types are described by patterns of categories of discrete variables that occur more often than expected from chance. Antitypes are described by patterns that occur less often than expected from chance. Application of CFA is of interest when the focus is on people rather than variables

## What Goes Together and What Does Not Go Together – The Person Perspective

Empirical research has a number of preferred perspectives. Most prominent is the causal perspective where researchers conduct investigations to identify the causes of the phenomena under study. For example, a number

[1] Please address correspondence to Alexander von Eye, Michigan State University, Department of Psychology, 119 Snyder Hall, East Lansing, MI 48824-1117.

of genetic predispositions have been identified as sufficient causes for the development of Alzheimer's disease. It is well known that the empirical identification of causes poses major challenges to research. Bollen (1989) stated that the following three conditions must be met for researchers to be able to label variables or events as causes of other events: (a) isolation, (b) association, and (c) directionality. Isolation is typically taken care of using experimental methodology. Directionality has proven largely elusive (see, e.g. , von Eye & Schuster, 1999). Association is the most frequently applied concept in empirical research. The present chapter is concerned with a particular facet of association, the local association (see later discussion; Havránek & Lienert, 1984; von Eye & Brandtstädter, 1982). There are associations that are present in a particular segment of the data space only. In other segments, the variables are independent.

Standard appraisals of association focus on variables. For example, researchers use measures of covariance or correlation to assess the association between two continuous variables. Examples of applications include methods for comparing scores from serial testing (see chap. 6, this volume). In the domain of categorical variables, researchers use log-linear models, methods of information theory, or coefficients of similarity between discrete variables to assess the association between variables, for example, in the assessment of malingering (see chap. 8, this volume). In either case, results are expressed in terms of *relationships among variables*.

The perspective that leads to data analysis focusing on variables has been termed *variable-oriented* (Bergman, Eklund, & Magnusson, 1991; Bergman & Magnusson, 1997). This perspective is complemented by the *profile-oriented perspective* (Bergman et al., 1991) which has also been called the *person-oriented* perspective (Magnusson, 1985). Here, individuals or groups of individuals are the focus of interest. More specifically, researchers ask whether there are individuals or groups of individuals that are unique in certain respects, and attempt to describe such unique groupings. Uniqueness can result from expectations concerning the a priori probability of occurrence, but also from expectations concerning the profile characteristic of group members and their changes over time.

Together with cluster analysis, CFA is a method for *person-oriented* evaluation. CFA differs from most methods of cluster analysis in that it allows one to consider (a) the a priori probability of occurrence of patterns of variable categories (Gutiérrez-Peña & von Eye, 2000; Spiel & von Eye, 1993; Wood, Sher, & von Eye, 1994 ), and (b) associations among variables (von Eye, 1988). The a priori probability of occurrence of patterns of variable categories is called the *CFA base model*. Patterns of variable categories, also termed *configurations*, constitute *types* if they occur at rates higher than expected from the base model. They constitute *antitypes* if they occur at rates lower than expected from the base model. CFA allows investigators to make statistical decisions concerning the existence of types and antitypes.

In standard description of associations, no constraints are placed on where in the data space the association between variables is supposed to hold. In contrast, types and antitypes are manifestations of *local associations*, that is, associations that manifest in specific sectors of the data space only. As such, they contradict the assumptions specified via the base model. However, rather than causing the base model to be rejected, they indicate where in the data space "the action is." In other sectors of the data space, the base model may not be contradicted. In this case, these sectors contain no configurations that appear more often or less often than expected from the base model (also called a chance model).

The following sections provide an overview of CFA as the main representative of the person perspective (for more detail see, e.g., von Eye, 1990; for CFA in applied research see von Eye, Spiel, & Wood, 1996a, 1996b. see also Lienert & Krauth, 1975).

## AN OVERVIEW OF CONFIGURAL FREQUENCY ANALYSIS

Consider the cross-tabulation, $Y = I \times J \times K \times \ldots = [y_{ijk\ldots}]$ , spanned by the variables, $Y_1, Y_2, Y_3, \ldots$, where $Y_1$ has $I$ categories, $Y_2$ has $J$ categories, $Y_3$ has $K$ categories, and so on. Let $\hat{m}_{ijk\ldots}$ be the cell frequencies that are estimated using some model, that is, the estimated expected cell frequencies. In the following sections we review CFA base models, significance testing in CFA, protection of the significance level, and recent developments of CFA as a method. In addition, we provide a data example.

### The CFA Base Model

Let $M$ be a statistical model for the cross-tabulation, $Y$. $M$ is a *CFA base model* if there is only one class of effects that can contradict the assumptions made in the base model. This includes any main effects and interactions not included as part of the base model. The following paragraphs describe three sample CFA base models.

To illustrate the concept of a CFA base model, we present three examples. Consider the three variables, $I$, $J$, and $K$. The cross-tabulation of these three variables is $Y = [y_{ijk}]$. The first base model is the Aclassical or first-order CFA main effect model of complete independence among variables. This model only considers that the categories of the variables $Y_i$ can occur at different rates. There are no terms for interactions. However, this model does contain all possible terms for main effects. Therefore, only one class of effects can contradict this model, specifically, the class of interactions. In other words, any interaction can cause this base model to fail, which may result in the detection of types and antitypes.

The second example is the second-order CFA base model, that is, the base model that considers both all main effects and all first-order interactions. The second-order CFA base model can be contradicted only by the existence of second-order interactions or, when more than three variables are investigated, the existence of second, or higher order interactions.

The CFA base models of first and second order can be contradicted by the existence of terms from a higher hierarchical level than the one used to specify the base model. In addition to this kind of base model, there are CFA base models for which the class of contradicting effects is defined at the substantive level. Consider, for example, the base model of prediction CFA. This model groups variables into predictors and criteria. Let the variables $Y_1$ and $Y_2$ be the predictors, and $Y_3$ and $Y_4$ the criteria. Then, the CFA base model for these two groups of variables includes (a) the main effect terms of all variables, (b) all possible interactions among the predictors, and (c) all possible interactions among the criteria.

This model can be contradicted by the class of effects that relates the predictors, $Y_1$ and $Y_2$, to the criteria, $Y_3$ and $Y_4$. These effects are all predictor-criteria interactions. However, they belong to the different hierarchical levels of first-, second-, and third-order interactions. These interactions share in common that they each involve both predictor and criterion variables (von Eye, 1988, 1990).

## CFA Types and Antitypes

In modeling approaches investigators pursue the goals of identifying a model that fits, is better than competing models, and is substantively meaningful. Interpretation of results typically proceeds in terms of the variable-oriented approach. That is, association patterns among variables, joint frequency distributions, or dependency structures among variables are depicted (Goodman, 1981). In contrast, when applying CFA, investigators attempt to identify those configurations that contradict the base model. These are the sectors of the data space where "the action is," that is, where there exist deviations from the base model that can only be explained using terms that are not part of the base model. Interpretation of CFA results proceeds in terms of the person-oriented approach. Groups of individuals are depicted by the configuration of characteristics that was observed more frequently or less frequently than expected from the base model.

It should be noted that the aforementioned "groups of individuals" can also be groups of data points. CFA is open as to the kind of information it processes. Specifically, there exist versions of CFA that allow one to search for types and antitypes in single-subject designs (von Eye, Indurkhya, & Kreppner, 2000; von Eye & Spiel, 1994). Types in single subject designs suggest that a particular behavior pattern is most typical and more likely than expected for this individual. Antitypes suggest that a particular behavior pattern is less likely than expected for the particular individual.

More specifically, CFA tests, for a given cell, $i$, whether $m_i = \hat{m}_i$, where $i$ indexes all cells in a cross-tabulation and $m_i$ is the observed frequency for Cell $i$. If, statistically, $m_i > \hat{m}_i$, the configuration of characteristics of cell $i$ describes a *CFA type*. If, in contrast, $m_i < \hat{m}_i$, the configuration of characteristics describes a *CFA antitype*. It should be noticed that CFA is the only person-oriented method that allows researchers to talk about sectors of the data space that are less densely populated than could be expected from some chance model.

**Significance Tests in CFA**

Many tests have been proposed for application in CFA. Three of these are reviewed here. The first test that was considered for use in CFA was the exact binomial test (Krauth & Lienert, 1973). This test is exact in the sense that the point probabilities for the extreme tails of a distribution are completely enumerated. There is no need to assume that some sampling distribution is approximated well. When $N$ is large (which it should be for CFA; one rule of thumb is that $N$ be at least twice as large as the number of cells in a table; types and antitypes are more likely to surface when $N$ is a multiple of that), the binomial test can be tedious to calculate. A good approximation to the normal distribution is provided by the rarely used Anscombe (1953) test (von Eye, 1998), which is supposedly more nearly normally distributed than the square root of the better-known Pearson $\chi^2$ component.

The binomial and the Anscombe tests can be applied under any CFA base model. In contrast, Lehmacher's test (1981) can be applied only under first- order CFA base models, that is, main effect models. In addition, this test presupposes fixed marginals. The test is asymptotic and is based on the hypergeometric distribution. Lehmacher's test is more powerful than the other two tests. However, it tends to suggest non conservative decisions unless sample sizes are very large. Therefore, a continuity correction has been proposed (Küchenhoff, 1986), which involves subtracting 0.5 from the numerator of the test statistic.

### Protection of the Experiment-wise $\alpha$ in Confirmatory and Exploratory Research

Although mostly applied in exploratory contexts, CFA can also be of use in confirmatory research. Exploratory CFA asks for each cell of a cross-tabulation, whether $m_i = \hat{m}_i$. Confirmatory CFA asks this question for an a priori specified set of cells. In each case (except if the a priori specified set of cells contains only one cell) testing involves application of multiple simultaneous tests to the same cross-classification. Multiple simultaneous tests carry the risks that (a) dependency exists among tests which can cause the nominal $\alpha$ error to differ dramatically from the factual $\alpha$ error, and (b) just because $\alpha > 0$ some tests will lead to erroneous rejection of null hypotheses.

Because of these two risks, protection of the experiment-wise $\alpha$ has become routine in CFA applications. Although many and complex procedures have been proposed for $\alpha$ protection, typically researchers resort to the classical Bonferroni procedure or to Holm's (1979) improved version of it. The Bonferroni procedure takes only the total number of tests, t, to be performed into account. The result of applying this procedure is a globally adjusted significance level, $\alpha^*$.

Holm's (1979) procedure considers, in addition to the total number of tests, the number of tests already performed before the ith test. For Holm's procedure to make sense, test statistics have to be arranged in descending order or, equivalently, tail probabilities have to be arranged in ascending order. For a description of more elaborate procedures, see von Eye (1990).

*A sample CFA application: Psychosomatic Symptomatology and Sleep Patterns.* The following example uses data from a study on sleep behavior (Görtelmeyer, 1988). One key result of this study was the description of six types of sleep behavior. These types had resulted from analyzing the data using first-order CFA. The six types describe respondents who sleep (a) short periods of time early in the morning, (b) symptom-free during normal night hours, (c) symptom-free but wake up too early, (d) short periods early in the morning and show all symptoms of sleep problems, (e) at normal night hours but show all symptoms of sleep problems, and (f) long hours from early in the evening on but show all symptoms of sleep problems. As occurs in most CFA investigations, only a part of the entire sample was assigned to one of the types. Specifically, a subsample of 107 respondents was a member of one of the types, and a subsample of 166 did not belong to any type. For the following analyses, the remaining 166 respondents are treated as if they belonged to a seventh type.

TABLE 7.1
CFA of Types of Sleep Problems as Predicted by Psychosomatic
Symptoms

| Configuration | Frequencies | | Significance Tests | | Result |
|---|---|---|---|---|---|
| SP | Observed | Expected | z | p(z) | |
| 11 | 19 | 11.04 | 3.31 | .0005 | Type |
| 12 | 3 | 10.96 | -3.31 | .0005 | Antitype |
| 21 | 20 | 12.04 | 3.18 | .0007 | Type |
| 22 | 4 | 11.96 | -3.18 | .0007 | Antitype |
| 31 | 16 | 9.54 | 2.83 | .0023 | Type |
| 32 | 3 | 9.47 | -2.83 | .0023 | Antitype |
| 41 | 5 | 4.52 | -0.01 | .4956 | |
| 42 | 4 | 4.48 | 0.01 | .4956 | |
| 51 | 4 | 7.03 | -1.38 | .0833 | |
| 52 | 10 | 6.97 | 1.38 | .0833 | |
| 61 | 8 | 9.54 | -0.49 | .3116 | |
| 62 | 11 | 9.47 | 0.49 | .3116 | |
| 71 | 65 | 83.30 | -4.41 | .00001 | Antitype |
| 72 | 101 | 82.70 | 4.41 | .00001 | Type |

After creating the six types of sleep problem behavior, Görtelmeyer (1988) examined their external validity. In one of these studies, he asked whether respondents who display psychosomatic symptoms while sleeping differ in type membership. For the following analysis, we cross-tabulate the six (+1) types of sleep problem behavior (*S*) and the two levels of psychosomatic symptomatology (*P*), above (= 2) and below median (= 1). The resulting 7 x 2 cross-tabulation (Görtelmeyer, 1988,) is analyzed using first-order Prediction CFA with *P* as the predictor and *S* as the criterion. The Lehmacher test (1981) was used with Küchenhoff's (1986) continuity correction. The $\alpha$-level was set to 0.05 and Bonferroni-adjusted, which led to $\alpha^* = 0.00357$.

In the following paragraphs we report results of first- order CFA of the cross-tabulation of types of sleep problem behavior and levels of psychosomatic psychopathology (for alternative analyses see Gutiérrez-Peña & von Eye, 2000; von Eye & Brandtstädter, 1997). Table 7.1 displays CFA results and suggests that there are four types and four antitypes. Reading from the top of the table, the first type, 1-1, suggests that below-median occurrence of psychosomatic symptoms predicts Sleep Pattern Type 1, that is, sleeping for short periods in the early morning. The corresponding antitype, 2-1, suggests that above-median occurrence of psychosomatic symptoms makes this sleep pattern unlikely. Type 2-1 suggests that below-median occurrence of psychosomatic symptoms leads also to frequent observation of symptom-free sleep during normal night hours. This type goes also hand-in-hand with an antitype, 2-2, suggesting that this pattern is unlikely for respondents with above-median psychosomatic symptomatology. The third type-antitype pair is for Sleep Pattern 3, that is, for symptom-free sleep that is shortened by early awakening. As for the first two pairs, below-median occurrence suggests high probability for this sleep pattern, and above-median occurrence suggests low probability.

The last type-antitype pair was observed for those respondents that did not belong to any of the Sleep Pattern Types. Antitype 7-1 suggests that respondents with below-median occurrence of psychosomatic symptoms are unlikely to belong to this group. In contrast, Type 7-2 respondents with above-median occurrence of psychosomatic symptoms are highly likely to belong to this group.

It should be noted that what looks like tied *z* tests in Table 7.1 is specific to the case where only two variables are analyzed, one of which is dichotomous. If one estimates a model where the marginal frequencies are retained (as is usually the case), deviations $\hat{m}_i < m_i$ are counterbalanced by deviations $\hat{m}_j > m_j$, with $i \ldots j$. The two deviations are symmetric. Thus, the marginal frequencies are reproduced, and the *z* test statistics assume the same value. This characteristic is exploited in two-sample CFA and in Prediction CFA (Lienert, 1971; von Eye, 1990).

**Models and Developments of CFA**

This section gives an overview of CFA models. There is an emphasis on recent developments and on models of possible relevance to neuropsychology. In the first years since Lienert (1969) proposed CFA, the method was chiefly used to detect deviations from log-linear main effect models. There were only a few special CFA models for more complex designs. Most important among these is Prediction CFA (PCFA). This variant of CFA assumes that variables are divided in two groups, the predictors and the criteria. The base model for PCFA is saturated in both predictors and criteria. Therefore, types and antitypes point by necessity to relationships between predictors and criteria.

*Developments of Prediction CFA.*    PCFA has been further developed chiefly in two directions. One line of development expands the number of groups of variables used. Lienert and von Eye (1988) discussed using more than two groups in research where variable relationships are assumed to be symmetric. This is not the case in PCFA, where the direction of variable relationships is of concern. However, the base models for the approach by Lienert and von Eye and the base models for extended PCFA are the same; that is, PCFA is saturated in all levels of interaction within predictors and within criteria. Therefore, the models discussed by Lienert and von Eye are applicable to multi group PCFA also.

The second line of development was initiated by Lienert and Netter (1987; see also Netter, 1996). Here, additional variants of prediction types were developed. This includes *bi-prediction types,* which allow researchers to test predictions of the kind "if a then b *and* if non-a then non-b."

*Deviation From Independence.*    A second area of development of CFA models concerns concepts of deviation from independence. A large number of CFA base models has been developed. However, there have been only two attempts to define different CFA types and antitypes depending on kind of deviation from independence. In the first attempt, von Eye, Spiel, and Rovine (1995) proposed three concepts of types and antitypes, based on Goodman's (1991) concepts of deviation from independence. Specifically, Goodman described five coefficients that assess degree of deviation from independence. These coefficients belong to three concepts of deviation from independence. The first is the *interaction type.* The second concept is the *correlation.* The third concept is the *weighted interaction.* Of the coefficients that assess deviations from independence, a subset is *marginal-free,* that is independent of marginals. The other coefficients are *marginal-dependent.* In the second attempt, Gonzáles Debén (1998) employed a new interaction-type definition of residuals.

Before von Eye et al.'s (1995) article, CFA types and antitypes were all defined in terms of marginal-dependent measures. The 1995 article presents simulation results and empirical data illustrations showing that different definitions of deviation from independence can lead to the detection of different types and antitypes. Thus, more than one concept of non independence is now available for the search for types and antitypes. Von Eye et al. showed that appraisals of type and antitype patterns can differ greatly, depending on the kind of deviation from independence CFA focuses on. Thus, users need to make one additional decision, that is, the decision concerning the concept of deviation from independence on which types and antitypes are based.

***Log-linear models of quasi-independence.*** A third line of CFA developments focused on the methodology used for estimating base models. Victor (1989) argued that it may be inappropriate to estimate base models including all cells of a contingency table if there is reason to believe that there may exist types and antitypes. Types and antitypes may belong to some other population than the rest of the table for which some base model applies. Therefore, Victor suggested using the more general quasi-independence log-linear models instead of standard hierarchical log-linear models as in most other CFA base models, in particular for confirmatory CFA.

***Using prior information.*** The fourth line of development of CFA methods discussed here deals with the exploitation of a priori existing information. Standard CFA as well as standard log-linear modeling estimate parameters and expected cell frequencies using only the information provided with the cross-tabulation. However, in many cases additional information is available, such as information on the occurrence rate of patterns of characteristics, that is, configurations in the population. In clinical contexts this may be the prevalence rates of syndromes or rates of spontaneous remissions. If sample information suggests that there may exist types and antitypes, taking into account this additional information may lead to different appraisals of data. Wood et al. (1994), Spiel and von Eye (1993), and Gutiérrez-Peña and von Eye (2000) therefore proposed methods that use information that exists about the relative frequencies or probabilities of types. Wood et al. and Gutiérrez-Peña and von Eye proposed conjugate methods that open the door to a Bayesian rendering of CFA. Spiel and von Eye (1993) stayed within the standard log-linear framework of most CFA models and used the existing information in the form of weights when estimating expected cell frequencies.

The following sections introduce two new facets of CFA. The first facet represents an extension that allows consideration of covariates in CFA. The second facet is concerned with effect size in PCFA.

## COVARIATES IN CFA

With only a few exceptions (these include, e.g., the conjugate methods proposed by Wood et al., 1994, and Gutiérrez-Peña and von Eye, 2000), CFA base models can be expressed in terms of log-frequency models (see von Eye, 1988, 1990). Most illustrative are representations in terms of the design matrix approach. Recent results (von Eye & Spiel, 1996) show that even symmetry models of CFA can be expressed this way.

In this section we propose extending CFA by including covariates (for technical details see Glück and von Eye, 2000). Covariates can be viewed as variables that are not part of a standard hierarchical log-linear model. In experimental research, covariates are often used to balance out weaknesses in design or sampling, for example, when possible predictors appear partially confounded with independent experimental variables. In the present context, covariates appear as aggregate scores that characterize cases in a cell. There can be more than one score per cell.

### Data Example

The data for the following example are taken from Khamis (1996). The data describe the use of Cigarettes $(C)$, Alcohol $(A)$, and Marijuana $(M)$ in a sample of $N = 2,276$ high school students. Each drug was scored as either used $(= 1)$ or not used $(= 2)$. These data can be analyzed using, for instance, log-linear modeling (Khamis, 1996) or CFA (see later discussion). Now suppose that, after a first analysis it becomes known in an imaginary reanalysis that all of those students that use both marijuana and alcohol also have police records for traffic violations $(V = 1)$, and none of the others is known for traffic violations $(V = 2)$. One may now ask whether knowledge of this covariate changes CFA results.

The cross-tabulation of $M$, $A$, and $C$ appears in Table 7.2, along with results for (a) CFA without and (b) CFA with the covariate, $V$. CFA was performed using the normal approximation of the binomial test with Bonferroni adjustment of the experimentwise $\alpha$. The adjusted $\alpha^*$ was 0.00625. Types are labeled with $T$; antitypes are labeled with $A$. The application of standard, first-order CFA with no covariate suggests that more high school students than expected from the assumption of variable independence use all three drugs, Marijuana, Alcohol, and Cigarettes (Type 111); fewer students than expected use only Marijuana and Alcohol

TABLE 7.2
CFA of Drug Use Data

| Config. MAC | Obs. Freq. | CFA Without Covariate | | | CFA With Covariate | | |
|---|---|---|---|---|---|---|---|
| | | $f_e$ | $z$ | $p(z)$ | $f_e$ | $z$ | $p(z)$ |
| 111 | 279 | 64.88 | 26.97 | $< \alpha^*; T$ | 110.49 | 16.44 | $< \alpha^*; T$ |
| 112 | 2 | 47.33 | -6.66 | $< \alpha^*; A$ | 1.72 | 0.22 | 0.414 |
| 121 | 456 | 386.70 | 3.87 | $< \alpha^*; T$ | 341.09 | 6.75 | $< \alpha^*; T$ |
| 122 | 44 | 282.09 | -15.15 | $< \alpha^*; A$ | 327.70 | -16.94 | $< \alpha^*; A$ |
| 211 | 43 | 124.19 | -7.49 | $< \alpha^*; A$ | 211.51 | -12.17 | $< \alpha^*; A$ |
| 212 | 3 | 90.60 | -9.39 | $< \alpha^*; A$ | 3.28 | -0.16 | 0.438 |
| 221 | 538 | 740.23 | -9.05 | $< \alpha^*; A$ | 652.91 | -5.33 | $< \alpha^*; A$ |
| 222 | 911 | 539.98 | 18.28 | $< \alpha^*; T$ | 627.30 | 13.31 | $< \alpha^*, T$ |

(Antitype 112); more students than expected use only Marijuana and Cigarettes (Type 121); fewer students than expected use only Marijuana (Antitype 122), only Alcohol and Cigarettes (Antitype 211), only Alcohol (Antitype 212), or only Cigarettes (Antitype 221); and more students than expected do not use any of the three drugs (Type 222).   Also considering the (hypothetical) citation record creates a different picture (cf. Mellenbergh, 1996). The antitypes 112 and 212 do not appear any longer. Thus, there are as many students as expected from the main effect model that use only Marijuana and Alcohol (Configuration 112) or only Alcohol (Configuration 212). In both cases, the additional information provided by the covariate helped identify these small observed frequencies as within expectation.

**Discussion**

This section illustrates the use of covariates in CFA applications. Embedding CFA and CFA base models within the framework of log linear modeling makes the use of covariates easy and straightforward. Ready-to-use software exists for log-linear modeling, for example, Eliason's CDAS (1990), and for CFA (von Eye, 1998), which allows researchers to consider covariates when estimating expected cell frequencies for CFA.

There is a natural upper limit for the number of covariates that can be included in CFA base models. Suppose the number of cells in a cross tabulation is $n_t$, and the number of vectors needed for the CFA base model, including the vector for the grand mean parameter, is $n_b$. Then the largest number of covariates that can exist simultaneously in a CFA base model is $n_c = n_t - n_b - 1$. Consider, again, the aforementioned data example. The maximum number of covariates that can be in this model is $n_c = 8 - 4 - 1 = 3$.

Recalling that the main use of CFA is in exploratory contexts, one may wonder why there is not one application where covariates are part of the model. In particular in exploratory research one often faces data that were collected without extensive randomization and control procedures in place. Therefore, the possibility to balance out uneven sampling, sampling errors, or partial confounds seems of utmost importance.

## THE BINOMINAL EFFECE SIZE DISPLAY
## AS A TOOL TO DETERMINE PREDICTION SUCCESS IN
## PREDICTION CONFIGURAL FREQUENCY ANALYSIS

This section introduces the Binomial Effect Size Display (BESD) for use in PCFA. Specifically, the BESD is proposed as a method to determine the amount of prediction success. The next two subsections present PCFA. and the BESD, respectively. The subsection that follows gives data examples.

### Prediction Configural Frequency Analysis

PCFA (Lienert & Krauth, 1973; cf. von Eye, 1990) is a method for cell-wise analysis of predictor-criterion relationships in cross-classifications. Let *P* denote the set of predictor variables under study, and *C* the set of criterion variables. Then, PCFA estimates expected cell frequencies using the log-frequency model described previously. This model is saturated within both the predictors and the criteria, and it proposes independence of predictors and criteria. Thus, it can be violated only if there are predictor-criteria relationships.

### The Binomial Effect Size Display

Thus far, researchers have used prediction types and antitypes as statistical concepts. The present chapter proposes enriching this concept by the BESD (Rosenthal & Rubin, 1982). The Binomial Effect Size (BES) is a measure of effect size in 2 x 2 cross classifications. The range of the BES is $-1 \leq BES \leq +1$.

The BES is equivalent to the correlation coefficient between the row and the column variables of the cross-classification, if the table is symmetric (axial symmetry) (Cohen, 1988; Rovine & von Eye, 1997). In addition, it allows statements concerning the *size of the prediction effect*. If the first column of the 2 x 2 table contains the targeted outcome category and the first row contains the training or experimental group of cases, large positive values of the BES indicate the proportionate increase in targeted outcomes that the experimental group has over the control group. In other words, the BES is the proportion by which the experimental group is more successful than the control group.

**Data Examples**

TABLE 7.3

2 x 2 Contingency Table for Creating Alliterations and Number of Mistakes Made During the Assessment for Patients with Pathological Scores in "Pointing at Objects"

| Total Number of Mistakes | Alliterations | | Row Sums $m_i$ |
|---|---|---|---|
| | + | - | |
| + | 5 | 28 | 33 |
| - | 37 | 2 | 39 |
| Column Sums $m_j$ | 42 | 30 | 72 |

The following two data examples, taken from Krauth and Lienert (1973) illustrate interpretation of the BES. In a sample of $N = 162$ inpatients with symptoms of aphasia, the following three variables were observed: $A$ = pointing at objects ("please point at the boat"), $D$ = creating alliterations ("please list as many words as you can that begin with an $M$"), and $E$ = number of verbal and phonemic mistakes made during the assessment procedure. Each of the variables was dichotomized at the median with + indicating pathological and - indicating quasi-normal behavior. In the following analyses we cross the variables $D$ and $E$ separately for patients in the $A+$ and the $A-$ categories. The prediction hypothesis is that the total number of mistakes made allows one to predict whether a patient shows a pathological score in Creating Alliterations. Table 7.3 resulted for the patients in the $A+$ category. The statistically significant $\chi^2 = 43.52$ can be interpreted as suggesting a *prediction type*. The total number of mistakes

TABLE 7.4
2 x 2 Table of Number of Mistakes and Alliteration Performance for
Patients with Nonpathological Scores in Pointing

| Total Number of Mistakes | Alliterations | | Row Sums $m_{i.}$ |
|---|---|---|---|
| | + | - | |
| + | 8 | 37 | 45 |
| - | 18 | 27 | 45 |
| Column Sums $m_{.j}$ | 26 | 64 | 90 |

seems to allow one to predict the pathological nature of patients performance in Creating Alliterations. Considering the sample size dependency of $\chi^2$-measures, one may wonder how big these improvements are. The BES = (5/33)-(28/30)= -.81 This value suggests that a high number of mistakes is predictive of *lack of pathology in Alliterations*, and the proportion of cases correctly predicted is over 80%. As is obvious from the comparison of the $\chi^2$ with the BES, the proportion and the direction of the relationship can be directly identified only using the BES.

The second data example asks whether the same relationship holds for patients with less than pathological performance in the pointing task. Table 7.4 displays the cross-tabulation of Number of Mistakes and Alliteration Performance for this group of patients.

The Pearson $\chi^2$ for this table is $\chi^2 = 3.64$. This value is statistically not significant (the critical value is $\chi^2_{1;0.05} = 3.84$). Nevertheless, one can ask how big the effects were. Inserting into (2) yields BES = -0.27. This suggests that the difference between pathological and nonpathological performance in the alliteration task is less than 30%. Again, the sign of the BES is negative. Thus, the direction of the prediction is the same as in the $A+$ group. However, in spite of the larger sample size, this negative association fails to reach significance. Interpretation of positive BES scores vary accordingly.

**Discussion**

In this section we proposed using the Binomial BESD for evaluation of size of effects associated with types and antitypes in PCFA. Using the BESD adds three important facets to PCFA:

1.  Types and antitypes of PCFA can be identified using a large number of measures and statistical tests (von Eye, 1990). Many of these tests approximate the same sampling distribution. Differences in results often stem from differences in approximation characteristics of tests. The BESD allows one to describe strength of effects regardless of statistical test used, and independent of sample size.
2.  In the analysis of continuous variables, power considerations are an integral part of planning and interpreting research. In the analysis of categorical variables, power considerations seem less popular. Specifically in CFA applications, power considerations are rarely made. This chapter is the first to introduce power considerations into the canon of CFA methods. (For the relationship of BESD to power analysis see Cohen, 1988).
3.  The paper by von Eye et al. (1995) introduced a new array of type/antitype definitions for CFA. Evaluation of cross-classifications can differ depending on the definition of type that invstigators use. The BESD is a model-independent measure of how strong effects are in two-sample or PCFA.

    Considering that the design of PCFA can be employed in designs of the kind shown in Tables 7.3 and 7.4, and to contrast pre post measurements with predictor configurations, it seems reasonable to also use the BESD for CFA designs of similar nature. Examples of such designs include two sample CFA, which compares two samples in regard to a number of discriminatory variable configurations (Lienert, 1971). Expected cell frequencies for 2-sample CFA are estimated using the same log-linear model as for PCFA (von Eye, 1990).

## SUMMARY AND DISCUSSION

Over the years, CFA has developed from a method that was hardly different than residual analysis in log-linear modeling, to a multifaceted multivariate method that allows researchers to make statistical decisions in person-oriented endeavors. This chapter provided an overview of concepts, methods, and recent developments of CFA as they can be pertinent to application in neuropsychology. In addition, this chapter introduced two new features for CFA. The first of these features provides the option to take covariates into account. The CFA base model with covariates was introduced in a way parallel to analysis of variance models with covariates (see, e.g., Neter, Kutner, Nachtsheim, & Wasserman, 1996).

   The role of covariates can be seen from several perspectives. Here, two perspectives seem of particular interest. First, covariates are *independent variables* that (a) are known to be related with the dependent variables, and (b) not part of the design variables. This is not necessarily a weakness of designs. It is very well conceivable, that researchers did not have the means to control all possible independent variables, or that certain variables are out of the control of experimenters, for instance for technical or ethical reasons. However, it may be possible to collect information on these variables. CFA now can accommodate this type of information.

Second, covariates can be either continuous or categorical. If they are continuous, the means on the covariates are the entries in the covariate vector(s) in the base model. If they are discrete, dummy coding may be needed to do justice to the nature of the covariates.

BES is the second feature proposed for use in CFA. Recently, the measure has come under critique (Thompson & Schumacker, 1997). Critics argue that (a) application of the measure is limited to 2 x 2 tables and therefore cannot be meaningfully applied to continuous data; (b) BES provides little information beyond raw percentages; and (c) it can distort results when binomial success deviates from 0.50. The first argument is not of relevance in the present context, because it was proposed applying the BES in 2 x 2 BESDs. The second argument is more serious. It is based on the characteristic of the BES that it does not take into consideration the main effects of the row and column variables. Thus, group sizes and binomial success rates have to be assumed to be equal, that is, 50%. When the data deviate from this assumption, the BES may overestimate effect sizes, relative to a model that does consider main effects. Put in different terms, the BES is a *marginal-free* measure.

In CFA it is virtually never the case that group sizes and success rates are equal. Therefore, the BES is of interest in particular if the use of marginal-free measures is considered appropriate. Otherwise, results can be enriched by using the measure of association, $\phi$ (which is sensitive to differences in margins itself). Alternatively, the unbiased estimates proposed by Thompson and Schumacker (1997) can be calculated. These, however, defy the purpose of having an intuitively appealing and visually plausible display of effect size. Therefore, the BES and the BESD are considered useful, in particular because they consider only specific parts of the information available in the 2 x 2 table.

## ACKNOWLEDGMENTS

Alexander von Eye's work on this chapter was supported in part by NIAAA Grant 2 RO1 AA07065. The authors are indebted to G. A. Lienert and Ronald D. Franklin for careful readings and constructive comments on earlier versions of this chapter.

## REFERENCES

Anscombe, F. J. (1953). Contribution to discussion of paper by H. Hotelling: New light on the correlation coefficient and its transform. *Journal of the Royal Statistical Society, B, 15*, 229 - 230.

Bergman, L. R., Eklund, G., & Magnusson, D. (1991). Studying individual development: Problems and methods. In D. Magnusson, L. R. Bergman, G. Rudinger, & B. Törestad (eds.), *Problems and methods in longitudinal research* (pp. 1 - 27). Cambridge, England: Cambridge University Press.

Bergman, L. R., & Magnusson, D. (1997). A person-oriented approach in research on developmental psychopathology. *Development and Psychopathology, 9*, 291 - 319.

Bollen, K. A. (1989). *Structural equations with latent variables.* New York: Wiley.

Cohen, J. (1988). *Statistical power analysis for the behavioral sciences* (2nd ed.). Hillsdale, NJ: Lawrence Erlbaum.

Eliason, S. R. (1990). *CDAS. Categorical Data Analysis System.* The University of Iowa, Department of Sociology.

Glück, J., & von Eye, A. (2000). Including covariates in Configural Frequency Analysis. *Psychologische Beiträge, 42*, 405-417.

Gonzáles Debén, A. (1998). *Experiencias con un nuevo indice de falta de adjuste en el analysis de tables de contigencia.* [Results from using a new index of lack-of-fit in contingency tables analysis]. Unpublished master's thesis, University of Havana. Havana, Cuba.

Goodman, L. A. (1981). Three elementary views of log-linear models for the analysis of cross-classifications having ordered categories. *Sociological Methodology*, 191 - 239.

Goodman, L. A. (1991). Measures, models, and graphical displays in the analysis of cross-classified data. *Journal of the American Statistical Association, 86*, (3), 1085 - 1111.

Görtelmeyer, R. (1988). *Typologie des Schlafverhaltens* [Typology of sleep behavior]. Regensburg, Germany: Roderer.

Gutiérrez Peña, E., & von Eye, A. (2000). A Bayesian approach to configural frequency analysis. *Journal of Mathematical Sociology, 24*, 151 - 174.

Havránek, T., & Lienert, G. A. (1984). Local and regional vs. global contingency testing. *Biometrical Journal, 26*, 483 - 494.

Holm, S. (1979). A simple sequentially rejective multiple test procedure. *Scandinavian Journal of Statistics, 6*, 65 - 70.

Khamis, H. J. (1996). Application of the multigraph representation of hierarchical log-linear models. In A. von Eye & C. C. Clogg (Eds.), *Categorical variables in developmental research: Methods of analysis* (pp. 215 - 229). Boston: Academic Press.

Krauth, J., & Lienert, G. A. (1973). *KFA. Die Konfigurationsfrequenzanalyse und ihre Anwendung in Psychologie und Medizin* [CFA. Configural Frequency Analysis and its application in psychology and medicine]. Freiburg, Germany: Alber.

Küchenhoff, H. (1986). A note on a continuity correction for testing in three-dimensional configural frequency analysis. *Biometrical Journal, 28,* 465 - 468.

Lehmacher, W. (1981). A more powerful simultaneous test procedure in configural frequency analysis. *Biometrical Journal, 23,* 429 - 436.

Lienert, G. A. (1969). Die AKonfigurationsfrequenzanalyse als Klassifikationsmethode in der Klinischen Psychologie [Configural Frequency Analysis as a method for classification in Clinical Psychology]. In M. Irle (Ed.), *Bericht über den 26. Kongreß der Deutschen Gesellschaft für Psychologie* (pp. 244 - 253)[Proceedings of the 26th congress of the German Psychological Association]. Göttingen, Germany: Hogrefe.

Lienert, G. A. (1971). Die Konfigurationsfrequenzanalyse III: Zwei- und Mehrstichproben KFA in Diagnostik und Differentialdiagnostik. [CFA: Two and more sample CFA in linquistics and differential psychology]. *Zeitschrift für Klinische Psychologie und Psychotherapie, 19,* 291 - 300.

Lienert, G. A., & Krauth, J. (1973). Die Konfigurationsfrequenzanalyse als Prädiktionsmodell in der angewandten Psychologie. [Configural frequency analysis as a prediction model in applied psychology]. In H. Eckensberger (Ed.), *Bericht über den 28.Kongreß der Deutschen Gesellschaft für Psychologie in Saarbrücken 1972* (pp. 219 - 228). Göttingen: Hogrefe.

Lienert, G.A., & Krauth, J. (1975). Configural Frequency Analysis as a statistical tool for defining types. *Educational and Psychological Measurement, 35,* 231 - 238.

Lienert, G. A., & Netter, P. (1987). Nonparametric analysis of treatment response tables by bipredictive CFA. *Methods of Information in Medicine, 26,* 89 - 92.

Lienert, G. A., & von Eye, A. (1988). Syndromaufklärung mittels generalisierter ISA. [Explaining syndromes using generalized interaction structure analysis.] *Zeitschrift für Klinische Psychologie, Psychopathologie, und Psychotherapie, 36,* 25-33.

Magnusson, D. (1985). Implications of the interactional paradigm for research on human development. *International Journal of Behavioral Development, 8,* 115 - 137.

Mellenbergh, G. J. (1996). Other null model, other (anti)type. *Applied Psychology: An International Review, 45,* 329 - 330.

Neter, J., Kutner, M. H., Nachtsheim, C. J., & Wasserman, W. (1996). *Applied linear statistical models* (4th ed.). Chicago: Irwin.

Netter, P. (1996). Prediction CFA as a search for types: History and specifications. *Applied Psychology: An International Review, 45,* 338 - 344.

Rosenthal, R., & Rubin, D. B. (1982). A simple, general purpose display of magnitude of experimental effect. *Journal of Educational Psychology, 74,* 166 - 169.

Rovine, M. J., & von Eye, A. (1997). A 14th way to look at a correlation coefficient: Correlation as the proportion of matches. *The American Statistician, 51,* 42 - 46.

Spiel, C., & von Eye, A. (1993). Configural frequency analysis as a parametric method for the search for types and antitypes. *Biometrial Journal, 35,* 151-164.

Thompson, K. N., & Schumacker, R. E. (1997). Evaluation of Rosenthal and Rubin's binomial effect size display. *Journal of Educational and Behavioral Statistics, 22,* 109 - 117.

Victor, N. (1989). An alternative approach to configural frequency analysis. *Methodika, 3,* 61 - 73.

von Eye, A. (1988). The General Linear Model as a framework for models in configural frequency analysis. *Biometrical Journal, 30,* 59-67.

von Eye, A. (1990). *Introduction to Configural Frequency Analysis - The search for types and antitypes in cross-classifications.* Cambridge, UK: Cambridge University Press.

von Eye, A. (1998). CFA. A program for 32 bit operation systems. *Methods of Psychological Research - Online, 3,* 1 - 3.

von Eye, A., & Brandtstädter, J. (1982). Systematization of results of configuration frequency analysis by minimizing Boolean functions. In H. Caussinus, P. Ettinger, & J. R. Mathieu (Eds.), *Compstat 1982, part II: Short communications, summaries of posters* (pp. 91-92). Vienna, Austria: Physica.

von Eye, A., & Brandtstädter, J. (1997). Configural Frequency Analysis as a searching device for possible causal relationships. *Methods of Psychological Research - Online, 2*(2), 1 - 23.

von Eye, A., Indurkhya, A., & Kreppner, K. (2000). CFA as a tool for person-oriented research - Unidimensional and within-individual analyses of nominal level and ordinal data. *Psychologische Beiträge, 42,* 353-401.

von Eye, A., & Schuster, C. (1999).  Modeling the direction of causal effects - an approach for manifest categorical variables. *Revista Multiclinica, 3,* 16-40.

von Eye, A.,  Spiel, C. (1994). Die Konfigurationsfrequenzanalyse als idiographische Methode zur Identifikation von Typen und Antitypen. [The identification of types and antitypes in configural frequency analysis]. *Zeitschrift für Differentielle und Diagnostische Psychologie, 15,* 201 - 210.

von Eye, A., & Spiel, C. (1996). Standard and non-standard log-linear symmetry models for measuring change in categorical variables. *The American Statistician, 50,* 300 - 305.

von Eye, A., Spiel, C., & Rovine, M. J. (1995). Concepts of nonindependence in configural frequency analysis. *Journal of Mathematical Sociology, 20,* 41 - 54.

von Eye, A., Spiel, C., & Wood, P. K. (1996b). CFA models, tests, interpretation, and alternatives - A rejoinder. *Applied Psychology: An International Review, 45,* 345 - 352.

von Eye, A., Spiel, C., & Wood, P. K. (1996a). Configural frequency analysis in applied psychological research. *Applied Psychology: An International Review, 45,* 301 - 327.

Wood, P. K., Sher, K., & von Eye, A. (1994).  Conjugate methods in configural frequency analysis. *Biometrical Journal, 36,* 387 - 410.

# *Actuarial Assessment of Malingering:*

## *Rohling's Interpretive Method*

**Martin L. Rohling**[1]
*University of South Alabama*

**Jennifer Langhinrichsen-Rohling**
*University of South Alabama*

**L. Stephen Miller**
*University of Georgia - Athens*

## CONSIDERATIONS IN THE DIAGNOSIS OF MALINGERING

In recent years, attorneys, physicians, and psychologists have had to become more familiar with the diagnosis of malingering. Patients who malinger are consciously choosing to feign or exaggerate symptoms, often in order to obtain compensation. These same professionals are often given the responsibility of determining the degree to which the expressed symptoms represent valid, exaggerated, or feigned deficits. For example, a substantial subgroup of individuals seeking compensation (20% to 25%) may warrant the diagnosis of malingering (Binder, Villanueva, Howieson, & Moore, 1993; Guilmette, Sparadeo, Whelihan, & Buongiorno, 1994). Recently, Binder and Rohling (1996) completed a comprehensive meta-analytic review of the effect of financial compensation on the experience and treatment of head injury. They found that patients who received economic incentives were significantly more likely to persist in their

---

[1]Please address correspondence to Martin Rohling, Ph.D. Assistant Professor Department of Psychology University of South Alabama 381 Life Science Building Mobile, AL 36688-0002. mrohling@usouthal.edu

complaints of sequelae, regardless of the severity of their injury. An earlier meta analysis by Rohling, Binder, and Langhinrichsen-Rohling (1995) found comparable results for chronic pain patients. Specifically, compensated chronic pain patients reported more pain than did noncompensated chronic pain patients even when the two groups' severity of injuries were comparible prior to receiving compensation. In a third meta analytic study, Binder, Rohling, and Larrabee (1997) found the effect size for residual cognitive deficits from mild head injury was nearly zero (e.g., few, if any deficits can be identified on neuropsychological measures following this type of trauma). One implication of these authors' body of work might be that, in the absence of financial incentives, few patients would experience sequella due to mild head injuries.

There are a number of reasons why it is important for professionals to accurately differentiate between malingers and individuals with detectable neurologically based impairments. First, accurate diagnosis is critical because it appears that awarding unnecessary financial compensation can make patients' symptoms worse (e.g., Binder and Rohling, 1996; Rohling et al., 1995). Second, compensating patients who are reporting undetectable impairments likely inflates insurance costs and inequitable distribute of health care dollars. Third, other iatrogenic disorders, such as depression and somatoform disorders may develop as a result of inappropriate distribution of health resources. Fourth, attorneys and neuropsychologists likely lose credibility when they pursue unfounded mild injury lawsuits (e.g., see Faust & Ziskin, 1988).

The focus of this chapter is on the difficulties inherent in diagnosing malingering in the population of individuals who have experienced a mild neurological event and who are seeking compensation for their impairments. We summarize human judgment research as it applies to this complex differential diagnosis and present an actuarial strategy that will facilitate neuropsychological detection of valid and feigned neurocognitive deficits.

**Diagnostic Problems Faced by Neuropsychologists When Feigning Occurs**

The assessment of malingering has increasingly become an expected component of neuropsychological assessment (Williams, 1998). As a result, neuropsychologists should be aware of the diagnostic criteria of malingering. *The Diagnostic and Statistical Manual of Mental Disorders* (4th ed.) [*DSM-IV*]; American Psychiatric Association, 1994) defines three criteria that must be met before a diagnosis of malingering should be applied. First, these criteria require the determination that a patient has feigned or exaggerated symptoms. Second, patient must have intentionally produced the symptoms. Finally, the patient's motivation for reporting symptoms has to be the acquisition of external incentives. Therefore, when neuropsychologists try to determine if these criteria have been met, several complex decisions must be made. These decisions can be conceptualized as following a two (symptoms are valid vs. feigned) by two (unintentional vs. intentional) by two (no incentives vs. incentives) by two (internal incentives vs. external incentives) matrix that results in sixteen possible outcomes. We offer suggestions that contrast with more traditional resolutions to each decision (e.g., Lezak, 1995; for a critic of traditional methods see Wedding, 1983). Particular attention is paid throughout this chapter to issues raised by Wedding and Faust (1989) in their research review of neuropsychologists' accuracy of assessment. We show how many of the standard assessment problems that they described are magnified when the differential diagnosis of malingering is involved.

### *Criterion 1: Determining If Symptoms Are False or Grossly Exaggerated*

First, the neuropsychologist attempts to determine whether a symptom is valid, grossly exaggerated, or feigned. Traditionally, this decision has been left to the clinical judgment of the evaluator. The judgment of symptom validity is most complex when the patient's complaint is a subjective experience (e.g., "My personality has changed."). When the neuropsychologist obtains abnormally low test scores, she or he must also judge whether the patient's objective performance is reasonable or exaggerated, given the severity of a lesion. Traditionally, standards of "reasonableness" are determined by the personal or professional judgment of the examiner, rather than by using an actuarial strategy (Wedding, 1983). Actuarial methods are appropriate for a number of acute measures such as a patient's post injury time to follow commands (Dikmen, Machamer, Winn, & Temkin, 1995). Research on human judgment has shown that trained professionals' clinical judgments are likely to be unreliable (Garb & Schramke, 1996; Oskamp, 1965; for an alternative view see McCaffrey & Lynch, 1992; Trueblood & Binder, 1997). In forensic cases, competent neuropsychologists often disagree about the "reasonableness" of a particular symptom, when the determination is based on their own experience and beliefs.

Normative data have been psychology's "gold standard" as a way of minimizing subjective bias. Epidemiological research data are available to determine the probability of a certain level of deficit being presented post trauma. From normative data, the likelihood or reasonableness of developing any particular symptom post injury can be calculated. Neuropsychologists can then use a standard procedure to determine the probability that a patient's complaint is valid and the likelihood that any particular symptom resulted from the alleged injury. Norm-based predictions can then be compared to the assessed deficits. Probability can then be assigned to the likelihood that the assessed complaint resulted from the alleged injury. This procedure would result in a uniform standard for determining the likelihood that a patient is feigning or grossly exaggerating a complaint.

***The Importance of Neuropsychological Signs as Opposed to Patient-Reported Symptoms.*** The definition of signs versus symptoms is relevant to the discussion of how neuropsychologists might objectively assess a patient's complaint. A symptom is a subjectively experienced problem that is believed to be causally related to a disorder. For example, a headache is a symptom because it cannot be objectively measured by a physician. We know that a person has a headache because they tell us so. Fever, on the other hand, can be verified by a physician by using an objective method of assessment (e.g., a mercury thermometer). Therefore, fever is considered a sign. Both symptoms and signs can be indications of a specific illness, as a headache and a fever can be a direct result of a cold or the flu. Although physicians may ask patients if they feel warm (i.e., Does the patient exhibit a symptom?), patients' responses to these questions can be considered independent of whether or not they have a fever. Traditionally, evaluation of feigning has been based on symptom complaints gathered during clinical interview, which are not easily verified.

Although it is more difficult to feign a sign than a symptom, it is easier to feign a neuropsychological sign than a physical sign. For example, a patient may intentionally withhold known answers to a psychometrically sound assessment of memory. When the chance of obtaining exceedingly low scores or an unusual pattern of errors is low, it is likely that factors other than the suspected dysfunction caused the patient's poor performance. Furthermore, a direct examination of test scores and item responses may give the neuropsychologist clues as to whether the patient consciously chose to do poorly on a task or not. It is on this basis that we believe that neuropsychologists have tools available to more objectively conclude whether the patient's test scores and symptomatic complaints are feigned or grossly exaggerated.

### Criterion 2:  Determining Whether Intention or Awareness Existed

*DSM-IV* requires that the patient intentionally (i.e., consciously) feign or exaggerate a symptom. How one defines the word "intentional" ultimately determines if the diagnosis of malingering is applied. A patient's intentions to feign and manipulate are typically not disclosed to the professional, particularly if the patient is attempting to manipulate the contingencies via the evaluation. Therefore, it is common to infer a patient's intentions from his or her behavior. This is the second complex judgment required for the diagnosis.

Neuropsychologists often infer patients' awareness on the basis of their "pattern of responding" to interview questions and test items. Rogers, Harrell, and Liff (1993) suggested methods to assist neuropsychologists with this complex inference process. They proposed that intention to deceive may be assumed if a patient (a) has symptoms with a late onset (b) is resistant to treatment or evaluation (c) has no obvious neurological findings or inconsistent findings on neurological exams (d) presents with bizarre signs or symptoms that are inconsistent with current models of cognitive functioning and/or (e) exhibits discrepancies between what is expected and what is observed. Unfortunately, Rogers et al. did not specify how neuropsychologists should determine when these behaviors have been exhibited by a patient. For example, no procedures were proposed for determining if a patient's results are significantly different from expectation. Furthermore, no recommendations were provided as to how neuropsychologists are to integrate inconsistent positive and negative findings from these methods. As a result, these excellent suggestions are not often utilized in a reliable manner.

Neuropsychologists' assessment of the intentionality of sign or symptom production has been further complicated by the changing nature of the attorney-client relationship. For example, recent evidence suggests that some attorneys believe it is their professional obligation to educate their clients about the assessment process prior to their being subjected to it (Youngjohn, 1995). Although little is known about the degree to which this educational process alters the validity of the obtained test results some have argued that this process may actually function as a method of "coaching" the client so as to avoid detection of malingering (Youngjohn, 1995).

To resolve the neuropsychologist's dilemma in assessing intention, we make several recommendations. First, neuropsychologists should view a client's intention to deceive on a continuum rather than as a totally present versus totally absent dichotomy. Using this continuum, malingering can be considered as a reasonable diagnosis even if the neuropsychologist has only enough evidence to show that a patient is beyond the midpoint of this continuum (e.g., it can be inferred that the patient has some level of intention to deceive in order to respond in the manner evident in the test results). Thus, the *DSM-IV* criterion of intentionality could be judged present when only two of Rogers et al.'s (1993) criteria appear to be present. Likewise, intentionality would still be judged as present in situations in which some of the patient's signs and symptoms appear to be valid, if it can be proven that the patient has intentionally feigned or exaggerated other signs and symptoms in order to increase their chances of receiving compensation.

### *Criterion 3:Determining If Incentives Exist*

Because malingering requires that incentives exist, it is not uncommon for patients to avoid disclosing that they are trying to obtain compensation for their alleged injury. If this deception is successful, the neuropsychologist may be less likely to infer malingering. For example, attorneys may inadvertently facilitate their clients' attempts at deception by having another professional preliminarily evaluate their clients (e.g., neurologist, chiropractor, family practitioner, physical therapist, etc.). This "middle person" then refers the client to a neuropsychologist for an assessment. The neuropsychologist has no direct contact with or knowledge of the attorney. Complex circumstances, including the use of professionals from various disciplines, pose several challenges to accurate diagnosis. First, if the neuropsychologist remains unaware of existing external incentives, their likelihood of accurately detecting malingering may be diminished. Second, when these circumstances occur, neuropsychologists may feel significant pressure to provide diagnoses other than malingering in borderline cases in order to ensure that they are reimbursed for their work. These real-world influences highlight the possibility that judgments made by clinicians can be biased and objective decision strategies are needed.

Consequently, neuropsychologists should directly question their patients about the nature of the referral and if they have retained an attorney. Answers to these questions should be well documented. Documenting patients' responses can minimize later problems if the patient has not been sincere in her or his answers. Neuropsychologists should make explicit agreements with clients regarding the need to access all pertinent medical records, high school records, and employment information. They should get consent for collateral interviewing. Refusal to agree to these stipulations should results in a refusal to evaluate a patient. These conditions are communicated to all referring professionals prior to evaluation.

### Criterion 4:  Determining If Incentives Are Internal or External

The *DSM-IV* requires that the clinician substantiate that any existing incentives to exaggerate symptoms or malinger be external rather than internal. Unfortunately, this concept, often referred to as locus of control, has long been debated by psychologists. At one extreme, behaviorists have argued that all incentives can be considered reinforcers and that all reinforcement is external. These psychologists would then view all incentives as external. In contrast, psychoanalytic theorists have argued that there is a real difference between external and internal incentives, with internal incentives being driven by unmet emotional needs that were frustrated during childhood. The acquisition of an external incentive would not satisfy these more primitive needs.

As a result of the ongoing professional debate, we recommend that neuropsychologists narrowly define external incentives as economic incentives (e.g., disability payments, health care insurance coverage, civil litigation settlements), making them more concrete and quantifiable. Despite our redefinition, we believe that the neuropsychologist should not have to prove that external incentives exist in order to diagnose malingering. Conversely, we also believe that the presence of these incentives should not be insufficient to establish the existence of malingering. Many seriously injured patients are justifiably seeking compensation for obvious and real impairments. Instead, the known existence of external incentives should be used to aid in establishing of a malingering diagnosis. Conversely, the lack of external incentives mitigate the diagnosis of malingering. Furthermore, the probability of diagnosing malingering should be directly related to the quantity, saliency, and economic value of potential incentives.

### The Problem of Mixed Results in the Examination of Multiple Symptoms.

Once primary decisions are established, their interaction must be considered. What is the diagnostic outcome when some signs or symptoms seem to have been feigned, whereas others seem legitimate? No techniques for determining the contribution of conflicting signs or symptoms to the final diagnosis have been specified in the literature. Consequently, this integration has also been left to clinical judgment. As a result, competent neuropsychologists with the same assessment results often come to opposite conclusions if they weigh the influence of these results differently.

To resolve this problem, we recommend that a neuropsychologist attempt to calculate the odds that a particular pattern of signs or symptoms would result from a particular lesion. If signs or symptoms have unusually low odds of presenting together (i.e., less than 5%), it should be assumed that conscious intention was required for such a pattern to be exhibited. These calculations can be used to give an objective measure of the patient's level of intention. Another objective strategy is to compare a patient's scores to the normative scores obtained from patients who truly suffer from the alternative disorders. This second strategy also gives the neuropsychologist a method of calculating the probability that conscious feigning of signs or symptoms occurred. Finally, comorbidity of disorders is relatively common in this population. Multiple signs and symptoms may not be generated from a single diagnosis. Instead, they may represent multiple disorders. Consequently, for most patients the integration process may best be resolved by diagnosing multiple disorders. The disorder that appears to account for the most variance within a pattern of signs or symptoms should also be identified as primary.

## ESTABLISHING CURRENT DIAGNOSIS

When neuropsychologists are asked to evaluate a patient, what if two disorders are suspected?  Several categories of psychiatric disorders are often considered during the diagnostic process. These disorders typically include: (a) factitious disorders, (b) somatoform disorders (e.g., pain disorder), ©) disorders of affect (e.g., major depressive episode), anxiety (e.g., panic disorder), and thought (e.g., paranoid schizophrenia), (d) other physical disorders (e.g., endocrine problems or other metabolic disorders); and (e) neurological dysfunction (e.g., closed head injury, stroke, Alzheimer's disease, learning disabilities). We specifically presented these alternative diagnoses in this order to reflect the underlying assumption about the neurological bases of each (i.e., from least neurologically based to most). Differential diagnosis then involves both determining the validity of patients' signs and symptoms, and basis for the expression of the symptoms. Neuropsychologists who diagnose malingering must also determine if a patient suffers concurrently from other disorders.

Many patients who malinger have valid psychiatric symptoms and may have had valid neurological symptoms at some point. Their psychiatric problems may lead them to misinterpret physical signs and poorly judge environmental contingencies. Consequently, neuropsychologists suspecting malingering should be acutely sensitive to other concurrent disorders, as they are likely to coexist.

**Traditional Methods of Detecting Signs of Feigning During Neuropsychological Assessment**

Two reviews of malingering (Rogers et al., 1993; & Williams, 1998) appear in recent scientific literature, with a combination of overlapping recommendations revealing nine methods of detecting feigning (i.e., floor effect; performance curve; magnitude of error; atypical presentation; psychological sequelae; inattention; slow responding; haphazard, systematic, random, or sequential responding; and symptom validity tests). The floor effect was defined by Rogers et al., who suggested that a patient who is attempting to feign dysfunction will even fail tasks that severely impaired patients get right. A second method advocated by Rogers et al. is based on the hypothesis that patients who are attempting to feign often fail easier items whereas they pass more difficult ones. This can be seen if a clinician were to examine a patient's performance curve across test items and compare that to the items' degree of difficulty. Rogers et al. also hypothesized that patients who are feigning respond with a magnitude of error that is uncommon for brain injured patients. For example, when asked "Who is the president of the United States?" a feigning patient might respond "George Washington," rather than with the more common error of "Ronald Reagan". Another method suggests that patients who feign are inconsistent or atypical in their presentation of signs and symptoms (Rogers et al., 1993). For example, a patient who shows up late for his or her appointment may claim to have forgot the appointment time. However, during the clinical interview, the same patient may give explicit details of the results of prior evaluations as well as the specific dates and times of when these evaluations were conducted. Rogers et al. also hypothesize that patients who feign neuropsychological deficits can be detected by examining their responses on noncognitive or personality inventories, as they give invalid responses to these personality inventories (e.g., Minnesota Multiphasic Personality Inventory, 2nd ed. [MMPI-2]).

Williams (1998) hypothesized that patients who are feigning attempt to do so by intentionally not paying attention. For example, when patients are told to listen to a series of digits that will be read to a patient, they may purposefully distract themselves so as not to hear the digits. Then, when asked to repeat the digits, they can sincerely report being unable to recall the correct series. Furthermore, Williams suggested that patients who feign impairment respond more slowly to questions than do truly brain-injured patients. Their longer response time is thought to result from the additional time it takes to generate an incorrect response while inhibiting a correct one. Williams also hypothesized that patients who are attempting to feign cognitive impairment often develop a strategy for responding that does not involve giving the correct answer (e.g., answering every third item as true). Therefore, if a neuropsychologist examines a patient's response pattern carefully and notices a haphazard, systematic, or random pattern, this should be considered a sign of malingering.

***Symptom Validity Tests***. The last method proposed by both Rogers et al. (1993) and Williams (1998) recommended the use of symptom validity tests. These are typically forced-choice tests in which 50% of the right answers should be achieved by chance alone (e.g., predicting heads every time a coin is flipped will typically result in half of the predictions being correct). Patients who perform significantly below chance on forced-choice tests (e.g., 20% correct with a probability of less than .05 from the binomial distribution) are assumed to have achieved such poor performance by intentionally giving incorrect responses to questions. Of the nine proposed methods of detecting feigning, this method is the least susceptible to problems in human judgment.

We believe that the methods reviewed by Rogers et al. (1993) and Williams (1998) are reasonable approaches to detecting feigning. If a neuropsychologist notices any of these signs or symptoms during an evaluation of a patient, the level of suspicion that the patient is feigning should be raised and greater scrutiny of the patient's responses should ensue. One challenge that faces the neuropsychologist, however, is that the statistical information needed to make the judgments is often missing. Another challenge is that many neuropsychologists fail to utilize available statistical procedures, even when data are provided, because calculations are time consuming and non reimbursable. The problem is, however, that without these statistical analyses, neuropsychologists must depend on their subjective clinical experience and judgment to utilize the malingering criteria. These judgments often require the neuropsychologist to interpret patients' data patterns. Research has shown that neuropsychologists make many mistakes when subjectively interpreting test scores and patterns (Arkes & Faust, 1987; Dawes & Corrigan, 1974). In part, this is because there is significant overlap between the patterns found in patients who are feigning and those found in neurologically impaired patients. These errors also occur because humans, in general, use simplified heuristics in their decision making that poorly detect complex patterns that exist in the data.

**Assessment Problems Faced by Neuropsychologists Who Diagnose Malingering:    Common Human Judgment Errors to Which Neuropsychologists Are Susceptible**

When a neuropsychologist has diagnosed malingering without having completed any statistical calculations related to the probability that the diagnosis is accurate, the diagnosis is open to a legal challenge of the evaluator's judgment. Wedding and Faust (1989) showed that neuropsychologists are just as likely as other humans to commit judgment errors. They also pointed out that these errors could be avoided if neuropsychologists were to take better advantage of their statistical training and if they would fully use the technology that is readily available (e.g., personal computers and statistical software). Failure to do so reduces neuropsychologists' probability of successfully detecting. Wedding and Faust (1989) described five common errors in human judgment that have been shown to apply to neuropsychologists' diagnostic decisions.

*Hindsight Bias.* The hindsight bias may cause a neuropsychologist who has reviewed a patient's medical record to diagnose only those disorders that have already been noted in the record. For example, if a computer-aided tomography (CT) scan is read by a radiologist as being indicative of cerebral atrophy caused by Alzheimer's disease, the neuropsychologist will make the same diagnosis. Tests will be administered and scores interpreted in such a way as to make the diagnosis of Alzheimer's disease appear to be correct.

*Confirmatory Bias.* When a neuropsychologist hypothesizes that a memory disorder was caused by a motor vehicle accident, questionnaires may be administered that ask the patient to rate his or her memory. Complaints of memory problems on these questionnaire are then used to support the original hypothesis. The problem with the strategy is that the neuropsychologist failed to recognize that complaints of memory problems are fairly common and may be due to other disorders that interfere with memory rather than to the traumatic brain injury (e.g., depression). The overlap between the two distributions may be unknown or ignored by the neuropsychologist. The selective gathering of evidence is particularly common if the hypothesis-testing model of assessment is followed (e.g., see Lezak, 1995).

*Overreliance on Salient Data.* Some neuropsychologists may believe that a certain test score is a pathognomonic sign of a disorder (e.g., Reitan, 1986). Thus, when a patient exhibits this sign, a neuropsychologist concludes that the disorder is present. Additional test scores that are inconsistent with the diagnosis are ignored. For example, if a neuropsychologist concludes that a patient has feigned memory impairment based on the patient's deceptive responses to questions regarding psychiatric history, s/he may ignore the patient's performance on more objective tests that are valid indicators of neurological dysfunction.

***Under Utilization of Base Rates.***   Neuropsychologists may underutilize base- rate information (Arkes, 1981). For example, if a patient's test scores fall into a range that is common for patients who suffer from a rare disorder, neuropsychologists may be inclined to diagnosis the patient with the rare disorder. The error is that, although patients with the rare disorder may always score in this low range, low scores may have also been obtained by patients who suffer from more common disorders. Typically, the most likely cause for the low score is the common disorder and not the rare disorder. For example, personality change and poor judgment in a male who is in his 50s may be due to Pick's disease a relatively rare disorder. However, this same pattern is also seen in patients suffering from Alzheimer's disease. Although Pick's disease tends to strike persons at an earlier age than does Alzheimer's disease, Alzheimer's disease is five times more common in this age range than is Pick's disease. Therefore, the abnormality is more likely caused by Alzheimer's disease than it is by Pick's disease.

***Failure to Analyze Co-Variation.***   A neuropsychologist may have administered one test that results in poor performance by the patient. To validate this finding, the neuropsychologist administers a second test that is highly correlated with the first. When a similar pattern of poor performance is found on the second test, the neuropsychologist assumes that his or her diagnosis of dysfunction has been confirmed. However, if the first test did not measure the construct of interest accurately, the correlated second test may simply replicate invalid findings rather than substantiate the diagnosis per se (Chapman & Chapman, 1969).

## A STATISTICAL AND ACTUARIAL PROCEDURE FOR THE ANALYSIS OF NEUROPSYCHOLOGICAL DATA

Williams (1997) noted that despite the research that shows how these common human biases in decision making also exist for neuropsychologists, awareness of these biases has not prevented them from occurring. Essentially, admonishing neuropsychologists to think better has not been found to alter their capacity to make diagnoses with any greater reliability or validity. Therefore, Williams recommended using technology as a decision aid. These decision aids would then help neuropsychologists correctly interpret psychometric test data and increase the accuracy of their diagnoses (Sicoly, 1989). Consistent with several researchers' recommendations (e.g., Garb & Schramke, 1996; Sicoly's, 1989; Williams, 1997), we have developed a process of data analysis, called the Rohling Interpretive Method (RIM), that can be programmed on most personal computers. This RIM will help neuropsychologists overcome common human judgment errors. The logic of the RIM has been presented in greater detail elsewhere (Miller & Rohling, 2001).

In this chapter, we highlight how the Rohling Interpretive Method (RIM) helps a neuropsychologist avoid the biases noted by Wedding and Faust (1989). The methodology used in the RIM is similar to that recommended for meta-analytic reviews of research literature (e.g., see Glass, McGaw, & M. L. Smith, 1981; Rosenthal, 1984). The linear combination of scores we recommend is supported by the research of Dawes (1979), Dawes and Corrigan (1974), and Heaton et al. (2001). It follows a model similar to that presented by Kiernan and Matthews (1976). We believe it to be a more statistically sound method of analysis which improves upon
the Impairment Index (II) of Reitan and Wolfson (1985), and the Average Impairment Rating (AIR) of Russell, Neuringer, and Goldstein (1970). A further advantage is that it does not restrict a neuropsychologist to a particular battery of tests.

The steps of the RIM are listed in Table 8.1. When these steps are conducted on an individual case basis with a calculator, they can be time consuming. However, by programming a personal computer with commonly available statistical software (e.g., Microsoft Excel; SPSS for Windows; Statview; sample program available from the authors), each of these steps is easily automated. Once automated for an initial case, the time it takes to complete future interpretations is reduced. In fact, it takes less time to conduct a RIM interpretation than it takes to complete a more traditional interpretation that does not require that these calculations be completed.

Each step of the RIM process is illustrated with two example cases. The tables and graphs that are presented for these cases are referred to throughout the case description. Steps 1 through 17 of the RIM process generate a table of summary statistics, which is also put in graphic form. Steps 18 through 24 describe the interpretation of the summary statistics.

Both case examples were referred for assessment by an attorney and litigation was expected. Issues of financial compensation existed in both cases and concern over malingering or symptom exaggeration also

TABlE 8.1

Steps of Rohling's Evaluation -

Miller's Interpretation of Neuropsychological Data (RIM).

| *Summary Statistics: Steps 1-17.* | 13. Determine the upper limit necessary for premorbid performance. |
|---|---|
| 1. Design and administer a flexible test battery. | 14. Conduct one-sample $t$ tests on each of the means generated. |
| 2. Estimate premorbid general ability (EPGA). | 15. Conduct a between-subjects ANOVA with domain means. |
| 3. Convert test scores to a common metric (e.g., T-scores with $M = 50$, *sd* $= 10$). | 16. Conduct a power analysis for each of the domains and the TBM scores. |
| 4. Assign each test score to the cognitive domain for which it has the highest factor loadings. | 17. Sort test scores in ascending order for qualitative inspection |
| 5. Calculate cognitive domain means, standard deviations, and sample sizes. | *Interpretation: Steps 18-24* |
| 6. Calculate test battery means (TBM), including an Overall, Domain, and Instrument TBM. | 18. Determine the test battery's validity by examining the symptom validity, sample size, and heterogeneity statistics. |
| 7. Calculate the heterogeneity probabilities for each domain. | 19. Determine if psychopathology influenced test scores. |
| 8. Assign categories of impairment. | 20. Use test battery means to determine if impairment exists. |
| 9. Determine the percentage of test scores that fall in the impaired range. | 21. Determine patterns of strengths and weaknesses across the domains. |
| 10. Graphically display all of the summary statistics in T-score format. | 22. Examine the mean T-scores from the noncognitive domains. |
| 11. Calculate effect sizes for all domains and TBM scores. | 23. Explore low power comparisons for Type II errors. |
| 12. Calculate a confidence intervals for all domains and TBM scores. | 24. Examine the response operating characteristics of sorted T-scores. |

applied. In the first case, a traumatic-brain-injured patient is presented who had clear evidence of neurological impairment (e.g., LOC [loss of consciousness] of 17 days, positive findings on CT scanning, MRI [magnetic resonance imaging] scanning, EEG [electroencephalogram] results, and neurological examination). Case 1 is presented to give the reader a clear understanding of how a brain-injured patient's RIM output is examined. Case 2 is that of a suspected malingering patient. In Case 2, in contrast to Case 1, there were no positive findings upon presentation at the emergency room, nor on CT scanning, MRI scanning, EEG readings, nor during the neurological exam. Case 2 is meant to illustrate the advantages of the RIM process over traditional interpretations when milder injures are involved.

**Case 1: Traumatic Brain Injury Caused by a Motor Vehicle Accident**

Case 1 is that of Truman Hurt, a 22-year-old white right-handed man who allegedly suffered a head injury in a motor vehicle accident (MVA). Mr. Hurt's attorney referred him for an evaluation. Litigation processes were begun when Mr. Hurt's insurance claims were denied. The assessment issues focused on Mr. Hurt's premorbid use of alcohol and illicit drugs. Mr. Hurt's attorney believed that the defense might argue that Mr. Hurt's cognitive deficits preceded his MVA and were due to alcohol and/or substance abuse. If this explanation were accepted, the insurance company could not be held responsible for Mr. Hurt's neuropsychological deficits; the company could then justify their denial of compensation.    Mr. Hurt was administered a battery of tests to assess the extent of his cognitive deficits, the likelihood that these deficits could be attributed to the MVA, and the truthfulness of his responses. Data generated from this test battery were then subjected to the RIM process. Tables 2a and 2b show the summary statistics generated by the RIM process. Figure 8.1 is a graphical portrayal of these same results. The mean for the symptom validity domain (SV) fell within the above-average range. This indicates that Mr. Hurt was probably responding truthfully to the assessment measures and that the results can be meaningfully interpreted as representing neurocognitive functioning. Sample sizes ($n$) appeared relatively adequate, particularly for those domains in which there was significant heterogeneity (see column headed Hetero. $p$ value). Finally, the heterogeneity of the test results could be explained by Mr. Hurt's lateralized left-hemisphere lesion, focused at the intersection of the frontal, parietal, and temporal lobes. When the variability of this lateralization was considered, the cause of the heterogeneity of his results seemed apparent.

TALBE 8.2a
RIM scores for Mr. Hurt

| | *M* | *sd* | *n* | *Hetero.* <br> *p value* | *Classify* | *%TI* |
|---|---|---|---|---|---|---|
| Sx Validity (SV) | 60.0 | 0.0 | 2 | --- | Superior | 0.00 |
| Emotion/Person (EP) | 55.4 | 12.3 | 11 | --- | High Avg. | 0.00 |
| Estimated Premorbid (EPGA) | 48.1 | 4.4 | 6 | --- | Average | 0.00 |
| Overall TBM (OTBM) | 37.2 | 11.4 | 63 | <.005 | Mild | 0.46 |
| Domain TBM (DTBM) | 35.5 | 6.8 | 7 | --- | Mild | 0.86 |
| Instrument TBM (ITBM) | 38.0 | 10.4 | 14 | --- | Mild | 0.50 |
| Verbal (VC) | 36.5 | 10.3 | 9 | --- | Mild | 0.56 |
| Performance (PO) | 45.0 | 13.5 | 8 | <.10 | Average | 0.25 |
| Executive (EF) | 38.1 | 8.1 | 11 | --- | Mild | 0.54 |
| Memory (ML) | 36.8 | 15.5 | 9 | <.025 | Mild | 0.33 |
| Attention (AW) | 35.8 | 7.5 | 14 | --- | Mild | 0.50 |
| Process Speed (PS) | 21.5 | 2.1 | 2 | --- | Mod-to-Sev | 1.00 |
| Language Aphasia (LA) | 36.0 | 13.3 | 10 | <.10 | Mild | 0.50 |

Regarding psychopathology, the mean score for the *emotional-personality (EP)* domain is in the high-average range and not indicative of be significant (PreM-Nec, Table 8.2b), all of the test battery means fell below the required 44.5. Finally, the one-sample *t*-test results (Table 8.2b) show significant impairment that is quite unlikely to have occurred by chance alone. These results strongly support the conclusion that Mr. Hurt significant psychopathology that might have influenced Mr. Hurt's test results. Looking at the tests score more closely, all validity indices were within the normal range and his pattern of scores did not suggest any obvious *DSM-IV* diagnostic category.

Mr. Hurt's *Estimated Premorbid General Ability (EPGA)* indicates that his general ability was within the average range. Furthermore, there is little variability in the *EPGA*. This indicates that it is unlikely that Mr. Hurt had a preexisting ability deficit (e.g., a learning disability). Small variability in the *EPGA* also increases the ease of interpreting the current assessment. Because there is little variability in the *EPGA* and the estimate is in the

normal range, it is unlikely that Mr. Hurt was showing significant impairments in his ability prior to the accident that could be attributed to drug and alcohol use.

TABLE 8.2b
RIM Scores for Mr. Hurt (continued)

| | ES | CI | PreM Nec. | 1-sample t Test | ANOVA S&W | Power (1-b) |
|---|---|---|---|---|---|---|
| Domain | | | | | | |
| SV | 1.00 | 0.0 | 60.0 | --- | --- | --- |
| EP | 0.54 | 6.7 | 62.1 | --- | --- | --- |
| EPGA | -0.19 | 3.6 | 44.5 | --- | --- | --- |
| OTBM | -1.09 | 2.4 | 39.6 | <.0001 | --- | --- |
| DTBM | -1.26 | 5.0 | 40.5 | <.0020 | --- | --- |
| ITBM | -1.01 | 4.9 | 42.9 | <.0000 | --- | --- |
| VCl | -1.16 | 6.4 | 42.9 | <.0050 | --- | --- |
| PO | -0.31 | 9.0 | 54.0 | --- | S | 0.32 |
| EF | -1.00 | 4.4 | 43.5 | <.0010 | --- | --- |
| ML | -1.13 | 9.6 | 46.4 | <.0300 | --- | 0.97 |
| AW | -1.23 | 3.6 | 39.4 | <.0030 | --- | --- |
| PS | -2.66 | 9.5 | 31.0 | <.0200 | W | --- |
| LA | -1.21 | 7.7 | 43.7 | <.0100 | --- | --- |

However, as depicted in Table 8.2a, Hetero *p* value, recall that there was significant variability in the *OTBM*. When this is the case, there is a possibility that the individual has significant cognitive strengths and weaknesses. This is the case for Mr. Hurt. Verbal Comprehension - Aphasia language measures on the right side of Fig. 8.1 display. Specifically, Mr. Hurt has a significant deficit in his processing speed. Conversely, his performance domain is a relative strength, showing less impairment than in other areas. Finally, as discussed previously in this chapter, interpretations of neuropsychological test data are enhanced by direct comparisons of the obtained results to the results that could be predicted from the literature. Using data from the nature of the injury Mr. Hurt sustained (e.g., time to follow commands of 17 days), and interpolating from data published by Rohling, Millis, and Meyers (2000), it was estimated that Mr. Hurt's *T*-score should be 35.8 (ranging from a *T*-score of 27.4 to 42.7 at the 90% confidence interval). Once again, the obtained *T*-scores (Table 8.2b) were exactly as would be expected, with the exceptions noted earlier (i.e., performance skills less impaired and processing speed more impaired).

The next three rows in Tables 8.2a and 8.2b (*Overall Test Battery Mean [OTBM], Domain Test Battery Mean [DTBM],* and *Instrument Test Battery Mean [ITBM]* depict an overall view of Mr. Hurt's performance on the assessment battery. Ideally, these three numbers should yield highly similar results. Specifically, when examining the *ES*s for each of these estimates (Table 8.2b), they are all of almost equal magnitude (-1.09, -1.26, and -1.01, respectively). Furthermore, as can be seen in Figure 8.1, all three global measures of performance on the test battery fall well below the average range. Finally, the percentage of tests impaired also suggests significant impairment across the test battery (46%, 86%, and 50%, respectively). Examining the premorbid level necessary for these results to has suffered a head injury that has resulted in residual cognitive deficits.

Looking next at Mr. Hurt's language domain, there was evidence of heterogeneity in his overall score. This was evident in his test scores that were most likely to be lateralized. That is, he demonstrated problems with naming, reading, writing, and fluency whereas there was no evidence of impairment in his gestural and graphic abilities.

No evidence of a learning disability or premorbid strengths or weaknesses was evident in Mr. Hurt's academic record. This came from several standardized test results he had been administered (e.g., Otis-Lennon Test, Stanford Achievement Test, ACT [American College Test], and high school grades). None of his prior records would have predicted a significant strength on the low power domain of performance skills (Power,

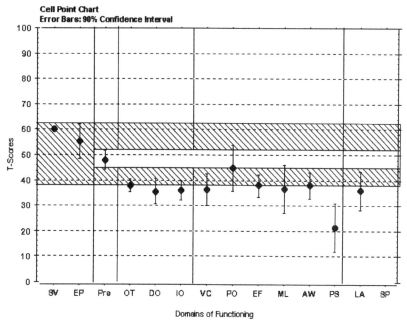

FIG 8.1. Graphic Profile of Mr. Hurt

Table 8.2b). Therefore, it is believed that this is a consequence of his accident and argues against impairments being due to alcohol or substance abuse, which tends to have a nonlateralized pattern of impairments.

Finally, in looking at the numerically sorted $T$-scores, there was no evidence that the pattern of scores found in the summary statistics was contradicted by the performance curve found in his numerically sorted $T$-scores. This is the same pattern described previously. Thus, there is no reason to believe that his test results were inadvertently misinterpreted by using inappropriate tests, norms, or caused by impaired motivation.

As a result of this interpretation, the neuropsychologist was confident in asserting that Mr. Hurt was experiencing impairment due to a neurological injury. Clearly, this individual was not malingering. Instead, his pattern of performance reflects sequella of head injury. Moreover, there was no evidence to support the insurance company's assertion that these deficits existed prior to the accident and were a result of Mr. Hurt's drug and alcohol use.

### Case 2: Malingering of Memory Impairment

Mea Fake was a 32-year-old white left-handed woman who claimed to have suffered a mild head injury at work. She was referred by a managed care company that was responsible for handling her workers' compensation claim. The primary issue in Ms. Fake's case was the determination of the cause of her persistent symptoms (e.g., headache and memory problems). Were these complaints due to (a) neurological injury, (b) preexisting psychiatric dysfunction (e.g., depression), or ©) malingering? This was the second referral of Ms. Fake's case; the first involved simply a review of records to determine the quality of her prior assessments and/or treatments, and to recommend what, if anything, should be done for her in the future. The only neuropsychological testing following her initial accident was with the Wechsler Adult Intelligence Scale -Revised (WAIS-R), Wechsler Memory Scale-Revised (WMS-R), and the D-scale of the MMPI-2. While reviewing Ms. Fake's records, it was noted that the prior evaluation was considered to have been inadequate for this type of case. First, there was no estimate of her premorbid general ability. Second, no tests were administered to assess the validity of her signs or symptoms. Third, the D-scale of the MMPI-2 was considered to have been an inadequate assessment of her emotional or personality status. Finally, although the psychologist's conclusions may have been correct, based on the available data, the potential for litigation in this case also caused concerned about the brevity of the evaluation.

As a result, the review of records resulted in a second assessment that was more comprehensive than that administered by the first psychologist. Consistent with the RIM process outlined previously, Ms. Fake was administered a battery of tests to assess symptom validity, personality functioning, and cognitive ability. Appendix A lists each of the test instruments administered and the scores obtained. Data were collected to derive estimates of Ms. Fake's premorbid level of functioning. Information was also collected about the work-related head injury in order to generate estimates of the extent of deficits that could be expected from this type of trauma.

Tables 8.3a, 8.3b, and Fig. 8. 2 show Ms. Fake's results as generated by the RIM process. The first thing to notice is Ms. Fake's symptom  validity results. Ms.Fake's SV domains core fell into the impaired range (Table 8.3a). This indicates that there is a strong probability that Ms. Fake was exaggerating or feigning signs and symptoms. The diagnosis of malingering should be considered at this point. In addition, the invalidity of these measures suggests that all other data generated from the assessment should be viewed with caution. According to Step 18 of the RIM process, it is important that the neuropsychologist next review the heterogeneity of variance (Hetero $p$ value). This tells the examiner whether the data from all the tests that were combined told the same story (e.g., did all the measures of personality have the same results?). Considerable variability was obtained on the symptom validity measures, the emotion/personality domain, the OTBM, as well as the performance skills, executive skills, and memory domains. A review of Ms. Fake's performance on the symptom validity tests indicates that although most of the symptom validity tests identified Ms. Fake as an invalid responder (i.e., 73% in %TI), she did less exaggerating on the more obvious tests of

TABLE 8.3a.
RIM scores of Ms. Fake

| | *M* | *sd* | *n* | *Hetero p value* | *Classify* | *%TI* |
|---|---|---|---|---|---|---|
| SV | 17.3 | 20.1 | 11 | <.0001 | Severe | 0.73 |
| EP | 44.4 | 13.5 | 10 | <.0500 | Below Avg. | 0.30 |
| EPGA | 44.9 | 1.2 | 6 | --- | Below Avg. | 0.00 |
| OTBM | 39.5 | 16.3 | 53 | <.0001 | Mild | 0.41 |
| DTBM | 42.8 | 11.2 | 6 | --- | Below Avg. | 0.33 |
| ITBM | 44.4 | 13.4 | 10 | --- | Below Avg. | 0.40 |
| VC | 39.4 | 7.4 | 6 | --- | Mild | 0.50 |
| PO | 43.2 | 13.2 | 8 | <.1000 | Below Avg. | 0.38 |
| EF | 59.3 | 16.8 | 7 | <.0500 | Superior | 0.14 |
| ML | 24.8 | 15.2 | 16 | <.0050 | Mod-to-Sev | 0.75 |
| AW | 43.5 | 6.4 | 15 | --- | Below Avg. | 0.27 |
| LA | 46.7 | --- | 1 | --- | Average | 0.00 |

malingering. The variability in Ms. Fake's emotional/personality data appeared to be due to Ms. Fake's higher scores on measures of hypochondriasis, depression, and hysteria on the MMPI-2.

TABLE 8.3b.
RIM scores of Ms. Fake continued

|  | ES | CI | PreM Nec. | 1-sample t Test | ANOVA S&W | Power (1- b) |
|---|---|---|---|---|---|---|
| SV | -3.27 | 11.0 | 28.3 | <.0002 | W | --- |
| EP | -0.56 | 7.8 | 52.2 | <.1100 | --- | 0.66 |
| EPGA | -0.51 | 1.0 | 44.0 | <.0001 | --- | --- |
| OTBM | -0.54 | 3.8 | 43.3 | <.0100 | --- | --- |
| DTBM | -0.21 | 9.2 | 52.0 | --- | --- | 0.21 |
| ITBM | -0.05 | 7.8 | 52.2 | --- | --- | 0.13 |
| VC | -0.55 | 6.1 | 45.5 | <.0700 | --- | 0.48 |
| PO | -0.17 | 8.8 | 52.1 | --- | --- | 0.20 |
| EF | 1.44 | 12.4 | 71.7 | <.0400 | S | --- |
| ML | -2.01 | 6.7 | 31.5 | <.0001 | W | --- |
| AW | -0.14 | 2.9 | 46.5 | --- | --- | 0.22 |
| LA | 0.18 | --- | --- | --- | --- | --- |

This led the neuropsychologist to be concerned that test scores may also have been influenced by the non-neurological factors of depression and somatosization. The variability in Ms. Fake's OTBM indicates that Ms. Fake is presenting a pattern of relative strengths and weaknesses on the cognitive data. As is evident from Fig. 8.2, Ms. Fake is performing significantly poorly on the memory and learning measures, but did particularly well on the measures of executive skills. All attempts to eliminate this heterogeneity were unsuccessful. That is, there were no signs of lateralization in her test scores; nor was there evidence of a preexisting learning disability. Furthermore, when the effect of a disproportionate number of tests that were administered in the domains of memory and attention were reduced by examining the ITBM (i.e., one mean score per instrument administered), the *ES* shrank from -.54 to -.05. This smaller effect size was not significantly different from her EPGA and raises doubt about the existence of residual cognitive deficits caused by a neurological injury.

Furthermore, Ms. Fake's EPGA clearly and consistently placed her in the low-average range of ability. Little variability was obtained in Ms. Fake's EPGA, estimate indicating that she probability had few noticeable strengths or weaknesses in her cognitive profile prior to the alleged head injury. In contrast, her current assessment results indicate a great deal of variability, both across the various domains and within domains, as there

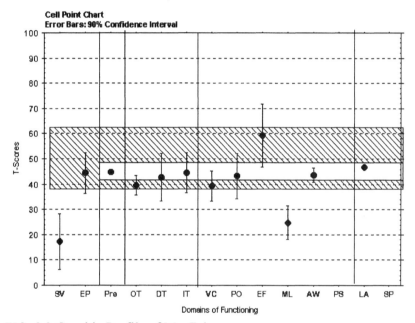

FIG. 8.2 Graphic Profile of Ms. Fake.

was also excess variability on Ms. Fake's performance skills, executive skills, and memory domains. A review of the specific test results suggests the following: Ms. Fake was an unsophisticated test taker. Consistent with her presenting complaint, she performed poorly on all obvious measures of memory. However, she did not perform nearly as poorly when memory functioning was assessed more subtly.

Using the OTBM results for Ms. Fake, and interpolating from data published by Rohling, Mills, and Myers (2000), it was expected that Ms. Fake should have been unconscious for four days, with a 90% confidence interval ranging from 16 hours to 9 days. Ms. Fake reported that she was unconscious for 10 minutes and recalls traveling in the ambulance to the emergency room. The amount of time she claimed to be unconscious is 500 times less than the mean that was predicted from her OTBM. This strongly suggests that Ms. Fake was feigning or exaggerating symptoms.

Several of the domains may have had insufficient statistical power to detect small residual deficits. This should raise the neuropsychologist's concern about making a Type II error (i.e., concluding no cognitive deficits exist when they actually do). The chances of detecting *ES*s in the range seen in Ms. Fake's data are quite low (i.e., see Power, Table 8.3b), ranging from .13 to .21 for her DTBM and ITBM, respectively. If the neuropsychologist were to try and administer enough tests for these *ES*s to be reliably detected, the number of tests administered would range between 165 and 2,650. Considering that the current test battery, with a sample size of 53, took approximately 8 hours to complete, this would mean that Ms. Fake would have to be assessed from between 3 days and 10 weeks. Clearly, this amount of time is an unreasonable solution to the problem of low power, particularly because the validity indices of the test battery raise serious doubt as to the motivation of Ms. Fake to perform to the best of her ability.

Finally, examining the numerically sorted *T*-scores, Ms. Fake performed particularly poorly on some of the more simple tests (e.g., PDRT, [Portland Digit Recognition Test]) and quite well on the more difficult tests (e.g., WCST, [Wisconsin Card Sorting Test]). This floor effect is further evidence of the probability that she was attempting to feign cognitive impairment.

As a result of this interpretation, the neuropsychologist should strongly consider a diagnose of malingering. Her obtained test scores were inconsistent with the alleged injury. Furthermore, given past research on the influence of compensation on mild head injury, it seems likely that awarding compensation to this patient would only enhance her experience of symptoms.

**Case Examples Summary**

Summarizing the findings of the two cases, it seems clear that Mr. Hurt and Ms. Fake each came to the evaluation sessions through similar referral mechanisms. Both had external incentives, however the resulting diagnoses were clearly different. Mr. Hurt did not receive a psychiatric diagnosis and all of his residual deficits were attributed to the injuries he suffered in his

MVA. On the other hand, Ms. Fake was given three psychiatric diagnoses, which included malingering, depression, and dependent personality disorder. None of her cognitive complaints were believed to be due to a neurological injury.

Competent neuropsychologists who use their statistical training, well-standardized test instruments, up-to-date knowledge of brain-behavior relationships, and technological aids such as personal computers and statistical software, can complete a state-of-the-art assessment that is both reliable and valid. A conscientious approach avoids most of the problems highlighted by Wedding and Faust (1989) – is objective, can be replicated, and is easy to present in court. It operationalizes many of the suggests made by other researchers (e.g., Rogers et al., 1993; Williams, 1998) in the assessment of malingering. The RIM process does not depend on the personal insight or experience to complete. Clear decision rules can be applied. It helps a neuropsychologist avoid overconfidence in his or her diagnoses. It facilitates the separation of statistical fact from artifact, without allowing a neuropsychologist to become biased by incomplete data analysis. It statistically considers covariation in test measures and facilitates the neuropsychologist's use of only the most valid of data. Finally, it assists the neuropsychologist in assessing alternative or concurrent diagnoses and the use of base rates of these diagnoses.

## REFERENCES

American Psychiatric Association. (1994). *Diagnostic and statistical manual of mental disorders*, (4ᵗʰ ed.). Washington, DC: Author.

Arkes, H. R. (1981). Impediments to actual clinical judgment and possible ways to minimize their impact. *Journal of Consulting and Clinical Psychology, 49*, 323-330.

Arkes, H. R., & Faust, D. (1987, August). Cue utilization in neuropsychology. In D. Faust (Chair), *Clinical judgment in neuropsychology. How good are we?* Symposium conducted at the annual convention of the american psychological association, New York.

Binder, L. M. (1993). *Portland Digit Recognition Test* (2nd ed.). Portland,OR: Author.

Binder, L. M., & Rohling, M. L. (1996). Money matters: A meta-analysis of the effect of financial incentives on recovery from closed-head injury. *American Journal of Psychiatry, 153*, 7-10.

Binder, L. M., Rohling, M. L., & Larrabee, G. (1997). A review of mild head trauma. Part I: A meta-analytic review of neuropsychological studies. *Journal of Clinical and Experimental Neuropsychology, 19*, 421-431.

Binder, L. M., Villanueva, M. R., Howieson, D., & Moore, R. T. (1993). The Rey AVLT Recognition Memory Task measures motivational impairment after mild head trauma. *Archives of Clinical Neuropsychology, 8*, 137-147.

Chapman, L. J., & Chapman, J. P. (1969). Illusory correlation as an obstacle to the use of valid psychodiagnostic signs. *Journal of Abnormal Psychology, 74*, 217-280.

Dawes, R. M. (1979). The robust beauty of improper linear models in decision making. *American Psychologist, 34*, 571-582.

Dawes, R. M., & Corrigan, B. (1974). Linear models in decision making. *Psychological Bulletin, 81*, 95-106.

Dawes, R. M., Meehl, P. E., & Faust, D. (1989). Clinical versus statistical prediction of human outcomes. *Science, 243*, 1668-1674.

Dikmen, S. S., Machamer, J. E., Winn, H. R., & Temkin, N. R. (1995). Neuropsychological outcome 1-year post head injury. *Neuropsychology, 9*, 80-90.

Dunn, L. M., & Dunn, E. S. (1997). *Peabody Picture Vocabulary Test-III*. Circle Pines, MN: American Guidance Service.

Faust, D., Hart, K., & Guilmette, T. J. (1988). Pediatric malingering: The capacity of children to fake believable deficits on neuropsychological testing. *Journal of Consulting and Clinical Psychology, 56*, 578-582.

Faust, D., Hart, K., Guilmette, T. J., & Arkes, H. R. (1988). Neuropsychologists' capacity to detect adolescent malingering. *Professional Psychology: Research and Practice, 19*, 508-515.

Faust, D., & Ziskin, J. (1988). The expert witness in psychology and psychiatry. *Science, 241*, 31-35.

Garb, H. N., & Schramke, C. J. (1996). Judgment research and neuropsychological assessment: A narrative review and meta-analysis. *Psychological Bulletin, 120*, 140-153.

Glass, G. V., McGaw, B., & Smith, M. L. (1981). *Meta-analysis in social research*. Beverly Hills, CA: Sage.

Goldberg, L. R. (1968). Simple models or simple processes; Some research on clinical judgments. *American Psychologist, 23*, 483-496.

Greene, R. L. (1979). Response consistency on the MMPI: The TR index. *Journal of Personality Assessment, 43*, 69-71.

Guilmette, T. J., Sparadeo, F. R., Whelihan, W., & Buongiorno, G. (1994). Validity of neuropsychological test results in disability evaluations. *Perceptual and Motor Skills, 78*, 1179-1186.

Heaton, R. K., Gladsjo, J. A., Palmer, B. W., Kuck, J., Maracotte, T. D., & Jeste, D. V. (2001). Stability and course of neuropsychological deficits in schizophrenia. *Archives of General Psychiatry, 58*, 24-32.

Ivnik, R. J., Malec, J. F., Smith, G. E., Tangalos, E. G., & Petersen, R. C. (1996). Neuropsychological tests norms above age 55: COWAT, BNT, Token, WRAT-R Reading, AMNART, Stroop, TMT, JLO. *The Clinical Neuropsychologist*, 10, 262-278.

Kiernan, R. J., & Matthews, C. G. (1976). Impairment index versus *T*-score averaging in neuropsychological assessment. *Journal of Consulting and Clinical Psychology*, 44, 951-957.

Lezak, M. D. (1995). *Neuropsychological Assessment* (3rd ed.). New York: Oxford University Press.

McCaffrey, R. J., & Lynch, J. K. (1992). A methodological review of method skeptic reports. *Neuropsychology Review*, 3, 235-248.

Miller, L. S., & Rohling, M. L. (2000). A statistical interpretive method for neuropsychological test data. *Neuropsychological Review, 11*, 141-167.

Millis, S. R. (1994). Assessment of motivation and memory with the Recognition Memory Test after financially compensable mild head injury. *Journal of Clinical Psychology, 50*, 601-605.

Oskamp, S. (1965). Overconfidence in case-study judgments. *Journal of Consulting and Clinical Psychology, 29*, 261-265.

Reitan, R. M. (1986). Theoretical and methodological bases of the Halstead-Reitan Neuropsychological Battery. In G. Grant & K. M. Adams (Eds.), *Neuropsychological assessment of neuropsychiatric disorders* (pp. 3-29). New York: Oxford University Press.

Reitan, R. M., & Wolfson, D. (1985). *The Halstead-Reitan Neuropsychological Test Battery. Theory and clinical interpretation.* Tucson, AZ: Neuropsychological Press.

Rogers, R., Harrell, E. H., & Liff, C. D. (1993). Feigning neuropsychological impairment: A critical review of methodological and clinical considerations. *Clinical Psychology Review, 13*, 255-274.

Rohling, M. L., Binder, L., & Langhinrichsen-Rohling, J. (1995). Money matters: A meta-analysis of the association between of financial compensation and the experience and treatment of chronic pain. *Health Psychology, 14*, 537-547.

Rosenthal, R. (1984). *Meta-analytic procedures for social research*. Beverly Hills, CA: Sage.

Russell, E. W., Neuringer, C., & Goldstein, G. (1970). *Assessment of brain damage: A neuropsychological key approach.* New York: Wiley-Interscience.

Sicoly, F. (1989). Computer-aided decisions in human services: Expert systems and multivariate models. *Computers in Human Behavior, 5*, 47-60.

Trueblood, W., & Binder, L. M. (1997). Psychologists' accuracy in identifying neuropsychological test protocols of clinical malingerers. *Archives of Clinical Neuropsychology, 12,* 13-27.

Wechsler, D. (1981). *Wechsler Adult Intelligence Scale-Revised.* San Antonio TX: The Psychological Corporation.

Wechsler, D. (1987). *Wechsler Memory Scale-Revised.* San Antonio, TX: The Psychological Corporation.

Wedding, D. (1983). Clinical and statistical prediction in neuropsychology. *Clinical Neuropsychology, 5,* 49-54.

Wedding, D., & Faust, D. (1989). Clinical judgment and decision making in neuropsychology. *Archives of Clinical Neuropsychology, 4,* 233-265.

Wiggins, N., & Hoffman, P. J. (1968). Three models of clinical judgment. *Journal of Abnormal Psychology, 73,* 70-77.

Williams, J. M. (1997). The prediction of premorbid memory ability. *Archives of Clinical Neuropsychology, 12,* 745-756.

Williams, J. M. (1998). The malingering of memory disorder. In C. R. Reynolds (Ed.), *Detection of malingering during head injury litigation. Critical issues in neuropsychology.* (pp 105-132). New York: Plenum.

Youngjohn, J. R. (1995). Confirmed attorney coaching prior to neuropsychological evaluation. *Assessment, 2,* 279-283.

## APPENDIX

All scores used published norms to compute T-Scores (Mn = 50, sd = 10). When these were not available, Heaton et al. (1991) norms were used. For those tests not in the Heaton et al. battery, norms from Spreen & Strauss (1998) were used.

| *Truman Hurt's Test Scores* | *Score* | *T* |
|---|---|---|
| **Estimated Premorbid General Ability** | | |
| Oklahoma Premorbid Intelligence Estimates | | |
|     VIQ | 87 | 41 |
|     PIQ | 99 | 49 |
|     FSIQ | 91 | 44 |
| Barona Regression Equations | | |
|     VIQ | 91 | 44 |
|     PIQ | 93 | 45 |
|     FSIQ | 91 | 44 |
| National Adult Reading Test | | |
|     VIQ | 91 | 44 |
|     PIQ | 102 | 51 |
|     FSIQ | 105 | 53 |
| Otis-Lennon | | |
|     FSIQ | 92 | 45 |
| California Achievement Test | | |
| Class Rank | | |
|     Upon Drop-Out (11th Grade) | | |
| | 92 | 45 |
| **Intelligence Tests** | | |
| Wechsler Adult Intelligence Scale-Revised | | |
|     Information | 29% | 45 |
|     Digit Span (F = 5; B = 5) | 8 | 43 |
|     Vocabulary | 6 | 38 |
|     Arithmetic | 7 | 40 |
|     Comprehension | 9 | 47 |
|     Similarities | 8 | 43 |
|     Picture Completion | 9 | 47 |
|     Picture Arrangement | 11 | 53 |

| *Truman Hurt's Test Scores* | *Score* | *T* |
|---|---|---|
| Block Design | 10 | 50 |
| Object Assembly | 13 | 60 |
| Digit Symbol | 8 | 43 |
| Verbal IQ | 81 | 37 |
| Performance IQ | 101 | 51 |
| Full Scale IQ | 87 | 41 |

## Executive Functioning

Wisconsin Card Sorting Test

| | | |
|---|---|---|
| # of Trials | 77 | |
| Total # Correct | 66 | |
| Total # of Errors | 11 | 62 |
| % Errors | 14% | 61 |
| Perseverative Responses | 6 | > 80 |
| % Perseverative Responses | 8% | 73 |
| Perseverative Errors | 6 | 74 |
| % Perseverative Errors | 8% | 66 |
| Nonperseverative Errors | 5 | 59 |
| % Nonperseverative Errors | 6% | 58 |
| Conceptual Level Responses | 65 | |
| % Conceptual Level Responses | 84% | 60 |
| # of Categories Completed | 6 | |
| Trials to Complete the 1st Category | 11 | |
| Failure to Maintain Set | 1 | |
| Learning to Learn | -1.5 | |

Stroop Color Word Test

| | | |
|---|---|---|
| Word Reading | 77 | 35 |
| Color Naming | 34 | 19 |
| Color-Word Reading | 24 | 29 |
| Interference Score | .4 | 50 |

## Attention/Working Memory

Trail Making Test (A & B)

| | | |
|---|---|---|
| Trails A  (Errors = 0) | 26 | 51 |
| Trails B  (Errors = 0) | 51 | 55 |

Digit Vigilance Test

| *Truman Hurt's Test Scores* | *Score* | *T* |
|---|---|---|
| Total Time | 523 | 29 |
| # of Errors | 1 | 59 |

**Memory & Learning**

Wechsler Memory Scale-Revised

| | Score | T |
|---|---|---|
| General Memory Index | 72 | 31 |
| Verbal Memory Index | 78 | 35 |
| Visual Memory Index | 74 | 33 |
| Attention/Concentration Index | 70 | 30 |
| Delayed Recall Index | 62 | 25 |
| Digit Span Forwards | 6 | 39 |
| Digit Span Backwards | 5 | 43 |
| Visual Memory Span Forwards | 6 | 37 |
| Visual Memory Span Backwards | 6 | 41 |
| Logical Memory I | 20 | 42 |
| Logical Memory II | 9 | 36 |
| % Savings | 45% | |
| Visual Reproduction I | 32 | 46 |
| Visual Reproduction II | 22 | 38 |
| % Savings | 69% | |

Rey-Auditory Verbal Learning Test

| | Score | T |
|---|---|---|
| Trial 1-5 Total Score | 36 | 28 |
| Trial 1 | 4 | 29 |
| Trial 5 | 8 | 29 |
| Trial B | 6 | 47 |
| Trial 6 (Delayed Recall) | 9 | 42 |
| % Savings | 112% | |
| Trial 7 (30 min. Delayed Recall) | 7 | 33 |
| % Savings | 87% | |
| Recognition Hits | 12 | 46 |
| False Positives | 9 | |
| Discriminability | 76% | |
| Response Bias | .50 | |

Rey-Osterrieth Complex Figure Test

| | Score | T |
|---|---|---|
| Copy | 31 | 31 |
| 3 min. Delay | 18 | 38 |
| 30 min. Delay | 16 | 33 |

| *Truman Hurt's Test Scores* | *Score* | *T* |
|---|---|---|
| **Symptom Validity** | | |
| Fifteen Items Test | | |
|     Total Recall | 15 | |
|     Location | 12 | |
| Word Memory Test | | |
|     Immediate Recognition | 67% | |
|     Delayed Recognition | 72% | |
|     Consistency 1 | 70% | |
|     Multiple Choice | 40% | |
|     Paired Associates | 40% | |
|     Free Recall | 35% | |
|     Long-Delay Free Recall | --- | |
| Portland Digit Recognition Test | | |
|     Easy Items (36) | 56% | |
|     Hard Items (36) | 72% | |
|     Total Items (72) | 60% | 32 |
| Dot Counting Test | | |
|     Intercept Grouped | .14 | |
|     Intercept Ungrouped | -1.1 | |
|     Slope Grouped | .19 | |
|     Slope Ungrouped | .50 | |
|     $R^2$ Grouped | .87 | |
|     $R^2$ Ungrouped | .96 | |
|     Time/Dot Grouped | .21 | |
|     Time/Dot Ungrouped | .41 | |
|     UG: G Ratio Time/Dot | 2.0 | |
| **Language Aphasia** | | |
| Peabody Picture Vocabulary Test | | |
|     Estimated VIQ | 102 | 51 |
| **Emotional/Personality** | | |
| Minnesota Multiphasic Personality Inv.-2 | | |
|     Lie (L) | 6 | 62 |
|     Frequency (F) | 2 | 44 |

| *Truman Hurt's Test Scores* | | *Score* | *T* |
|---|---|---|---|
| Defensiveness (K) | | 20 | 61 |
| Hypochondriasis (Hs)   (K-corr) | | 22 | 69 |
| Depression (D) | | 20 | 70 |
| Hysteria (Hy) | | 34 | 77 |
| Psychopath. Deviate (Pd)  (K-corr) | | 24 | 53 |
| Masculinity-Femininity (Mf:) | | 34 | 55 |
| Paranoia (Pa) | | 7 | 39 |
| Psychasthenia (Pt) | (K-corr) | 33 | 61 |
| Schizophrenia (Sc) | (K-corr) | 26 | 50 |
| Hypomania (Ma) | (K-corr) | 13 | 37 |
| Social Introversion (Si) | | 23 | 45 |

| *Mea Fake's Test Scores* | *Score* | *T* |
|---|---|---|

**Estimated Premorbid General Ability**

Oklahoma Premorbid Intelligence Estimates

| | | |
|---|---|---|
| VIQ | 87 | 41 |
| PIQ | 104 | 53 |
| FSIQ | 93 | 45 |

Barona Regression Equations

| | | |
|---|---|---|
| VIQ | 98 | 48 |
| PIQ | 98 | 48 |
| FSIQ | 97 | 48 |

National Adult Reading Test

| | | |
|---|---|---|
| VIQ | 86 | 41 |
| PIQ | 99 | 49 |
| FSIQ | 90 | 43 |

Otis-Lennon

| | | |
|---|---|---|
| VIQ | 94 | 46 |
| PIQ | 97 | 48 |
| FSIQ | 95 | 46 |

Stanford Achievement Tests

| | | |
|---|---|---|
| Test Battery Total Score | 99 | 49 |

**Intelligence Tests**

Wechsler Adult Intelligence Scale-Revised

| *Mea Fake's Test Scores* | *Score* | *T* |
|---|---|---|
| Information | 8 | 43 |
| Digit Span (F = 5; B = 5) | 6 | 38 |
| Vocabulary | 7 | 40 |
| Arithmetic | 7 | 40 |
| Comprehension | 8 | 43 |
| Similarities | 6 | 38 |
| Picture Completion | 9 | 47 |
| Picture Arrangement | 14 | 63 |
| Block Design | 11 | 53 |
| Object Assembly | 12 | 57 |
| Digit Symbol | 5 | 33 |
| Verbal IQ | 80 | 37 |
| Performance IQ | 100 | 50 |
| Full Scale IQ | 86 | 41 |

## Executive Functioning

Wisconsin Card Sorting Test

| | | |
|---|---|---|
| # of Trials | 116 | |
| Total # Correct | 74 | |
| Total # of Errors | 42 | 40 |
| % Errors | 36% | 39 |
| Perseverative Responses | 32 | 33 |
| % Perseverative Responses | 28% | 31 |
| Perseverative Errors | 28 | 32 |
| % Perseverative Errors | 24% | 31 |
| Nonperseverative Errors | 14 | 47 |
| % Nonperseverative Errors | 12% | 48 |
| Conceptual Level Responses | 60 | |
| % Conceptual Level Responses | 52% | 39 |
| # of Categories Completed | 6 | |
| Trials to Complete the 1st Category | 11 | |
| Failure to Maintain Set | 0 | |
| Learning to Learn | -1.3 | |

Stroop Color Word Test

| | | |
|---|---|---|
| Word Reading | 64 | 28 |
| Color Naming | 51 | 31 |

| *Mea Fake's Test Scores* | *Score* | *T* |
|---|---:|---:|
| Color-Word Reading | 22 | 27 |
| Interference Score | 2.4 | 52 |

**Attention/Working Memory**

Trail Making Test

| | | |
|---|---:|---:|
| Trails A  (Errors = 0) | 53 | 26 |
| Trails B  (Errors = 2) | 173 | 27 |

Digit Vigilance Test

| | | |
|---|---:|---:|
| Total Time | 525 | 32 |
| # of Errors | 0 | 72 |

**Memory & Learning**

Wechsler Memory Scale-Revised

| | | |
|---|---:|---:|
| General Memory Index | 88 | 42 |
| Verbal Memory Index | 88 | 42 |
| Visual Memory Index | 90 | 43 |
| Attention/Concentration Index | 69 | 29 |
| Delayed Recall Index | 83 | 38 |
| Digit Span Forwards | 7 | 46 |
| Digit Span Backwards | 3 | 29 |
| Visual Memory Span Forwards | 9 | 52 |
| Visual Memory Span Backwards | 5 | 30 |
| Logical Memory I | 25 | 49 |
| Logical Memory II | 17 | 43 |
| % Savings | 68% | |
| Visual Reproduction I | 31 | 45 |
| Visual Reproduction II | 27 | 42 |
| % Savings | 87% | |

Rey-Osterrieth Complex Figure Test

| | | |
|---|---:|---:|
| Copy | 29 | 22 |
| 3 min. Delay | 22.5 | 45 |
| 30 min. Delay | 17 | 31 |

**Symptom Validity**

Fifteen Items Test

| | | |
|---|---:|---|
| Total Recall | 12 | |

Dot Counting Test

| *Mea Fake's Test Scores* | *Score* | *T* |
|---|---|---|
| Intercept Grouped | .36 | |
| Intercept Ungrouped | -4.0 | |
| Slope Grouped | .28 | |
| Slope Ungrouped | .96 | |
| R^2 Grouped | .66 | |
| R^2 Ungrouped | .95 | |
| Time/Dot Grouped | .31 | |
| Time/Dot Ungrouped | .63 | |
| UG: G Ratio Time/Dot | 2.0 | |

**Language Aphasia**

Boston Naming Test

| | | |
|---|---|---|
| # Correct | 27 | 43 |

Peabody Picture Vocabulary Test

| | | |
|---|---|---|
| Estimated VIQ | 109 | 56 |

Basic Aphasia Exam (BAE; Modified RIAS)

| | | |
|---|---|---|
| Verbal Mean (PICA Scoring 1-15) | 13.1 | 42 |
| Graphic Mean (PICA Scoring 1-15) | 13.2 | 48 |
| Gestural Mean (PICA Scoring 1-15) | 15.0 | 59 |
| Overall Score (PICA Scoring 1-15) | 13.7 | 48 |

Letter and Category Fluency

| | | |
|---|---|---|
| Total # for Letter F | 3 | 23 |
| Total # for Letter A | 3 | 29 |
| Total # for Letter S | 3 | 23 |
| Total for Animals | 11 | 33 |
| Total for Foods | 5 | 17 |

**Psychomotor Speed**

Finger Oscillation Test

| | | |
|---|---|---|
| Right (Dom.) | 31 | 20 |
| Left (Non-Dom.) | 33 | 23 |

**Academic Achievement**

Wide Range Achievement Test-Revised

| | | |
|---|---|---|
| Reading | 72 | 31 |

| *Mea Fake's Test Scores* | *Score* | *T* |
|---|---|---|
| Spelling | 60 | 23 |
| Arithmetic | 65 | 26 |

**Emotional/Personality**

Inventory to Diagnose Depression

| | | |
|---|---|---|
| Total Score | 23 | 29 |

Minnesota Multiphasic Personality Inv.-2

| | | |
|---|---|---|
| Lie (L) | 5 | 56 |
| Frequency (F) | 5 | 51 |
| Defensiveness (K) | 7 | 33 |
| Hypochondriasis (Hs) (K-corr) | 4 | 31 |
| Depression (D) | 11 | 34 |
| Hysteria (Hy) | 13 | 35 |
| Psychopath. Deviate (Pd) (K-corr) | 22 | 48 |
| Masculinity-Femininity (Mf) | 23 | 44 |
| Paranoia (Pa) | 11 | 53 |
| Psychasthenia (Pt) (K-corr) | 18 | 34 |
| Schizophrenia (Sc) (K-corr) | 18 | 36 |
| Hypomania (Ma) (K-corr) | 23 | 56 |
| Social Introversion (Si) | 25 | 49 |

# Recovery of Function

**Aarne Kivioja**
*Department of Orthopaedics and Traumatology, Helsinki University Central Hospital, Finland*

**Ronald D. Franklin**[1]
*St. Mary's Medical Center and Florida Atlantic University*

## Purpose

This chapter provides an overview of evaluation and measurement used in the prediction of recovery from brain injury. We also include a glossary of key terms in Appendix B. We include those rating scales, checklists, and norm-referenced tests that have been associated with recovery in the medical and neuropsychological literatures. We compare the statistical robustness of those measures reported as having the greatest predictive validity. Finally, we offer recommendations for improving the prediction of functional outcomes.

## Background

Recovery can refer to a wide variety of outcomes ranging from survival to complete return of premorbid abilities. Kolb and Whishaw (1990) made three generalizations regarding recovery of function and the chronic effects of brain damage on adults. First, complex behaviors that are composed of many functions appear to recover as a consequence of behavioral compensation. Second, incomplete lesions (i.e., traumatic brain injuries) produce the most pronounced recovery. Third, when a complete localized brain area controlling specific skills or abilities is damaged or removed, significant recovery is unlikely. They went on to report that between 65% and 75% of war veterans who sustained traumatic brain injuries show no

---

[1] Please address correspondence to PO Box 246, Candor, NC, 27229, rdfphd@yahoo.com

recovery whatsoever, but they recognized that the data on which these observations were made are not quantitative. What is more, in patients showing evidence of recovery, data do not adequately reflect the extent of recovery. Laurence Binder (1995) reported that significant variance is observed in the return to work within a year when return to work is evaluated using medical classifications of mild, moderate, and severe. Between 80% and 100% of patients sustaining mild head injuries are back at work. Approximately half (56%) of the patients with moderate injuries and just over a quarter (26%) of patients with severe head injuries returned to work within 12 months.

Researchers and clinicians operationally define recovery in ways that are difficult to compare across studies. For example, Little, Templer, Persel, and Ashley (1996) followed a well-practiced pattern of predicting outcome rather than return to function. For them, outcome means scores on psychological or neuropsychological tests.

Prigatano (1997) noted that a patient's ability to return to work may be societies' definition of successful cognitive rehabilitation. And, if rehabilitation efforts fail to attain this end, then the cost of rehabilitation will not be justified. Neuropsychological tests have been used to predict competitive employment (Boake et al., 1997). Yet, Barbara Wilson's (1997) review of approaches to cognitive rehabilitation does not include return to work as a goal of rehabilitation as defined by the World Health Organization or Dr. Wilson.

When all types of injuries are considered, recovery from an accident or assault is generally a time-consuming but well-ending process. Tales about ancient warriors and sportsmen often describe full recovery. Injuries of ancients usually resulted from stab wounds, low-energy blows, or sprains. Recuperation was based mainly on spontaneous recovery with modern surgical repair of serious wounds (viz., heart) appearing relatively recently (Rehn, 1897). In the 20th century the development of cars and high buildings have changed the pattern of injuries from the low-energy injuries of the ancients toward high-energy ones. The treatment of high-energy injuries from traffic accidents and falls in patients with multiple injuries has required considerable innovation in medicine during this century. The practice of starting an intra venous line on scene dates from the late 1950s. The possibility of detailed injury imaging with either ultrasound, computerized tomography, or magnetic resonance imaging originated in the 1970s. Advances in imaging have virtually replaced the need for neuropsychological assessment in many settings, especially for the localization of function for which the Reitan tests were designed (Ammerman & Campo, 1998).

The development of trauma surgery has given many more victims of accidents the chance to survive their injuries. The treatment chain begins with adequate initial care and fluid resuscitation at the scene of injury, with fast transport to the appropriate hospital capable of surgical interventions. There, all the injuries have to be assessed without delay and restorative measures taken. The initial resuscitative measures and operative treatment are often followed by lengthy rehabilitation.

Most injuries sustained in accidents can be grouped in two categories, blunt and penetrating. Blunt injuries result from decelerating forces, for example, car accidents and falls. In blunt injuries, any part of the body can sustain damage with corresponding sequella. Penetrating injuries result mainly from assaults or self-inflicted injuries with guns or knives. In penetrating injuries the body parts injured lie close to the wounds. Determining the category of injury poses a challenge in the early phases of diagnosis, occasionally resulting in delays that are beyond medically acceptable standards and increasing risk of sequella (Rehn, 1897). Diagnostic delays are more common in patients with multiple injuries and those involved in road crashes (Janjua, Sugrue, & Deane, 1998).

## Presentation

Within this chapter we consider three broad areas. The section Rating of Traumatic Injury, deals with methods and instruments useful in evaluating survival, cognition, and functional abilities. The Capacity for Independent Living section addresses a patient's ability to return to work or school, drive, and integrate socially. The section entitled Disability Determination reviews definitions and rating methods used to determine the degree of disability experienced by patients following brain injury.

## RATINGS OF TRAUMATIC INJURY

### Survival Ratings

Immediately following trauma, the challenge is keeping the patient alive. Two evaluation methods are commonly used to aid triage and guide treatment: rating scales and physical examination. Ratings provided by emergency medical technicians and emergency room attendants provide information regarding survival likelihood. A variety of rating scales have been developed to aid in early triage; some of them have shown efficacy in predicting later recovery and minimizing functional impairment.

*Rating Scales*

A number of scales have been constructed to predict survival in patients sustaining traumatic injury. We present the most commonly used scales in Table 9.1, correlated with patient survival.

TABLE 9.1
Mortality Ratings for Select Trauma Scales

| Scale | Authors | r | p |
|---|---|---|---|
| APACHE II | Vassar et. al. (1992) | .94 | |
| | Wong et. al. (1996) | .93 | |
| ASCOT | Champion et. al. (1996) | .69 | |
| GCS | Meredith et. al. (1998) | | .001 |
| ISS | Cheadle et. al. (1989) | | .050 |
| | Osler et. al. (1997) | .87 | |
| | Osler et. al. (1997) | .89 | |
| NISS | Osler et. al. (1997) | .89 | |
| | Osler et. al. (1997) | .91 | |
| TRISS | Wong et. al. (1996) | .67 | |
| | Milham et. al. (1995) | | .004 |
| | Champion et. al. (1996) | .64 | |

***Glasgow Coma Scale (GCS).*** The Glasgow Coma Scale (GCS) ranks three responses: eye-opening, verbal, and motor responses on a 15-point scale (see Lezak, 1995, p 755) and is perhaps the most studied of survival ratings. Zandbergem, de Hann, Stoutenbeek, Koelman, and Hijdra (1998) provided an excellent review of the GCS and its ability to predict survival for patients in anoxic-ischemic coma (see Table 9.2). Others have cited its general ability to predict survival and mortality (Signorini,Andrews, Jones, Wardlaw, & Miller, 1999; Sloan, et al. (1998). The GCS is a critical component of broader rating scales as well (viz., T-RTS ). Researchers have also correlated the GCS with a variety of outcome measures as reported in Table 9.3. Unfortunately, its ability to predict outcome beyond survival is poor.

TABLE 9.2
Predictive Value of Glasgow Coma Scores
Following Anoxic-Ischemic Coma[a]

| Factor | N | #Pts. | Sensitivity | Specificity |
|--------|---|-------|-------------|-------------|
| *Pupillary reactions* | 7 | 643 | 0.30-0.50 | 0.60-1.00 |
| *Motor response* | | | | |
| M1-3 first 24 hrs. | 4 | 269 | 0.63-0.95 | 0.30-0.79 |
| M1-3 Day 1 | 2 | 087 | 0.85-0.87 | 0.42-0.59 |
| M1-3 Day 3 | 3 | 307 | 0.70-1.00 | 0.29-1.00 |
| M1-2 Day 3 | 3 | 171 | 0.56-0.92 | 0.93-1.00 |
| M1 Day 3 | 3 | 171 | 0.11-0.58 | 1.00 |
| *GCS* 3-5 first 24 hrs. | 3 | 137 | 0.63-0.82 | 0.54-1.00 |

[a]Summary of Studies Reported by Zandbergen et al.(1998)

*Triage-Revised Trauma Score.* On-scene grading is possible with the Triage-Revised Trauma Score (T-RTS; Champion, Sacco, Copes, et al. 1989) where the parameters assessed are physiological data including systolic blood pressure, respiratory rate, and GCS. The actual Trauma Score, is the sum of weighted rankings for each of these variables, in contrast to the Triage Trauma Score which represents the sum of unweighted rankings. Theorists speculated that addition of the physiologic variables to the GCS might provide a more accurate predictor of long-term outcome. When Zafonte, Hammond, Mann, Wood, Millis, and Black (1996) compared GCS and T-RTS scores at rehabilitation admission with scores on the Disability Rating Scale (DRS), concordance was better for the GCS alone than for the T-RTS, but both were poor (-.25 vs. -.18 respectively).

*Injury Severity Score.* The Injury Severity Score (ISS) is a grading developed and updated by the American Association of Automotive Engineering that is more accurate than the T-RTS. To calculate the ISS number, six body regions are used: head or neck; face; chest; abdominal or pelvic contents; extremities or pelvic girdle; external. The individual injuries are graded from 1 (minor injury) to 5 (critical injury).

The ISS is obtained by squaring the three highest numbers from six regions and summing them (Baker, O'Neill, Haddon, & Long , 1974). Thus, the Injury Severity Score varies between 0 and 75. The score correlates with mortality, and no patient with an ISS of 75 survives.

TABLE 9.3
Pearson Correlations of Glasgow Coma Ratings
With Other Measures.

| Outcome Measure | r | Authors |
|---|---|---|
| Glasgow Outcome Scale | .31 | Zafonte, Hammond, Mann, Wood, Black, & Millis (1996) |
| Detailed Outcome Scale | .19 | van  der Naalt,van Zomeren, Sluiter, & Minderhoud (1999) |
| Disability Rating Scale | .25- | Zafonte, Hammond, Mann, Wood, Black, & Millis (1996) |

The ISS is not well validated in assessing long-term functional impairment (Hannan, Farrell, & Cayten, 1997; van der Sluis, tenDuis, & Geertzen , 1995). Also, the spine often is not included separately thereby making the assessment of neurologic recovery more difficult. In addition severe solitary brain injuries with relatively low ISS (16 or 25) tend to skew the otherwise linear correlation of ISS to mortality. Also, in a comparison of ratings from 15 observers, interrater agreement was poor, .28 for rater agreement and .50 for severity (Zoltie & de Dombal, 1993).

Osler, Baker, and Long (1997) proposed creation of a new version (NISS) of the severity score in order to take into account multiple injury sites. Using retrospective calculations from 6,575 cases at two sites, they reported that NISS provided a better data fit throughout the range of prediction than did the ISS with correlations between .896 and .907 for the NISS compared to .869 and .896 for the ISS. Brenneman, Boulanger, McLellan, and Redelmeier (1998) found both versions were accurate predictors of short-term mortality, although the NISS was slightly superior (.85 vs. .80), but noted the NISS can increase the severity of an injury.

*TRISS.* A combination of Trauma Score and Injury Severity Score called the, Trauma Injury Severity Score (TRISS; Boyd, Tolson, & Copes, 1987) is even more accurate in predicting survival for groups of patients than either scale alone. The TRISS has been widely used since 1986. However, its use was predicated on retrospective data and findings offer poor precision when describing anatomic injuries. The overall misclassification rate is 4.3% (Demetriades, Chan, & Velmahos, 1998). Errors in subgroups of patients older than 54 years are problematic and inconsistent, leading to recommendations for more accurate classifications (Champion et al., 1996; Rutledge, Osler, Emery, & Kromhout-Schiro, 1998). Addition of pH values improves the survival statistic (Milham, Malone, Blansfield, LaMorte & Hirsch, 1995). But, Wong, Barrow, Gomez, and McGuire (1996) noted that neither the TRISS, nor a similar measure, Acute Physiology and Chronic Health Evaluation (APACHE II), allow physicians to confidently predict the survival of individual patients. What is more, the APACHE system significantly overestimates the risk of death (Vassar, Wilkerson, Duran, Perry, & Holcroft, 1992) and TRISS underestimates deaths from infection (Cheadle et al, & Polk, (1989.)

*A Severity Characterization of Trauma.* A Severity Characterization of Trauma (ASCOT) was introduced in a multicenter study between 1987 and 1989 in the hopes of providing greater predictive validity and sensitivity. The ASCOT offered sensitivity similar to the TRISS (64.3 and 69.3, respectively) but the hoped-for enhancements in outcome prediction were not realized (Champion et al., 1996). ASCOT demonstrated stronger correlations with cognitive ability scores and behavior rating scores than the GCS when used with children, but neither scale correlated significantly with behavior ratings (Papero, Snyder, Gotschall, Johnson, & Eichelberger, 1997).

**Physical Examination**

The assessment of recovery of function should be started with anatomical body regions. One possibility is to look separately at the nine anatomical regions. Refinements including pelvic bones and urogenitals as separate regions have been suggested in foreign literature as well as the division of the back into upper and lower spine. Although chest and abdominal injuries require the most immediate attention, they very seldom cause permanent disability to surviving patients with blunt injuries, although surgical complications can result in brain injuries (viz., ischemia and anoxia.) In the long run most handicaps come from injuries to the pelvis, spine, extremities, and brain (Braithwaite, Boot, Patterson, & Robinson, 1998; Kivioja, Myllynen, & Rokkanen, 1990; van der Sluis, Eisma, Groothoff, & ten Duis, 1998). Brain injuries are serious in initial treatment and also cause permanent disability.

*Spinal Cord Injuries.* The recovery from spinal injury is first of all mainly dependent on the extent of injury to the spine at the very moment of the accident. The motor and sensory deficits can be grouped coarsely into Frankels groups A to E. In the NASCIS study, a more detailed assessment was made with pinprick and light sensation analyzed in 29 segments and motor function graded with six scores in each of 14 muscles with a maximum score of 70 (Bracken, Shepard, & Collins, 1990). After the first 24 hours of the spinal shock, the grouping in the Frankels classes can predict the recovery to full function or to walking with aids, the ability for self-care in a wheelchair, or constant dependence on personal assistance. In the early phases the neurologic damage can be slightly diminished by the use of massive amounts of methylprednisolone, which must be initiated within 8 hours from the injury (Bracken, 1998). Later, rehabilitation to keep the joints with a full range of motion, to train the remaining functioning muscles and to control the bladder and bowel function is essential. In the group of paralyzed patients, the prevention of complications (ulcers, pneumonia, urinary tract infections) remains a life-long task.

*Injuries to the Extremities.* Grade III open fractures of the tibia often cause a lengthy period of recuperation with problems of neuro-vascular reconstruction, wound coverage, and fracture healing. The question of meaningful limb-sparing surgery versus amputation should be considered along with the impact of retaining the limb if sensory perception or meaningful motor function cannot be restored (Rosenberg & Paterson, 1998).

*Trunk Injuries.* Chest injuries usually cause little impairment, but may result in a lower cardiorespiratory performance and even marked dyspnea after a prolonged tracheostomy with tracheal wall softening. Abdominal injuries occasionally cause late problems with bowel occlusion tendency. The risk of the sometimes fatal pneumococcal pneumonia after splenectomy is elevated if the patient does not receive adequate postinjury vaccination. The most common long-term problems after flail chest injury were persistent chest wall pain, chest wall deformity, and dyspnea on exertion (Beal & Oreskovich, 1985).

*Face and Neck Injuries.*  These injuries may cause cosmetic problems that upset the patient and those in his surroundings. Thus even fractures with only a slight dislocation should be treated actively. A typical example is a slight dislocation of the nasal bone.  Facial injuries are associated with occult frontal lobe injuries that may not be evident early in the course of treatment.  The most problematic sequels are related to soft-tissue injuries causing long-standing neck pain after a whiplash injury (Deyo, 2000;  Sullivan, Stanish, Waite, Sullivan, & Tripp, 1998).

*Brain Evoked Potentials.*  During the past two decades evoked potentials (EPs) have been correlated with admission GCS scores and the Disability Rating Scale (Rappaport, 1982) one year after injury as displayed in Table 9.4.    The similarities between several of the measures on admission and at one year are quite striking if the absolute values are considered (viz., auditory cortex, auditory total, visual cortex, and somatosensory cortex).  Although the correlations are generally low, some of them compare favorably with neuropsychological measures.  Greenberg et al. (cited in Zafonte, Hammond, and Peterson, 1996) predicted a Glasgow Outcome Score one year later with 80% accuracy using Multimodality Evoked Potentials (MEP).

TABLE 9.4
Brain evoked potentials

| Evoked Potentials Test | Admit CGS | Disability Rating @ 1 Year |
|---|---|---|
| Auditory brainstem | .08- | .26 |
| Auditory intermediate latency | .32- | .25 |
| Auditory cortex | .37- | .37 |
| Auditory total | .31- | .36 |
| Visual cortex | .28- | .24 |
| Auditory and visual cortex | .33- | .37 |
| Somatosensory intermediate latency | .59- | .32 |
| Somatosensory cortex | .38- | .34 |
| Somatosensory total | .54- | .35 |
| Auditory, visual, somatosensory cortex | .59- | .40 |
| Auditory, visual, somatosensory total | .62- | .37 |

## Cognition Ratings

For patients emerging from coma who need intensive treatment, orientation and mental status become important predictors of rehabilitation potential. A variety of rating scales are used with these patients and most have been studied for outcome.

*Galveston Orientation and Amnesia Test.* The Galveston Orientation and Amnesia Test (GOAT) provides a level of responsiveness in patients with recent brain injuries. Orientation to time, person, place, and date are serially queried along with memories for events immediately preceding and following the traumatic event. A score of $\leq 66/100$ denotes coma, and loss of consciousness (LOC) as measured by the GOAT has been useful in retrospectively distinguishing "good recovery" for patients in coma less than 8 days from "moderate to severe disability" when coma persists (Levin, O'Donnell, & Grossman, 1979). See also the next subsection on "Posttraumatic Amnesia."

*Glasgow Outcome Scale.* The Glasgow Outcome Scale (GOS) was originally designed for used in head injury research (Jennett, Snoek, Bond, & Brooks, 1981). This scale has also been cited in recent literature to measure physical and mental disabilities in both adult and pediatric trauma patients. The scaling is 1 = death; 2 = persistent vegetative state; 3 = severe disability (requires assistance with activities of daily living); 4 = moderate disability (independent, but disabled); 5 = mild or no disability (capacity to resume normal occupational and social activities). Some have reported the GOS as a good predictor of long-term disablement (Jennett et. al., 1981). The GOS provides a more comprehensive assessment of disability than either the Disability Rating Scale or the Activities of Daily Living Index (Pettigrew, J. T. Wilson, & Teasdale, 1998). Four neuropsychological tests have shown satisfactory concordance with GOS scores of Traumatic Coma Bank patients; Controlled Oral Word Association, Grooved Pegboard, Trailmaking Part B, and Rey-Osterrieth Complex Figure Delayed Recall were the most predictive of the 19 tests evaluated. The Grooved Pegboard accounted for 80% of the total variance (Clifton et al., 1993). Others believe that it lacks the specificity to accurately predict complex posttraumatic outcomes even though coma duration is a good predictor of severe injuries when the coma lasts more than 30 minutes (Carney & Gerring, 1990; Wilson, 1986). Alcohol use can spuriously lower initial GCS scores as well (Jagger, Fife, Vernberg, & Jane, (1984).

*Post-Traumatic Amnesia.*    Although not a rating scale, the duration of posttraumatic amnesia (PTA) has also been used to estimate head injury severity (Lezak, 1995).   Duration of less than one hour constitutes mild injury with moderate injury suggested when the duration spans one to twenty-four hours.  Severe injury is indicated by amnesia of a day or more.  Unfortunately, concordance with specific outcome markers has not been described and there is some difficulty obtaining agreement regarding when to start and end measurement.  At best, duration of PTA provides a gross marker for severe injury.   Zafonte, Hammond, and Peterson (1996) reported that 82% of patients who were comatose between 1 and 7 days resumed employment versus 47%, 18%, and 11% for persons unconscious 2-4, 5-7, and >8 weeks respectively.

In the absence of serial GOAT measures, it may be difficult to discriminate between LOC duration, PTA, and time under chemical restraint.  Intensive-care patients frequently receive chemical restraint, and data evaluating differential effects of LOC, PTA, and chemical restraint lack clear delineation.   In practice, PTA and LOC are often estimated as the interval between a patient's last "clear memory" preinjury and the first "clear memory" postinjury.  This practice has the obvious pitfalls of being subject to malingering as well as exaggeration of symptoms.

## Outcome Ratings

Patients surviving traumatic head injury often receive one or more evaluations of neuropsychological functions while in rehabilitation programs.  In a Denmark study, slight but significant increases in scores on neuropsychological tests administered at the beginning and end of rehabilitation have shown no association with return to employment (Teasdale, Skovdahl Hansen, Gade, & Christensen, 1997).

Five patterns of recovery have been documented during rehabilitation (Shiel, B. A. Wilson, McLellan, Horn, & Watson, 1998). Recovery curves revealed patients experience minimal recovery, slow even recovery, uneven recovery, a long period of minimal recovery followed by rapid change, and rapid recovery. However, no long-term predictors were identified, and methods for matching patients to specific recovery curves were anecdotal.

An array of psychometric tools were used to support the construct of "neuropsychological spectrum" by Little et. al (1996).   The "neuropsychological spectrum" was an attempt to "go beyond the literature" by fabricating a spectrum extending from biological foundations of behavior to acquired educational, vocational, and social skills. Diagnostic tools were selected in correspondence with the patient's place within this continuum. Correlation methods were then applied to scores within the spectrum as a method for predicting later performance at more advanced positions along the spectrum. Functional outcome, attainment of basic life skills, was best measured by motor, sensory, language, and academic achievement tests.

*The Sickness Impact Profile.* The Sickness Impact Profile (SIP) includes 12 subscores of ambulation, sleep/rest, household management, recreation, emotional well-being, work, and capacity for independent living. It is a tedious questionnaire that the patient must be able to complete independently. Consequently, patients with moderate to severe cognitive deficits would be unsuitable for evaluation using this profile. SIP may be most useful for patients with mild head injuries as well as for those with other traumatic injuries such as lower extremity fractures (MacKenzie, Burgess, & McAndrew, 1993).

*The Functional Independence Measure.* The Functional Independence Measure (FIM) is based on six sections of self care, sphincter control, mobility, locomotion, communication, and social cognition. These sections are divided into 18 separate items and graded 1-7. The range of FIM is from 18 (dependent) to 126 (fully independent) (Emhoff, McCarthy, & Cushman, 1991; Hetherigton, Earlam, & Kirk, 1995). However, FIM does not include physical activity beyond walking and stairs. As many trauma victims are young, we should also assess the disability to perform different leisure activities (e.g., sporting). Hall et al., (1996) reported a "substantial" ceiling effect from the FIM that is evident in half of the 612 individuals in their review by time of discharge.

Dombovy, Drew-Cates, and Serdans (1998) compared FIM scores to cognitive and adaptive skills in 32 patients averaging 28 months postdischarge from inpatient rehabilitation. Although FIM scores improved significantly, 40% of patients demonstrated cognitive impairments and 40% to 50% required assistance with activities around the house. None had returned to work.

Ratings from the FIM were compared to findings of the Halstead-Reitan Neuropsychological Test battery by Smith-Knapp, Corrigan, and Arnett (1996). Both methods predicted motor disability, but neither predicted cognitive function.

*Functional Assessment Measure.* The Functional Assessment Measure (FAM) expands the 18 FIM items by the addition of 7 measures to assess dependence and 5 to evaluate performance constitute the Functional Assessment Measure (FAM; Tesio & Cantagallo, 1998). Good reliability is reported for the motor items, but items assessing cognitive function have shown mixed results (Alcott, Dixon, & Swann, 1997; McPherson, Pentland, Cudmore, & Prescott, 1996). Hall et al. (1996) reported ceiling effects in one third of 612 traumatic brain injury patients, some of which were evident by the time of discharge from inpatient rehabilitation.

*Moderator Variables.* Moderator variables of head injury were also described by Lezak (1995) and include age, repeated head trauma, polytrauma, and preinjury alcohol abuse. She viewed the precision of moderator variables as poor, although MacKenzie, Siegel, and Shapiro (1988) disagreed. Lezak argued that age considerations limited to adult samples skew data and complications of repeated trauma are undefined in terms of inter-trauma duration or the interaction effects of severity per occurrence. Likewise, clear definitions and descriptions of polytrauma (affecting multiple sites per occurrence) and a measurable definition of alcohol abuse remain elusive. Factors influencing outcome, in addition to age, include family support and site of lesion (Lezak, 1995). Kalechstein, van Gorp, and Rappoport (1998) noted that moderator variables may affect discrepancies across norms that can affect neuropsychological interpretation. Others (e.g., Johnstone, Pinkowski, Farmer, & Hagglund, 1995) viewed moderator variables in adolescent TBI as having a more direct relationship with outcome than do objective neuropsychological test scores.

Patients' awareness of their impairment serves as a moderator variable that successfully predicts employment outcome, as does clinician impressions of the degree of impairment in the patients' awareness of their deficits (Sherer, Bergloff, High, Levin, & Oden, 1996). Intelligence has also been shown to affect scores on neuropsychological tests (Wiens, Fuller, & Crossen, 1997).

The effects of moderator variables on clinical outcome is a topic of debate among statistical theorists. Aguinis, Stone, and Eugene (1997) reported that moderator variables have "profound" effects on statistical power in multiple regression, both for main effects and interactions. What is more, the presence of moderator variables may result in violation of assumptions for linear modeling, thereby requiring the use of nonlinear estimates, especially when large numbers of groups (i.e., age cohorts) are considered (Neale, 1998).

## CAPACITY FOR INDEPENDENT LIVING

We have chosen to define independent living in terms of three interdependent realities of contemporary life. First, the ability to work or attend school is essential to personal independence in contemporary society.  Second, driving an automobile may not be necessary, but the abilities needed to drive constitute a cluster of near essential skills for independent survival in much of the developed world.  Third, the ability to function in social intercourse contributes substantially to one's quality of life as well as one's ability to obtain essential services.

**Return to Work**

Still too little is known about the final functional outcome of patients with multiple injuries, how fast they recover, and how many of them have residual disabilities.  Even patients with the most severe injuries are astonishingly capable of returning to work.  The percentage of reemployment has been from 76% to 79% in studies of injured patients with a mean ISS of 29 to 34 (Frutiger et al., 1991;  Seekamp, Regel, Tscherne, 1996).  Injuries most
likely to hinder employment are brain injuries and injuries to the spine, pelvis, and extremities.  Of the 79 brain-injured patients studied by Rao  et al. (1990), 66% returned to work or school by an average 16.5 months postdischarge from inpatient rehabilitation.  Even obvious signs of impairment in severely brain-injured patients (such as aphasia) have shown no diagnostic signs that have been consistently linked to occupational outcome (Gill, Cohen, Korn, & Groswasser, 1991).  After serious (multiple) injuries the recuperation period is long. It is not unusual for the ability to return to work to be one year in severe injuries with the recuperation period close to two years (Boyer & Edwards, 1991;  Kivioja et. al., 1990; van der Sluis et. al., 1995).
In a study of outcome predictors taken from the Traumatic Coma Data Bank (Ruff et al., 1993) 242 patients ranging in age from 12 to 65 received baseline and 6-month neuropsychological assessments (see Author R, Tables 9.5 & 9.6).  Unfortunately, the sample was not large enough for statistical analysis appropriate to the isolation of predictor variables using linear methods.  As a consequence, the authors "selected" predictors based on reviews of earlier literature.  The numbers of subjects varied for each group, with the largest pool (age) containing 93 and the smallest (Withdrawal/Depression at 6-12 months) containing 32.
Ezrachi, Ben-Yishay, Kay, Diller, and Rattok (1991) evaluated 59 clients in a neuropsychology rehabilitation program and compared data obtained at the start and end of treatment with both employability at discharge and employment status in six months (see Author E,  Tables 9.5 & 9.6).  Both at the end of treatment and six months later, staff ratings of a patient's acceptance of injury and limitations was the most important variable in predicting what a patient would be doing in six months.  The study included moderator variables described as "acceptance ratings" and

TABLE 9.5
Neuropsychological Test Variables
Correlated With Return to Work  => |.30|

| Variable | Author[a] | Pearson Correlation Back-to-work | | |
|---|---|---|---|---|
| | | <= 6 Months | 6-12 Months | 3-8 Years |
| Depression | C | na | .29 | na |
| | R | .10 | .36 | na |
| "involvement with others" | E | .53 | .46 | na |
| Verbal skills: | | | | |
| WAIS-R Vocabulary | R | .30- | .03 | na |
| categorical reasoning | E | .38 | na | na |
| verbal abilities | E | na | .38 | na |
| Finger Tapping | R | .16- | .33- | na |
| Attention        2&7 speed | R | .24- | .34- | na |
| Block Design (WAIS-R) | R | .25- | .42- | na |
| Trail Making | R/A | .28 | .30 | .22 |
| | G | .23- | na | na |
| visual processing | E | .40 | na | na |
| Purdue Pegboard | E | na | .30 | na |
| Motor-Free visual perception | A | na | na | .36- |
| Quick Test IQ | A | na | na | .31- |
| Raven WAIS estimate | A | na | na | .32- |
| STROOP color names | A | na | na | .40- |
| STROOP color recognition | A | na | na | .40- |
| WAIS Full-Scale IQ | A | na | na | .30- |
| | G | .20 | .27 | .29 |
| WMS Memory Quotient | | na | na | .43- |
| Categories | G | na | na | .30- |
| Symbol-Digit Mod. Written | G | .31 | na | na |

[a]A = Anke, Stanghelle, & Finset  (1997); C = Crépeau & Scherzer (1993); E = Ezrachi, Ben-Yishay, Kay, Diller, & Rattok (1991); R = Ruff, Marshall, Crouch, Klauber, Levin, Barth, Kreutzer, Blunt, Foulkes, Eisenberg,   Jane & Marmarou (1993); G = Girard, Brown, Burnett-Stolnack, Hashimoto, Heir-Wellmer, Perlman & Seigerman (1996)

described as compliance to therapy, participation in therapy, publically accepting problems and limitations, and a willingness to endorse staff recommendations.

The largest study to evaluate indicators for work status following TBI was conducted by Crépeau and Scherzer (1993). Their meta-analysis included French- and English-language articles appearing in electronic databases between 1967 and 1990. Their criteria required that articles report at least one quantitative predictor defined as using a homogeneous concept for both predictor and work variables. The 41 studies meeting these criteria contained 119 predictors and 192 indicators of return-to-work capabilities. Tables 9.5 & 9.6 (Author C) display variables containing correlation coefficients of .30 or greater. Duration of coma is the most studied variable, representing eight studies. Data from neuropsychological testings are conspicuously missing from this analysis. It is unclear why neuropsychological data are not represented unless the authors did not view neuropsychological constructs as homogeneous and excluded them.

TABLE 9. 6
Moderator Variables Correlated with Return-to-Work => |.30|

| Variable | Author[1] | Pearson Correlation Back-to-Work | | |
|---|---|---|---|---|
| | | <= 6 Months | 6-12 Months | 3-8 Years |
| coma length | E | .26- | .36- | na |
| regulation of affect | E | .40 | na | na |
| patient acceptance:MACC | R | .49 | .46 | na |
| staff global assessment | C | na | .35 | na |
| abnormal CT | C | na | .35 | na |
| Uni vs bilateral lesion | C | na | .30 | na |
| GCS first 24 hours | C | na | .35 | na |
| lower activity at 1 month post coma | C | na | .38 | na |
| sluggish vs agitated | C | na | .49 | na |
| PTA duration | C | na | .48 | na |
| aggression | C | na | .33 | na |
| Vocational Rehabilitation | C | na | .51 | na |
| litigation in low severity patients | C | na | .42 | na |
| family support | C | na | .43 | na |
| Mechanism of Injury | G | na | na | .31- |

[1]C=Crépeau & Scherzer (1993); E=Ezrachi, Ben-Yishay, Kay, Diller, & Rattok (1991);R=Ruff, Marshall, Crouch, Klauber, Levin, Barth, Kreutzer, Blunt, Foulkes, Eisenberg, Jane & Marmarou (1993); G=Girard, Brown, Burnett-Stolnack, Hashimoto, Heir-Wellmer, Perlman & Seigerman (1996)

In a separate report, patients admitted to one of three rehabilitation facilities ($n = 241$) received neuropsychological test batteries (an average of 44 days postinjury) with follow-up staggered at one, two, three, and four years post injury for employment evaluations (Boake et al. 1997). Ten neuropsychological measures (viz., GOAT, Token Test, Digit Span, Logical Memory I and II, Rey Auditory Verbal Learning Test, Block Design, Trail Making, Visual Form Discrimination test, and Wisconsin Card Sorting Test) were reported as statically significant predictors of either full-time competitive employment or education in regular classes based on their risk ratios (Ruff, et al., 1993). Critical scores for the tests included 95 for the GOAT and sixteenth percentile for the others. Acker and Davis (1989) have described several measures as predictive of outcome 3.8 years post injury by correlating neuropsychology scores taken during rehabilitation with the Social Status Outcome rating scale (SSO; see Table 9.7). In a separate study by Bayless, Varney, and Roberts (1989), Tinkertoy Test comp-o scores were directly correlated with successful employment ® = .44). Linear regressions linking neuropsychological test scores with successful employment outcomes were calculated for patients within seven years of injury (Brooks, Campsie, Symingron, Beattie, & McKinlay, 1987). Whereas poor coefficients of determination were obtained for Logical Memory and the Paced Auditory Serial Addition Test, stronger indicators were found for moderator variables of age, gender, and the absence of communication deficits. Long-term prognosis for patients who received multi-disciplinary rehabilitation was predicted using linear regression methods for 100 Michigan patients by Putnam & Adams (1992). Their findings revealed statistically significant correlation between prognosis and degree of improvement ($p < .005$, $r = .55$) and neuropsychological functioning ($p < .001$, $R = .42$). Unfortunately, data were not reported for specific neuropsychological tests.

Lezak (1995) cited findings from Gronwall (1977), who reported that the PASAT scores effectively indicate when concussion patients can resume vocational and social activity without experiencing undue stress.

Outpatients have also been compared using serial neuropsychological testing (see Author G Tables 9.6 & 9.7). Girard et al., (1996) evaluated six levels of productivity in three settings – home, school, and work – for 153 patients ages 13-70. In addition to performance on tests of information-processing speed, memory, and simultaneous processing, positive outcomes were related to educational level, absence of substance abuse, level of insurance funding, and mode of injury.

Although researchers have considered a variety of markers in predicting recovery, only recently have interaction and cumulative effects of these markers been considered together. In a pilot study, Martelli, Zasler, & Braith (1998) tested a composite approach to prediction with 28

TBI patients. By considering length of post traumatic amnesia, premorbid neurologic status, premorbid psychiatric status, estimated premorbid IQ, the presence of posttraumatic seizures, marital status, collateral injuries and accident victimization in linear regression analysis, they claimed a coefficient of determination of .51 in predicting posttraumatic vocational status and .69 in predicting disability status.

TABLE 9.7

Neuropsychology Correlates With Social Status Outcome

| Test | SSO Total | |
| --- | --- | --- |
| | _n_ | _r_ |
| Bender Gestalt errors | 086 | .30 |
| Draw A Person credit points | 080 | .25- |
| Motor Free Visual Perception Test | 057 | .44- |
| Quick Test IQ | 090 | .38- |
| Raven Matrices estimated WAIS IQ | 080 | .37- |
| Stroop Reading Color Names | 032 | .49- |
| Stroop Color Recognition | 032 | .36- |
| Stroop Interference raw score | 032 | .33- |
| Trail Making A time in seconds | 096 | .31 |
| Trail Making B time in seconds | 090 | .33 |
| WAIS VIQ | 062 | .28- |
| WAIS PIQ | 053 | .37- |
| WAIS FIQ | 054 | .41- |
| Wechsler Memory Scale MQ | 101 | .48- |
| Wisconsin Card Sort # categories | 022 | .27- |

Olfactory function was correlated with employability by Varney (1988). He looked at three groups of head injury patients who had been cleared for return to work at least two years earlier. From the 164 patients evaluated, 40 claimed total anosmia and 24 claimed partial anosmia. Of the total anosmics, 93% met criteria for vocational disability compared to 54% of the partial anosmia group. Varney viewed anosmia as an indicator of frontal lobe damage because of its proximity to the cribiform plate. For his sample at least half presented normal neurological and neuropsychological findings but were vocationally disabled. Their behavior deficits could only be identified from interviews with relatives.

## Return to Driving

The ability to drive should be discussed more often between the patient and the doctor. The need to drive is obvious in modern society, and some patients drive before they are fit to do so. The legal aspects of driving postinjury are poorly organized, as in most countries there is no obligation to consider the temporary withdrawal of the driving license in case of recuperation from injury or illness. Three methods for evaluating an individual's capacity to drive are in use: road testing, simulator testing, and neuropsychological testing. These methods were evaluated in a single study wherein evaluation of driving in simulators was compared to road driving for 29 "socially well recovered" patients and 29 matched controls (Lundqvist et al.,1997). Concomitant neuropsychological testing revealed that overall cognitive capacity, rather than attentional or perceptual-motor capacity, predicted driving performance with 78% confidence.

### *Road Testing*

The road test typically requires a patient to drive under nonstress conditions where safety factors are optimized. Frequently required functions, such as preparing to drive, driving at intersections, tracking (driving in a lane and changing lanes), speed, traffic observation, maintaining distance, attention to bicyclists and pedestrians, and parking, are usually addressed (Kroj & Pfeiffer, 1973). Road tests of this type require the examiner, usually a government employee, to make gross judgments regarding driving safety. Road tests evaluate the driving and emergency conditions that are most likely to create problems for individuals with brain impairment. The assessment is important because of the risk driving poses to persons and property. Niemann and Bavaria (2000) compared findings from road test with neuropsychological tests of alertness and Trails A and B with 92 inpatients who had sustained one of three categories of head injury. Their findings indicate greater sensitivity, specificity, and positive and negative predictive power for the road test alone when compared with either the neuropsychological measures or a combination of best predictors from road test, neuropsychology, and demographic data.

## Simulator Testing

Unlike road tests, simulators can create a variety of road conditions and emergency situations. An evaluator then uses mathematical models to predict the consequences of a patient's responses. Simulator testing may offer the safest and most complete evaluation of a patient's abilities. However, the availability of simulator testing is limited and the cost of purchasing hardware is often prohibitive to many psychologists. At the time of writing the costs for purchasing a simulator ranged from around $3,500 (Life Science Associates, 2000) to more than $60,000 (Systems Technology, 2000). Also, there is no way to know how accurately computer models predict actual emergency circumstances that could be life threatening. Driving simulators have been cross-referenced on the Internet (*http://www.inrets.fr/ur/sara/Pg_simus_e.html*), although most of the listings address research rather than applied uses.

## Neuropsychological Testing

In *The Neuropsychology of Everyday Life*, Tupper and Cicerone (1990) recommended a "typical" assessment paradigm for operating motor vehicles. In addition to neuropsychological assessment, they identified 9 components of vision and 11 other parameters as essential to the paradigm. Included in other parameters were tests of hearing, reaction time, functional strength, and simulator and full-scale vehicle operation. They also recommended using a multistage decision model having two conditional acceptance nodes.

When all groups of brain injury are considered, the recuperation from TBIs has been studied the most. About 60% of patients with moderate or severe TBI injuries return to driving (Fisk, Schneider, & Novack, 1998). In the state of Washington, inadequate support was found for the belief that individuals who have sustained a brain injury would be at increased risk of motor vehicle crashes. Building on the recommendations of Tupper and Cicerone (1990), several study methods have been developed to assess recuperation from TBI with respect to driving safety (see e.g., Brooke, Questad, Patterson, & Valois, 1992; Galski, Bruno, Ehle, 1993).

Duchek, Junt, Karlene, and Morris (1998) evaluated driving in Alzheimer's patients. They reported predictors of driving performance based on error rate and reaction time during visual search tasks. Unfortunately, their data are insufficient for development of predictive equations.

Perhaps as a consequence of poor prediction from theoretical proposals, several test batteries have been developed for the explicit purpose of testing driving abilities. We briefly describe these batteries and other measures available at the time of writing, noting the efficacy of each when data are available.

***Reaction Times.*** Robert Anderson's (1994) review of neuropsychological assessment of driving skills cautioned against the use of neuropsychological measures for predicting driving fitness. Even though reaction time shows moderately high correlation with driving a slalom course (Stokx & Gillard, 1986; cited in Anderson, 1994) it is unclear if or how driving under controlled conditions relates to road driving. A test battery proposed by Nouri & Lincoln (1993) demonstrated an 81% prediction rate for British stroke victims, but norms were poor and almost half of the patients in older groups failed. Simms & O'Toole (1994) also claimed an 80% specificity in a battery almost no examinee failed. Consequently, McKenna (1998) dismissed both studies, recommending in their stead a battery evaluating shape perception, visual-spatial relationships, and visual attention. She recommended use of the Stroop and Trail-Making tests, but provided no empirical support for their use.

***The Cognitive Behavioral Driver's Inventory.*** This test battery (known as the CBDI) was constructed in order to evaluate important components of driving such as reaction time, vision, and attention (Psychological Software Services, 1990). The inventory contains data from 232 brain-injured patients and 42 controls who were classified by various rehabilitation professionals for driving safety. Test-retest reliability scores ranged from .32 to .83. Pass-fail criteria used for validity measures were based on judgments of therapists compared with judgments of driving instructors. Incorporated into the inventory are scores from Wechsler Adult Intelligence Scale Picture Completion and Digit Symbol, Trails A & B, Brake Pedal Reaction Time, and Left/Right Periometers. Examinees then complete computer testing with a joy stick. The manual provides copious data tables and descriptions of the normative population. Unfortunately, the large number of abbreviations and lack of an index can easily confuse readers who are unfamiliar with the test and the statistical methods reported. Nonetheless, the CBDI contains excellent face validity.

A number of papers have been published in *The Journal of Cognitive Rehabilitation* describing the standardization and construct validity of the CBDI (Antrim & Engum, 1989; Engum, Cron, Hulse,

Pendergrass, & Lambert, 1988; Engum & Lambert, 1990; Engum, Lambert & Scott, 1990; Engum, Lambert, Womac, & Pendergrass, 1988). These authors are commended for including information about the skew of their samples as well as complete descriptions of their normative procedures. The CBDI's General Driving Index shows good discriminant validity for "passing" scores on actual driving tests as well as concordance with "readiness to drive" ratings of treating psychologists. Unfortunately, the authors provided no correlational data that might prove helpful in predicting later performance. Likewise, none of the studies compare ratings with the driving histories of patients following their return to driving. The testing appears time consuming, raises the ecological question of cost-effectiveness above and beyond the driving road test. Dr. Odie Bracy (personal communication October 3, 1999) reported an administration time of about 40 minutes, producing a 4-page computer-generated report that is well received by referring physicians.

***The d2 Test of Attention.***   This test was developed for the German Institute for Safety in Mining, Industry, and Transportation as a test to evaluate driving proficiency (Brickenkamp & Zillmer, 1998). Since its appearance in 1962, the test has been widely used in Europe and includes a number of translations including American English and Brazilian Portugese. Spreen and Strauss (1998) described the test as a measure of sustained attention and visual scanning ability. They reported test-retest reliabilities of .89-.92 and practice effects for 25% for normal subjects but none for brain- damaged subjects. Age, gender, and education effects have been reported but undefined.

***Traffic Psychological Test Battery.***   Computer-aided assessment of driving abilities is available from *Vienna Test System* (Schuhfried, 1995). The Schuhfried company develops traffic psychological tests and this offering  is an integrated testing system that allows evaluators to define, and then administer, a complete test battery. In addition to tests of reaction time, spatial testing, and vigilance tasks that are necessary for safe driving, there is a tachistoscopic traffic test. The tachistoscopic traffic test presents photographs for 1 second then requires the examinee to determine if there were people, cyclists, motor vehicles, traffic signs, or traffic signals in the photograph. Photographs sometimes contain all five stimuli and at other times only one. Norms are published in the software and tests can be administered as a standalone Windows application or through a network server. A printed report of percentile and $T$-scores for correct and incorrect answer entries is available.

At the time of writing the *Vienna Test System* contained 74 tests including many "standards" such as State-Trait, Minnesota Multiphasic Personality Inventory (MMPI), Social Adjustment, Mechanical-Technical Abilities, Corsi Block Tapping, and Alcoholism Selection Procedure. Although some of the tests were available only in German, others offered a choice of French, Spanish, or English. Once all of the tests are available in English, the system will be quite a bargain! If the software package included important validity studies and Web updates, it would be a "must have" system for for assessment psychologists.

The driving section, *Traffic Psychological Test Battery*, provides a variety of normative data that allows comparison with test records of 1,400 susceptible traffic board clients. Table 9.8 lists reliability data for the individual tests. The *determination test* has also been correlated with driving behaviors such as "incorrect slowing down" $r = .45$; "problems staying within a lane," $r = .42$; and "not safeguarding at crossings" $r = .39$. The *taschistoscopic traffic perception test mannheim* has also been correlated (® = .42 and .74 ) with "driving road tests." Specialty norms are also available for commercial drivers (Neuwirth, 1999).

TABLE 9.8
Vienna Test System: Traffic Psychology Test Battery Reliability

| Test | Duration | IC [a] | SH [b] | n |
|------|----------|--------|--------|---|
| Vienna Reaction Test | 06 | .99 | | 849 |
| Cognitrone | 15 | .98 | | 323 |
| Line-Tracking Test | 15 | .96 | | 448 |
| Vienna Determination Test | 06 | .99 | | 849 |
| Tachistoscopic Traffic Perception Test | 10 | .86 | | 303 |
| Corsi-Block-Tapping-Test | 10 | .96 | | 448 |

[a] IC - internal consistency, [b] SH - split-half.

None of the driving assessment instruments currently available systematically evaluate all of the parameters discussed by Tupper and Cicerone (1990). The *Traffic Psychological Test Battery* and the CBDI come closest. Many of the most important concerns raised by Tupper and Cicerone can be addressed in the hour or two required for administration of either the CBDI or the *Traffic Psychological Test Battery*.

**Return to School.**

Historically, many neuropsychologists considered a child's ability to return to school in much the same way they viewed an adult's capacity for return to work. In children, a direct relationship has been found between postinjury intelligence scores and duration of coma (Carney & Gerring, 1990). However, in addition to the issues germane to adult assessment, school reentry must be planned for a child. Additional evaluation considerations for school reentry include adapting the environment, transition from rehabilitation to school, developmental functioning, and teaching variables (Savage & Mishkin, cited in Haak and Livingston, 1997).

Since the passage of the Individuals with Disabilities Education Act[2] in 1975, and its revision[3] in 1990, TBI has become a disability category for students *requiring* special education services in public schools (*Federal Register*, 1992, p. 44802). The Act's revision addresses 14 domains of potential impairment: cognition; language; memory; attention; reasoning; abstract thinking; problem solving; sensory, perceptual, and motor abilities; psychosocial behavior; physical functions; information processing; and speech. Haak and Livingston (1997) described six issues relevant to appropriate educational programming for TBI students: information coordination between schools and medical facilities, assessment, programming, school reentry, family support, and transitions from school to community reintegration. Specific instructional procedures have also been proposed for brain-injured students (Cohen, 1991).

Determining when a child should return to school can be difficult. In addition to considering the readiness of the child, effects on and by family members and school programming can interact with motivation and emotion. Children having good family support and a well-thought-out school placement can become overwhelmed and withdrawn if they prematurely resume a demanding schedule. Likewise, children demonstrating near-complete recovery can falter academically if family or school expectations support poor performance. As with adults, age is an

[2]U.S. Public Law 94-142.
[3]U.S. Public Law 101-476.

important factor of recovery but there is growing evidence suggesting that children who sustain insults in areas of the brain that are "undeveloped" may subsequently fail in the attainment of important developmental milestones (Fletcher-Janzen & Kade, 1997).      Ylvisaker (1986) acknowledges that attention and motor problems are common sequella early in recovery from head injuries. However, motor and attention deficits tend to be transient, whereas more subtle problems in word retrieval, comprehension, verbal organization, verbal learning, and conversation skills remain.

Children recuperate more rapidly than adults and most children are able to return to school. In one series, cognitive impairments were found in 42% of child patients, but only 10% were in receipt of disablement allowances (van der Sluis, Kingma, Eisma, & ten Duis, 1997). Children evaluated between four and five years following severe TBI demonstrated reduced rates of learning new information, which were most apparent with verbal material. Others report that no significant recognition differences were observed between injury groups and matched controls as measured by the Wide Range Assessment of Memory (Nelson, Kelly & Stringer, 1998).

The validity of standardized testing with school children has been questioned by Ammerman and Campo (1998), because structured test settings providing one-to-one supervision in a distraction-free environment rarely reflect conditions of daily living for school-age children. What is more, many of the tests available to neuropsychologists were developed to evaluate adult abilities and then modified. Even those with the best norms and most thorough research base (Halstead - Reitan series) can muster only "satisfactory" reliability. Many of the tests are cited as "problematic." Ammerman and Campo acknowledged that most neuropsychological assessment procedures, especially the Reitan tests, were developed to localize head injury; but, this function has been replaced by other more accurate measurements and is of little importance in evaluating most severely injured children.

Adults do not have to return to work. But, most children must return to school. Sattler (1998) advised using a three-step process in the return of children to a school environment. First, consider the child's deficits and the effects their impairments in cognition may have on the learning experience. Second, evaluate the classrooms recommending environmental modifications that will facilitate the child's learning. Third, work with teachers to modify interactions and curricula. Children are highly susceptible to the interaction of brain damage and environmental factors. Memory and cognitive function were shown as correlated with many factors among 29 consecutive acute postinjury admissions to a university hospital (Max et al., 1999). Bivariate correlations (see Table 9.9) were significant for the variables studied.

In children 6-12 years of age no significant change was observed in test scores taken between 6 and 12 months postinjury for 42 severe and 52 moderate TBI patients (Taylor, Wade, Yeates, Drotar & Klein, 1999). At six months the authors reported multiple predictive measures (see Table 9.10), including modest associations with family status. The repeated measures evaluation began when children performed at 2 *SD*s (standard deviations) below their age mean on the Children's Orientation and Amnesia Test (COAT). Consequently, both time since injury and type of injury constitute uncontrolled error.

With the numbers of students sustaining head injuries increasing (Carney & Gerring, 1990) and the criteria for meeting educational needs expanding, a need for specialized and multidisciplinary evaluation of students with TBI has been recognized (Carney, 1991). Issues involving return to and reintegration into school are so complex, that consultation with a pediatric neuropsychologist should be made for each child. At the time of writing, the best evidence of qualifications as a pediatric neuropsychologist is board certification by the American Board of Pediatric Neuropsychology.

**Social Integration**

Restrictions in the ability to take care of oneself or in getting around are considered to be most debilitating and often render the person dependent on someone else for meeting the requirements of everyday living. Restrictions in physical activities, on the other hand, although not as limiting, have been shown to affect the amount and type of work one can perform at or outside the home.

Patients with multiple injuries are often discharged from hospitals to other types of institutions, 60% as geriatric patients and 40% in other patient groups (Zietlow, Capizzi, Bannon, & Farnell, 1994). This practice reflects the long time required for these people to be able to return to normal daily activities at home. Generally, it is good clinical practice to divide the burden between the acute care hospital and the rehabilitation center.

Usually even after most serious injuries, if the patient survives there is very little need for permanent help in ADL (activities of daily In the long run, most patients gain social independence and are able to return to work or at least are capable of independent living. The percentage of the permanently institutionalized lies around 2% (Rhodes, Aronson, Moerkirk, & Petrash, 1988). This is despite the fact that more than 80% have some prevailing disabilities even after 3 years (Seekamp et. al., 1996).

TABLE 9.10
Correlations Between COAT Stability
and 6 months Follow-Up

| Measure | Family Status $R^2$ | Total $R^2$ |
|---|---|---|
| VIQ | .02 | .44[b] |
| PIQ | .02 | .27[b] |
| TONI-2 | .02 | .29[b] |
| BNT | .01 | .43[b] |
| COWA | .03 | .16[b] |
| Token Test, Part V | .03 | .16[b] |
| CELF-R Sentence Structure | .02 | .15[a] |
| CELF-R Recalling Sentences | .00 | .16[a] |
| VMI | .01 | .22[b] |
| Grooved Pegboard Test | .08[b] | .21[b] |
| CVLT Total Words 1-5 | .03 | .29[b] |
| CPT-3  Respond Condition | .01 | .21[b] |
| CPT-3 Inhibit Condition | .02 | .09[a] |
| Underlining Test | .06 | .18[b] |
| Contingency Naming Test, time | .05 | .11[a] |
| Contingency Naming Test, errors | .02 | .33[b] |
| WJ Reading Cluster | .01 | .37[b] |
| WJ Writing Cluster | .00 | .44[b] |
| WJ Math Cluster | .00 | .37[b] |
| TRF School Performance | .01 | .59[b] |
| CDC Behavior Problems | .06[b] | .65[b] |
| TRF Behavior Problems | .01 | .38[b] |
| CBC Total Competence | .07[b] | .56[b] |
| WM Teacher-Related Social | .02 | .39[b] |
| WM Peer-Related Social | .01 | .30[b] |
| VABS | .06[b] | .63[b] |

[a] $p < .05$.        [b] $p < .01$.living) activities (Anke et al., 1997).

Acker's (1982) summary of the Head Injury Rehabilitation Project provided correlations between neuropsychological test scores and three categories of independent living: employment, community skills, and kitchen skills. Occupational therapists rated each catetory at six and twelve months following injury (see Table 9.11). For measures of community and kitchen skills, the WAIS PIQ is clearly the superior predictor at one year postinjury, as it is for employability.  Social status outcome (SSO; Mackworth, Mackworth, & Cope, 1982) was best predicted by a cognitive-visual battery, and to a lesser degree by components of the battery as described in Table 9.12.

TABLE 9.11

Comparisons between test measures and
occupational therapy independence ratings

| Psychological Test | *Employment* | | *Community* | | *Kitchen* | |
|---|---|---|---|---|---|---|
| | *6 mo* | *12 mo* | *6 mo* | *12 mo* | *6 mo* | *12 mo* |
| WAIS VIQ | .73 | .66 | .77 | .81 | .85 | .73 |
| WAIS PIQ | .88 | .87 | .63 | .87 | .74 | .92 |
| Trails A & B | .67 | .65 | .45 | .60 | .52 | .56 |
| Wechsler MQ | .65 | .64 | .63 | .73 | .71 | .63 |
| MFVPT[a] | .64 | .58 | .67 | .71 | .77 | .61 |

[a] Motor Free Visual Perception Test

***Social Status Outcome.***  Cope (cited in Acker & Davis, 1989) reported on a survey used in a 1977-1981 project that was developed to assess functioning levels of head-injured people in the community.  The instrument rated categories of living situations and functional level using four point rankings (0-3) for each category (see Table 9.13). M. D. Acker (personal communication, July 6, 1999) notes that the SSO is an "impairment" measure and as such produces higher scores for dysfunction Consequently, it produces higher positive correlations with other types of "impairment" ratings and negative scores when patients depend less on others. Pearson correlations between the SSO and neuropsychological tests appear in Table 9.14.

TABLE 9.12
*Social Status Outcome Correlated With Functional Tasks*

| Functional Task | R |
| --- | --- |
| Object Naming Time | .73 |
| Reading Time / 100 words | .67 |
| Sequence Memory Pictures | .65 |
| Motor Weakness | .71 |
| Word Finding / minute | .70 |
| Overall | .80 |

Moderator variables including age of injury, age at testing, age at follow-up, and education were meager predictors of social outcome (-.02 to -.12) in contrast to demonstrations by others (Lamport-Hughes, 1995; MacKenzie et al., 1988; Sherer, Bergloff, High, Levin, & Oden , 1996) that moderator variables can be as predictive of outcome as neuropsychological test scores.

Use of other instruments such as the Injury Impairment Scale (IIS),Functional Capacity Index (FBI), Rancho los Amigos Scale, and the Vineland Adaptive Behavior Scales (VABS) have been reported in studies evaluating capacity for independent living. However, predictive values have not been established for this purpose to date.

## DISABILITY DETERMINATION

In ancient times, recovery meant you had to survive the initial blood loss and the septic phase, and then return to your previous occupation or combat position. Modern recovery can be assessed in general terms of return to driving, return to school, return to work, and capacity for independent living. Another division would be the return to ADL, to nonwork activities, and to work. Disability was defined by the World Health Organization (WHO, 1980) as "any restriction or lack of ability to perform an activity in a manner or within the range considered normal for a human being (p. 174)." After the analysis of single impairments, an overall level of functional disability can be estimated. In Finland a national list of functional impairments updated by the Ministry of Health is used. From this list one can obtain the residual functional impairment in percentage values. The description begins with individual injuries, where the assessment is most accurate. If that list is not applicable, then a description of functional impairment in more general terms and larger body areas is used. The American Medical Association (AMA)

TABLE 9.13
*Social Status Outcome Ratings*

*Living situation:*

    0 = independent living
    1 = needs supervision, but not physical assistance
    2 = requires physical assistance or nursing care
    3 = needs acute care setting.

*Functional level:*

    0 = competitively employed or engaged in other independent avocational activity
    1 = in a special school program
    2 = requires a long-term care program
    3 = nonparticipating in an active program

provides guides to the evaluation of impairment in the United States, where percentage impairment of the whole person is used for establishing disability. A portion of the impairment ratings appear in Table 9.15 (American Medical Association, 1993).

In general, a disability can be considered permanent if it persists for two years after the trauma. Variations occur depending on the type of injury and the therapeutic responses of the patient. A number of rating instruments have been developed to aid in quantifying disability independent of the AMA ratings. The most widely cited are summarized as follows.

TABLE 9.14
Social Status Outcome Concordance $\geq |.30|$
With Neuropsychological Test Data.

| Test | n | r |
|------|---|---|
| Bender Gestalt errors | 86 | .40 |
| Motor Free Visual Perception Test | 57 | .40- |
| Quick Test IQ | 90 | .34- |
| Raven Matrices estimated IQ | 80 | .34- |
| Stroop Color Names | 32 | .33- |
| Trails   Time    A | 96 | .40 |
|                       B | 90 | .30 |
| WAIS   *PIQ* | 53 | .31- |
|              *FSIQ* | 54 | .39- |
| Wechsler Memory Scale MQ | 101 | .37- |
| Wisconsin Card Sort[a] | 22 | .46- |

[a]Number of categories.

***Injury Impairment Scale.***    The developers of the Injury Impairment Scale (IIS) differentiate between impairment and disability. Impairment, following the WHO model refers to "the loss of function or abnormal function of an organ, tissue, or organ system resulting after healing has occurred" (Champion, Sacco, Copes, 1991, p. 627). Disability is the effect or consequences of an impairment. Disability and impairment have been assessed with the multiple impairments on the whole person that restricts an individual from performing at or near the preinjury capability. Age, education, family and community support, personal financial resources, the availability of rehabilitation programs, and pre-existing conditions are determinants of disability relative to impairment. The IIS provides a basis for comparing reported disability for work or school, household activities, and ADLs during the first 18 months after injury (Waller, Skelly, & Davis, 1995). The IIS has seven ordinal levels: 0 = Normal function, no impairment; 1 = Impairment detectable, but does not limit normal function; 2 = Impairment level compatible with most, but not

TABLE 9.15
Examples of Disability Impairment Ratings
From the American Medical Association

| Impairment | Impairment Percentage | |
|---|---|---|
| | Visual Field | Whole Person |
| *Visual field loss* | | |
| Dense congruous, complete, homonymous, hemianopia, or bitemporal hemianopia. | 66 | 62 |
| Dense, congruous, complete, superior quadrantanopia. | 25 | 24 |
| Dense, congruous, complete, inferior quandrantanopia. | 30 | 28 |
| *Mental status impairments* | | |
| Impairment exists, but ability remainsto perform satisfactorily most activities of daily living. | | 1 - 14 |
| Impairment requires direction and supervision of daily living activities. | | 15 - 29 |
| Impairment requires directed care under continued supervision and confinement in home or other facility. | | 30 - 49 |
| Individual is unable without supervision to care for self and be safe in any situation. | | 50 - 70 |

all, normal function; 3 = Impairment level compatible with some normal function; 4 = Impairment level significantly impedes some normal functions; 5 = Impairment level precludes most useful function; 6 = Impairment level precludes any useful function. It has not been validated for pelvic or lower limb fractures (Massoud &Wallace, 1996).

*Disability Rating Scale.* The Disability Rating Scale (DRS) was developed for the ambitious task of establishing one rating instrument capable of quantitatively assessing disability severity from coma to recovery. It contains four categories, each with two items assessing arousal, self-care, physical dependence, and psychosocial adaptability (Rappaport, Hall, Hopkins, Belleza, & Cope, 1982). It is commonly used as the benchmark against which other disability ratings are compared (Cifu et al., 1996; Gouvier, Blanton, LaPorte, & Nepomuceno, 1987; Torenbeek, van der Heijden, de Witte & Bakx, 1998). Ditunno (1992) described the DRS as having greater reliability than the GOS, yet the ability of the DRS to predict discharge status ® = .40) has been modest (Eliason & Topp, 1984).

*Rand SF36.* The Rand Short Form (Rand SF) is a widely used instrument that measures self-reported health status in a number of domains, including general health, mental health, and physical function. The SF36 subscales are standardized to a 100-point scale, with higher scores representing better function. A low score on the general health scale indicates that the patient has the perception of poor personal health and the belief that it is likely to get worse. On the mental health scale, a low score measures feelings of nervousness and depression. The physical functioning scale evaluates limitations in performance of physical activities. Each of the subscales is composed of separate questions, and their scores are not mathematically linked. Outcome SF36 mental health was related to baseline mental health, 12-month PTSD and BDI depression scores, and increased drug and alcohol use (Michaels et al., 2000).

## DISCUSSION

Few scoring systems have focused on function, which is the true measure of trauma morbidity. A scoring scale useful in the trauma setting as a true measure of morbidity needs to address all areas of function, such as cognition, communication, mobility, self-care, and so forth (Emhoff et al., 1991). Anderson's (1994) brief review of return to academic and vocational function implies that each case is so unique that it is difficult to predict a person's return to work from test scores alone. Yet few systematic attempts at improving predictions by combining test scores with moderator variables exist. Those available offer inadequate information for replication or use in clinical practice. All of the studies located for review in this chapter are retrospective and lack integrated use of single-subject and group research designs. In combination, extant studies suggest that neuropsychological data have limited predictive validity for functional outcome with several exceptions. However, studies intimate that highly accurate predictive models are possible.

## High Predictive Validity

The prediction of mortality from screening instruments available in acute care is highly accurate as early as one day postinjury. The ability to predict relative independence from intelligence testing is also high. Prediction of driving abilities is adequate, when measures are taken postrecovery. Data suggest that gains in the abilities of adults are largely realized during the first year postinjury and gains for children maximize in about 6 months.

## Poor Predictive Validity

The prediction of functional outcome (i.e., return to work or school, etc.) from acute-care screening instruments is poor and contradictory. The ability of outcome forecasting from neuropsychological test data is about chance and roughly comparable to findings from evoked potentials or the duration of impaired consciousness taken early in the course of recovery. Simple tests (i.e., Bender Gestalt errors) appear almost as effective as test batteries in predicting SSO. Moderator variables such as age, gender, and family history may be as predictive of outcome as entire neuropsychological test batteries. Given these findings, it is difficult to support the efficacy of extensive neuropsychological batteries for the prediction of functional outcome following TBI.

## Barriers to the Efficacy of Findings

Researchers appear more interested in providing support for particular tests, or specific points of view, than in developing meaningful predictive instruments. Studies often "mine" hospital data by corralling a group of patients and "giving every test available" in hopes of "finding a diamond." Funding practices likely encourage neuroscience researchers in this regard. For the most part, research designs and data analysis methods appear "frozen" in models developed half a century ago. There is almost no use of the nonlinear, Bayesian, or neural network models that have proven so beneficial to computer and industrial sciences. This seems particularly unfortunate, given the plethora of data available that appear amenable to these methods. Perhaps researchers have become so specialized that they have few opportunities for interspecialization dialogue.

The language of head injuries appears problematic as well. Definitions and terms used in TBI research lack precision and clarity. Perhaps this difficulty is most evident in return-to-work research. Some studies base predictions on subjective classifications (viz., mild, moderate, or severe) and others use psychometric tests. Patients evaluated by psychometric tests must have a minimum level of ability. Therefore, psychometric scores are *always* skewed toward the highest functioning inpatients. What is more, the skew is truncated because the vast majority of inpatient admissions are rationed by health care administrators to patients with either very serious head injuries or multiple traumas. Outpatient research involving mild TBI most often studies malingering rather than functional abilities. Different populations are often described using similar terms. For example, "brain damage" rehabilitation patients are quite different from "brain damage" patients who require no rehabilitation. Yet, the patient who does not qualify for inpatient rehabilitation may experience a greater sense of loss in cognitive abilities, and in fact may have a more "damaged brain" than the inpatient. Inpatients are much more likely to sustain multiple traumas than patients experiencing only closed-head injuries. Within rehabilitation "brain damage" groups, data rarely discriminate between the locus of the injury or the degree of physiologic damage; and, sample sizes are usually to small for "averaging effects" to "smooth out" error variance. Studies of "war veterans" are likely contaminated by the secondary gain afforded from their disability or veteran status. Many conscientious and dedicated researchers spanning numerous professional disciplines have collaborated on head trauma research. Consequently, a national clearinghouse has been established to aid in the pooling and sharing of data between member groups. Unfortunately, reliance on established research data forces retrospective studies.

## Recommendations

Four changes in the national approach to head injury research are indicated. First, we need prospective studies that obtain support from police, emergency medical teams, community hospitals, and the private health care sector. This support would facilitate early identification of patients with milder head injuries who very rarely participate in rehabilitation or data-sharing programs. These data should be integrated into extant databases and the patients made available for prospective, longitudinal research. Second, research protocols should be developed that include data collections suitable for both single-subject and group comparisons of patients. There is a serious scarcity of single-subject research. And, if each patient is unique (as has been suggested), then the group design and analysis models that permeate the literature will offer little information useful for predicting individual cases (as is the current status). Third, a broader range of analysis tools should be routinely incorporated into research designs. The thousands of hours devoted to data analysis using linear modeling have produced disappointing and often contradictory findings. Given the markedly abnormal characteristics of these patients, perhaps it is time to look for predictive models that are better matched to the data and the clinical imperatives of patients. Fourth, specific psychometric tests and measures need to be selected for these patients that are independent of the ongoing revisions common in other areas of psychometrics. Measures should be culture-free, bound to neurologic processes, and appropriate for administration within a wide variety of environmental conditions. Incorporation of multiple analysis tools, such as the Bayesian model presented in Appendix B, should be included in the predictive model.

## REFERENCES

Acker, M. D., & Davis, J. R. (1989). Psychology test scores associated with late outcome in head injury. *Neuropsychology, 3,* 1-10.

Acker, M. D. (Ed.). (1982). *Head Injury Rehabilitation Project: Final report.* San Jose, CA: Santa Clara Valley Medical Center.

Aguinis, H., Stone, R., & Eugene, F. (1997). Methodological artifacts in moderated multiple regression and their effects on statistical power. *Journal of Applied Psychology, 82*(1), 192-206.

Alcott, D., Dixon, K., & Swann, R. (1997). The reliability of items of the Functional Assessment Measure (FAM): Differences in abstractness between FAM items. *Disability Rehabilitation, 19*(9), 355-358.

American Medical Association. (1993). *Guides to the evaluation of permanent impairment.* (4th ed.). Washington, DC: Author.

Ammerman, R. T. & Campo, J. V. (Eds.). (1998). *Handbook of pediatric psychology and psychiatry* (Vol. 2). Boston: Allyn & Bacon.

Anderson, R. M. (1994). *Practitioner's guide to clinical neuropsychology.* New York: Plenum.

Anke, A. G., Stanghelle J., & Finset, A. (1997). Long-term prevalence of impairments and disabilities after multiple trauma. *Journal of Trauma, 42,* 54-61.

Antrim, J. M. & Engum, E. S. (1989). The driving dilemma and the law: Patients' striving for independence vs. public safety. *Journal of Cognitive Rehabilitation, 7*(2), 16-19.

Association for the Advancement of Automotive Medicine. (1990). *The Abbreviated Injury Scale.* Des Plaines, IL: Author.

Baker, S. P., O'Neill, B., Haddon, W., & Long, W. B. (1974). The Injury Severity Score: A method for describing patients with multiple injuries and evaluating emergency care. *Journal of Trauma, 14*, 187-196.

Bayless, J. D., Varney, N. R., & Roberts, R. J. (1989). Tinker Toy Test performance and vocational outcome in patients with closed head injuries. *Journal of Experimental Neuropsychology, 11*, 913-917.

Beal, S. L., & Oreskovich, M. R. (1985). Long-term disability associated with flail chest injury. *American journal of Surgery, 150*(3), 324-326.

Binder, L. (1995, November). *Assessment of functional problems* [in neuropsychology]. Paper presented at the meeting of the National Academy of Neuropsychology, San Francisco, CA.

Boake, C., Millis, S. R., High., W. M., Delmonico R., Kreutzer, J. S., Rosenthal, M., Sherer, M., & Ivanhoe, C. (1997). Using early neuropsychological testing to predict long-term productivity outcome from traumatic brain injury. *Journal of the International Neuropsychological Society, 3*(12), 74-75.

Boyd C. R., Tolson, M. A., & Copes, W. S. (1987). Evaluating trauma care: The TRISS method. Trauma Score and the Injury Severity Score. *Journal of Trauma 27*, 370-378.

Boyer, M. G., & Edwards, P. (1991). Outcome 1 to 3 years after severe brain injury in children and adolescents. *Injury, 22*, 315-320.

Bracken, M. B. (1998). Pharmacologic treatment of acute spinal cord injury (Cochrane Review). In *The Cochrane Library, 3*,[CD-ROM]. Oxford, England: Update Software.

Bracken, M. B., Shepard, M. J., & Collins, W. F. (1990). A randomized, controlled trial of methylprednisolone or naloxone in the treatment of acute spinal cord injury. *New England Journal of Medicine, 322*, 1405-1411.

Braithwaite, I. J., Boot, D. A., Patterson, M., & Robinson, A. (1998). Disability after severe injury: Five year follow up of a large cohort. *Injury, 29*, 55-59.

Brenneman, F. D., Boulanger, B. R., McLellan, B. A., & Redelmeier, D. A. (1998). Measuring injury severity: Time for a change? *Journal of Trauma, 44*(4), 580-582.

Brickenkamp, R., & Zillmer, E. (1998). *D2 Test of Attention.* Seattle: Hogrefe & Huber.

Brooke, M. M., Questad, K. A., Patterson, D. R., & Valois, T. A. (1992). Driving evaluation after traumatic brain injury. *American Journal of Physical Medicine and Rehabilitation, 71*, 177-182.

Brooks, N., Campsie, L., Symington, C., Beattie, A., & McKinlay, W. (1987). Return to work within the first seven years of severe head injury. *Brain Injury, 1*, 5-19.

Buechler, C. M., Blostein, P. A., Koestner, A., Hurt, K., Schaars, M., & Mckernan, J. (1998). Variation among trauma centers' calculation of Glasgow Coma Scale score: results of a national survey. *Journal of Trauma, 45*(3), 429-432.

Carney, J. (1991, June). *Educational assessment of students with traumatic brain injury.* Unpublished paper presented at a Seminar on education and rehabilitation of children with acquired brain injury. Baltimore: Johns Hopkins University.

Carney, J., & Gerring, J. (1990). Return to school following severe closed head injury: A critical phase in pediatric rehabilitation. *Pediatrician, 17*, 222-229.

Champion, H. R., Copes, W. S., Sacco, W. J., Frey, C. F., Holcroft, J. W., Hoyt, D. B., & Weiglt, J. A. (1996). Improved predictions from a severity characterization of trauma (ASCOT) over Trauma and Injury Severity Score (TRISS): The result of an independent evaluation. *Journal of Trauma, 40*, 42-49.

Champion, H. R., Sacco, W. J., & Copes, W. S. (1991). Trauma scoring. In E. E. Moore, K. L., Mattox, & D. V. Feliciano (eds). *Trauma* (2nd ed., pp. 47-65). Norwalk, CT: Appleton & Lange.

Champion, H. R., Sacco, W. J., Copes, W. S., Gann, D. S., Gennarelli, T. A., & Flanagan, M. E. (1989). A revision of the trauma score. *Journal of Trauma-Injury and Critical Care, 29*(5), 623-629.

Cheadle, W. G., Wilson, M., Hersman, M. J., Bergamini, D., Richardson, J. D., & Polk, H. C. (1989). Comparison of trauma assessment scores and their use in prediction of infection and death. *Annals of Surgery, 209*(5), 541-545.

Cifu, D. X., Kreutzer, J. S., Marwitz, J. H., Rosenthal, M., Englander, J., & High, W. (1996). Functional outcomes of older adults with traumatic brain injury: A prospective multicenter analysis. *Archives of Physical Medicine Rehabilitation, 77*(9), 883-888.

Clifton, G. L., Kreutzer, J. S., Choi, S. C., Devany, C. W., Eisenberg, H. M., Foulkes, M. A., Jane, J. A., Marmarou, A., & Marshall, L. F. (1993). Relationship between Glasgow Outcome Scale and neuropsychological measures after brain injury. *Neurosurgery, 33*(1), 34-38.

Cohen, S. B. (1991). Adapting educational programs for students with head injuries. *Journal of Head Trauma Rehabilitation, 6*(1), 56-63.

Crépeau, F. & Scherzer, P. (1993). Predictors and indicators of work status after traumatic brain injury: A meta-analysis. *Neuropsychological Rehabilitation, 3*(1), 5-35.

Demetriades, D., Chan, L. S., & Velmahos, G. (1998). TRISS methodology in trauma: The need for alternatives. *British Journal of Surgery, 85*, 379-384.

Deyo, R. A. (2000). Pain and public policy [Editorial comment]. *New England Journal of Medicine, 342*(16), 1211-1213.

Ditunno, J. F., Jr. (1992). Functional assessment measures in CNS trauma. *Journal of Neurotrauma, 9*(1), 301-305.

Dombovy, M. S., Drew-Cates, J., & Serdans, R. (1998). Recovery and rehabilitation following subarachnoid hemorrhage: Part II. Long-term follow-up. *Brain Injury, 12*(10), 887-894.

Duchek, J. M., Junt, L. B., Karlene, B. B., & Morris, J. C. (1998). Attention and driving performance in Alzheimer's disease. *Journal of Gerontology, 53B*(2), 130-141.

Eliason, M. R., & Topp, B. W. (1984). Predictive validity of Rappaport's Disability Rating Scale in subjects with acute brain dysfunction. *Physical Therapy, 64*(9), 1357-1360.

Emhoff, T. A., McCarthy, M., & Cushman, M. (1991). Functional scoring of multi-trauma patients: who ends up where? *Journal of Trauma, 31,*1227-1232.

Engum, E. S., Cron, L., Hulse, C. K., Pendergrass, T. M., & Lambert, W. (1988). Cognitive Behavioral Driver's Inventory. *Cognitive Rehabilitation, 6*, 34-50.

Engum, E. S., Lambert, E. W. (1990). Restandardization of the Cognitive Behavioral Driver's Inventory. *Cognitive Rehabilitation, 8*, 20-27.

Engum, E. S., Lambert, E. W., & Scott, K. (1990). Criterion-related validity of the Cognitive Behavioral Driver's Inventory: Brain-injured patients versus normal controls. *Cognitive Rehabilitation, 8*, 20-26.

Engum, E. S., Lambert, E. W., Womac, J., & Pendergrass, T. (1988). Norms and decision making rules for the Cognitive Behavioral Driver's Inventory. *Cognitive Rehabilitation, 6*, 12-18.

Ezrachi, O., Ben-Yishay, Y., Kay, T., Diller L., & Rattok, J. (1991). Predicting employment in traumatic brain injury following neuropsychological rehabilitation. *Journal of Head Trauma, 6*(3), 71-84.

Faust, D. (1991). Forensic neuropsychology: The art of practicing a science that does not yet exist. *Neuropsychology Review, 2*(3), 205-231.

Fisk, G. D., Schneider, J., & Novack, T. A. (1998). Driving following traumatic brain injury: prevalence, exposure, advice and evaluations. *Brain Injury, 12*, 683-695.

Fletcher-Janzen, E., & Kade, H. D. (1997). Pediatric brain injury rehabilitation in a neurodevelopmental milieu. In C. R. Reynolds & E. Fletcher-Janzen (Eds.), *Handbook of clinical child neuropsychology* (pp. 452-481). New York: Plenum.

Frutiger, A., Ryf, C. H., Bilat, C. H., Rosso, R., Furrer, M., Cantieni, R., Rüedi T., & Lautenegger, J. (1991). A five years' follow-up of severely injured ICU patients. *Journal of Trauma, 3*, 1216-1225.

Galski, T., Bruno, R. L., & Ehle, H. T. (1993). Prediction of behind-the-wheel driving performance in patients with cerebral brain damage: a discriminant function analysis. *American Journal of Occupational Therapy, 47*, 391-396.

Gill, M., Cohen, M., Korn, C., & Groswasser, Z. (1991). Vocational outcome of aphasic patients following severe traumatic brain injury. *Brain Injury, 10*(1), 39-45.

Girard, D., Brown, J., Burnett-Stolnak, M., Hashimoto, N., Heir-Wellmer, S., Perlman, O. Z., & Seigerman, C. (1996). The relationship of neuropsychological status and productive outcomes following traumatic brain injury. *Brain Injury, 10*(9), 663-676.

Gouvier, W. D., Blanton, P. D., LaPorte, K. K., & Nepomuceno, C. (1987). Reliability and validity of the Disability Rating Scale and the Levels of Cognitive Functioning Scale in monitoring recovery from severe head injury. *Archives of Physical Medicine Rehabilitation, 68*(2), 94-97.

Gronwall, D. M. A. (1977). Paced Auditory Serial-Addition Task: A measure of recovery from concussion. *Perceptual and Motor Skills, 44*, 367-373.

Haak, R. A., & Livingston, R. B. (1997). Treating traumatic brain injury in the school: Mandates and methods. In C. R. Reynolds & E. Fletcher-Janzen (Eds.), *Handbook of clinical child neuropsychology* (pp. 482-505). New York: Plenum.

Hall, K. M., Mann, N., High, W. M., Wright, J., Kreutzer, J. S., & Wood, D. (1996). Functional measures after traumatic brain injury: Ceiling effects of FIM, FIM+FAM, DRS, and CIQ. *Journal of Head Trauma Rehabilitation, 11*(5), 27-39.

Hannan, E. L., Farrell, L. S., & Cayten, G. C. (1997). Predicting survival of victims of motor vehicle crashes in New York State. *Injury, 28*(9-10), 607-615.

Hetherigton, H., Earlam, R. J., & Kirk, C. J. (1995). The disability status of injured patients measured by the functional independence measure (FIM) and their use of rehabilitation services. *Injury, 26*, 97-101.

Jagger, J., Fife, D., Vernberg, K., & Jane, J. A. (1984). Effect of alcohol intoxication on the diagnosis and apparent severity of brain injury. *Neurosurgery, 15*, 303-306.

Janjua, K. J., Sugrue, M., Deane, S. A. (1998). Prospective evaluation of early missed injuries and the role of tertiary trauma survey. *Journal of Trauma, 44*, 1000-1007.

Janke, M. K., & Eberhard, J. W. (1998). Assessing medically impaired older drivers in a licensing agency setting. *Accident Analysis & Prevention, 30*(3), 347-361.

Jennett, B., Snoek, J., Bond, M. R., & Brooks, N. (1981). Disability after severe head injury: Observations on the use of the Glasgow Outcome Scale. *Journal of Neurology, 4*, 285-293.

Johnstone, B., Pinkowski, M., Farmer, J., & Hagglund, K. J. (1995). Neurobehavioral deficits, adolescent traumatic brain injury, and transition to college. *Journal of Clinical Psychology in Medical Settings, 1*(4), 375-386.

Kalechstein, A. D., van Gorp, W. G., & Rappoport, L. J. (1998). Variability in clinical classification of raw test scores across normative data sets. *Clinical Neuropsychologist, 12*(3), 339-347.

Kivioja, A. H., Myllynen, P. J., & Rokkanen, P. U. (1990). Is the treatment of the most severe multiply injured patients worth the effort? A follow-up examination 5 to 20 years after severe multiple injury. *Journal of Trauma, 30*, 480-483.

Kolb, B. & Whishaw, I. Q. (1990). *Fundamentals of human neuropsychology (3rd ed.). New York: Freeman.*

Kroj, G., & Pfeiffer, G. (1973). Der Köiner Fahrverhaltens-Test (K-F-V-T). Erfahrungen mit einer Fahrprobe im Rahmen der verkehrspsychologischen Eigunugsbegutachtung. Schriftenreihe Faktor mensch im Verkehr . [The Köiner traffic behavioral test (KFVT). Experiences from a test in traffic psychology. Factors describing people in traffic. Frankfurt, Germany: Tetzlaff-Verlag.

Lambert, E. W., & Engum, E. S. (1990). The Cognitive Behavioral Driver's Inventory: Item scatter and organic brain damage. *Cognitive Rehabilitation, 8*, 34-43.

Lamport-Hughes, N. (1995). Learning potential and other predictors of cognitive rehabilitation. *Journal of Cognitive Rehabilitation, 13*(4), 16-21.

Levin, H. S., O'Donnell, V. M., & Grossman, R. G. (1979). The Galveston Orientation and Amnesia Test. A practical scale to assess cognition after head injury. *Journal of Nervous and Mental Disease, 167*, 675-684.

Lezak, M. D. (1995), *Neuropsychological assessment* (3rd ed.). New York: Oxford University Press.

Life Science Associates. (2000). *Elemental Driving Simulator. Http://lifesciassoc.home.pipeline.com.* [Computer software, hardware, documentation and seminar package].

Little, A. J., Templer, D. I., Persel, G. S., & Ashley, M. J. (1996). Feasibility of the neuropsychological spectrum in prediction of outcome following head injury. *Journal of Clinical Psychology, 52*(4), 455-460

Lundqvist, A., Alinder, J., Alm, H., Gerdle, B., Levander, S. & Roennberg, J. (1997). Neuropsychological aspects of driving after brain lesion: Simulator study and on-road driving. *Applied Neuropsychology, 4*(4), 220-230.

MacKenzie, E. J., Burgess, A. R., & McAndrew, M. P. (1993). Patient-oriented functional outcome after unilateral lower extremity fracture. *Journal of Orthopedic Trauma, 7*, 393-401.

MacKenzie, E. J., Siegel, J. H., & Shapiro, S. (1988). Functional recovery and medical costs of trauma: Analysis by type and severity of injury. *Journal of Trauma, 28*, 281-297.

Mackworth, N., Mackworth, J., & Cope, D. N. (1982). Discipline report: Cognitive-visual. In M. D. Acker (Ed.). *Head Injury Rehabilitation Project: Final Report.* (Vol. 2, pp. 56-84). San Jose, CA: Santa Clara Valley Medical Center.

Martelli, M. F., Zasler, N. D., & Braith, J. A. (1998). Predicting outcome following rraumatic brain injury (TBI): Utility of a composite prognostic indicator checklist. *Archives of Clinical Neuropsychology, 12*(4), 362-366.

Massoud, S. N. & Wallace. W. A. (1996). The injury impairment scale in pelvic and lower limb fractures sustained in road traffic accidents. *Injury, 27*, 107-110.

Max, J. E., Roberts, M. A., Koele, S. L., Lindgren, S. D., Robin, D. A., Arndt, S., Smith, W. L., Jr., & Sato, Y. (1999). Cognitive outcome in children and adolescents following severe traumatic brain injury: Influence of psychosocial, psychiatric, and injury-related variables. *Journal of the International Neuropsychological Society, 5*, 58-68.

McKenna, P. (1998). Fitness to drive: A neuropsychological perspective. *Journal of Mental Health, 7*(1), 9-18.

McPherson, K. M., Pentland, B., Cudmore, S. F., & Prescott, R. J. (1996). An inter-rater reliability study of the Functional Assessment Measure (FIM+FAM). *Disability Rehabilitaion, 18*(7), 341-347.

Meredith, W., Rutledge, R., Fakhry, S. M., Emery, S., & Kromhout-Schiro, S. (1998). The conundrum of the Glasgow Coma Scale in intubated patients: a linear regression prediction of the Glasgow verbal score from the Glasgow eye and motor scores. *Journal of Trauma, 44*(5), 839-844.

Michaels, A. J., Michaels, C. E., Smith, J. S., Moon, C. H., Peterson, C. & Long, W. B. (2000). Outcome from injury: General health, work status, and satisfaction 12 months after trauma. *Journal of Trauma-Injury Infection & Critical Care,48*(5), 841-850.

Milham, F. H., Malone, M., Blansfield, J., LaMorte, W. W., & Hirsch, E. F. (1995). Predictive accuracy of the TRISS survival statistic is improved by a modification that includes admission pH. *Archives of Surgery, 130*(3), 307-311.

Neale, M. C. (1998). Modeling interaction and nonlinear effects with Mx: A general approach. In R. E. Schumacker (Ed.) *Interaction and nonlinear effects in structural equation modeling* (pp. 68-94). Mahwah, NJ: Lawrence Erlbaum Associates.

Nelson, J. E., Kelly, T. P., & Stringer, P. (1998). Long-term outcome of learning and memory in children following traumatic brain injury. *Journal of the International Neuropsychological Society, 4*, 205.

Neuwirth, W. (1999). *Traffic Psychology Test Battery International*. Lafayette, IN: Lafayette Instrument Company.

Niemann, H. & Bavaria, K. (2000, February). *Driving ability after brain damage: Predictive validity of neuropsychological tests*. Paper presented at the 28th Annual Meeting of the International Neuropsychological Society, Denver, CO.

Nouri, F. M., & Lincoln, N. B. (1993). Predicting driving performance after stroke. *British Medical Journal, 307*, 482-483.

Osler, T., Baker, S. P., & Long, W. (1997). A modification of the injury severity score that both improves accuracy and simplifies scoring. *Journal of Trauma, 43*(6), 922-925.

Ota, T., Akaboshi, K., & Nagata, M. (1996). Functional assessment of patients with spinal cord injury: measured by the motor score and the functional independence measure. *Spinal Cord, 34*, 531-535.

Papero, P. H., Snyder, H. M., Gotschall, C. S., Johnson, D. L., & Eichelberger, M. R. (1997). Relationship of two measures of injury severity to pediatric psychological outcome 1-3 years after acute head injury. *Journal of Head Trauma Rehabilitation, 12*(3), 51-67.

Pettigrew, L. E., Wilson, J. T., & Teasdale, G. M. (1998). Assessing disability after head injury: Improved use of the Glasgow Outcome Scale. *Journal of Neurosurgery, 89*(6), 939-943.

Ponzer, S., Bergman, B., Brismar, B. & Johansson, S. E. (1997). Women and injuries–factors influencing recovery. *Women and Health, 25*(3), 47-62.

Prigatano, G. P. (1997). Learning from our successes and failures: Reflections and comments on "Cognitive rehabilitation: How it is and how it might be." *Journal of the International Neuropsychological Society, 3,* 497-499.

Psychological Software Services. (1990). *Manual for the Cognitive Behavioral Driver's Inventory.* Indianapolis, IN: Author.

Putnam, S. H., & Adams, K. M. (1992). Regression-based prediction of long-term outcome following multidisciplinary rehabilitation for traumatic brain injury. *Clinical Neuropsychologist, 6*(4), 383-405.

Rao, N., Rosenthal, M., Cronin-Stubbs, D., Lambert, R., Barnes, P., & Swanson, B. (1990 ). Return to work after rehabilitation following traumatic brain injury. *Brain Injury, 4*(1), 49-56.

Rappaport, M. (1982). Discipline report: Brain evoked potentials. In M. D. Acker (Ed.). *Head Injury Rehabilitation Project: Final Report* (Vol. 2, pp 1-75). San Jose, CA: Santa Clara Valley Medical Center.

Rappaport, M., Hall, K. M., Hopkins, K., Belleza, T., & Cope, D. N. (1982). Disability rating scale for severe head trauma: Coma to community. *Archives of Physical Medicine Rehabilitation, 63*(3), 118-123.

Rehn L. (1897). Über penetrierende herzwunde und herznaht. [Experiences from penetrating heart injuries.] *Archiv fur Klinische Chirugie, 55,* 315-317.

Rhodes, M., Aronson, J., Moerkirk, G., & Petrash, E. (1988). Quality of life after the trauma center. *Journal of Trauma, 28,* 931-938.

Rosenberg, G. A., & Paterson, B. M. (1998). Limb salvage versus amputation for severe open fractures of the tibia. *Orthopedics, 21,* 343-349.

Ruff, M. R., Marshall, L. F., Crouch, J., Klauber, M. R., Levin, H. S., Barth, J., Kreutzer, J., Blunt, B. A., Foulknes, M. A., & Eisenberg H. M. (1993). Predictors of outcome following severe head trauma: Follow-up data from the Traumatic Coma Data Bank. *Brain Injury, 7,* 101-111.

Rutledge, R., Osler, T., Emery, S., & Kromhout-Schiro, S. (1998). The end of the Injury Severity Score (ISS) and the Trauma and Injury Severity Score (TRISS): ICISS, an International Classification of Diseases, Ninth Revision-Based Prediction Tool, outperforms both ISS and TRISS as predictors of trauma patient survival, hospital charges, and hospital length of stay. *Journal of Trauma, 44,* 41-49.

Sattler, J. M. (1998). *Clinical and Forensic Interviewing of Children and Families*. San Diego: Author.

Schuhfried, G. (1995). *Traffic Psychological Test Battery / Vienna Test System: Computer-Aided Psychological Diagnosis*. Lafayette, IN: Lafayette Insturment Company.

Seekamp, A., Regel, G., & Tscherne, H. (1996). Rehabilitation and reintegration of multiply injured patients: An outcome study with special reference to multiple lower limb fractures. *Injury, 27*, 133-138.

Sherer, M., Bergloff, P., High, W., Levin, E., & Oden, K. (1996, February). *Clinician rating of patients' impaired awareness after traumatic brain injury and employment outcome*. Paper presented at the 17th Annual Meeting of the International Neurolopsychological Society, Orlando, FL.

Shiel, A., Wilson, B. A., McLellan, D. L., Horn, S., & Watson, M. (1998). Patterns of recovery after severe head injury. *Journal of the International Neuropsychological Society, 4*, 209.

Signorini, D. F., Andrews, P. J., Jones, P. A., Wardlaw, J. M., & Miller, J. D. (1999). Predicting survival using simple clinical variables: A case study in traumatic brain injury. *Journal of Neurology, Neurosurgery, and Psychiatry, 66*(1), 20-25.

Simms, B., & O'Toole, L. (1994). *The contribution of cognitive and visual assessment to the prediction of driving performance* (TRL Project Report PR 50). Crowthorac, England: Transport Research Laboratory.

Sloan, M. A., Sila, C. A., Mahaffey, K. W., Granger, C. B., Longstreth, W. T., Jr., Koudstaal, P., White, H. D., Gore, J. M., Simoons, M. L., Weaver, W. D., Green, C. L., Topol, E. J., & Califf, R. M. (1998). Prediction of 30-day mortality among patients with thrombolysis-related intracranial hemorrhage. *Circulation, 98*(14), 1376-1382.

Smith-Knapp, K., Corrigan, J. D., & Arnett, J. A. (1996). Predicting functional independence from neuropsychological tests following traumatic brain injury. *Brain Injury, 10*(9), 651-661.

Spreen, O. & Strauss, E. (1998). *A Compendium of Nueorpsychological Tests*. (2nd ed.). NY: Oxford University Press.

Sullivan, M. J., Stanish, W., Waite, H., Sullivan, M., & Tripp, D. A. (1998). Catastrophizing, pain, and disability in patients with soft-tissue injuries. *Pain, 77*(3), 253-260.

Systems Technology. (2000). *STISIM Drive Model 500W*. *Http://www.systemstech.com/stidrsml.htm*.

Taylor, H. G., Wade, S. L., Yeates, K. O., Drotar, D., & Klein, S. K. (1999). Influences on first- year recovery from traumatic brain injury in children. *Neuropsychology, 13*(1), 76-89.

Teasdale, T. W., Skovdahl Hansen, H., Gade, A., & Christensen, A. L. (1997). Neuropsychological test scores before and after brain-injury rehabilitation in relation to return to employment. *Neuropsychological Rehabilitation, 7*(1), 23-42.

Tesio, L., & Cantagallo, A. (1998). The functional assessment measure (FAM) in closed traumatic brain injury outpatients: A Rasch-based psychometric study. *Journal of Outcome Measures, 2*(2), 79-96.

Torenbeek, M., van der Heijden, G. J., de Witte, L. P., & Bakx, W. G. (1998). Construct validation of the Hoensbroeck Disability Scale for Brain Injury in acquired brain injury rehabilitation. *Brain Injury, 12*(4), 307-316.

Tupper, D. E. & Cicerone, K. D. (1990). *The psychology of everyday life.* Boston: Kluwer.

van der Naalt, J., van Zomeren, A. H., Sluiter, W. J., & Minderhoud, J. M. (1999). One year outcome in mild to moderate head injury: Their predictive value of acute injury characteristics related to complaints and return to work. *Journal of Neurology, Neurosurgery, and Psychiatry, 66*(2), 207-213.

van der Sluis, C. K., Eisma, W. H., Groothoff, J. W., & ten Duis, H. J. (1998). Long-term physical psychological and social consequences of severe injuries. *Injury, 29,* 281-285.

van der Sluis, C. K., Kingma, J., Eisma, W. H., & ten Duis, H. J. (1997). Pediatric polytrauma: short-term and long-term outcomes. *Journal of Trauma, 43,* 501-506.

van der Sluis, C. K., tenDuis, H. J., Geertzen, J. H. B. (1995). Multiple injuries: An overview of the outcome. *Journal of Trauma, 3,* 681-686.

Varney, N. R. (1988). Prognostic significance of anosmia in patients with closed-head trauma. *Journal of Clinical and Experimental Neuropsychology, 10*(2), 250-254.

Vassar, M. J., Wilkerson, C. L., Duran, P. J., Perry, C. A., & Holcroft, J. W. (1992). Comparison of APACHE II, TRISS, and a proposed 24-hour ICU point system for prediction of outcome in ICU trauma patients. *Journal of Trauma, 32*(4), 490-499.

Waller, J., Skelly, J., & Davis, J. (1995). The injury impairment scale as a measure of disability. *Journal of Trauma, 39,* 949-954.

Wiens, A. N., Fuller, J. H., & Crossen, J. R. (1997). Paced auditory serial addition test: Adult norms and moderator variables. *Journal of Clinical and Experimental Neuropsychology, 19*(4), 473-483.

Wilson, B. A. (1986). Future directions in the rehabilitation of brain injured people. In A. L. Christensen & P. P. Uzzell (Eds.), *Neuropsychological rehabilitation* (pp 69-86). Boston: Kluwer.

Wilson, B. A. (1997). Cognitive rehabilitation: How it is and how it might be. *Journal of the International Neuropsychological Society, 3*, 487-496.

Wong, D. T., Barrow, P. M., Gomez, M., & McGuire, G. P. (1996). A comparison of the acute physiology and chronic health evaluation (APACHE) II score and the Trauma-Injury Severity Score (TRISS) for outcome assessment in intensive care unit trauma patients. *Critical Care Medicine, 24*(10), 1642-1648.

World Health Organization. (1980). *International classification of impairment, disability and handicap: A manual of classification relating to the consequences of disease*. Geneva, Switzerland: Author.

Ylvisaker, M. (1986). Language and communication disorders following pediatric head injury. *Journal of Head Trauma Rehabilitation, 1*(4), 48-56.

Zafonte, R. D., Hammond, F. M., Mann, N. R., Wood, D. L., Black, K. L., & Millis, S. R. (1996). Relationship between Glasgow Coma Scale and functional outcome. *American Journal of Physical Medicine and Rehabilitation, 75*(5), 364-369.

Zafonte, R. D., Hammond, F. M., Mann, N. R., Wood, D. L., Millis, S. R., & Black, K. L. (1996). Revised trauma score: An additive predictor of disability following traumtic brain injury? *American Journal of Physical Medicine and Rehabilitation, 75*(6), 456-461.

Zafonte, R. D., Hammond, F. M., & Peterson, J. (1996). Predicting outcome in the slow to respond traumatically brain-injured patient: Acute and subacute parameters. *NeuroRehabilitaion, 6*, 19-32.

Zandbergem, E. G. J., de Hann, R. J., Stoutenbeek, C. P., Koelman, J. H. T. M., & Hijdra, A. (1998). Systematic review of early prediction of poor outcome in anoxic-ischemic coma. *Lancet, 352*(9143), 1808-1812.

Zietlow, S. P., Capizzi, P. J., Bannon, M. P., & Farnell, M. B. (1994). Multisystem geriatric trauma. *Journal of Trauma, 37*, 985-988.

Zoltie, N., & de Dombal, F. T. (1993). The hit and miss of ISS and TRISS. Yorkshire Trauma Audit Group. *British Medical Journal, 307*(6909), 906-909.

## APPENDIX A

### Glossary

| Acronym | Definition |
| --- | --- |
| ADL | Activities of Daily Living |
| AIS | Abbreviated Injury Scale |
| AMA | American Medical Association |
| APA | American Psychological Association |
| APACHE | Acute Physiology and Chronic Health Evaluation |
| ASCOT | A Severity Characterization of Trauma |
| BNT | Boston Naming Test |
| CBC | Child Behavior Checklist |
| CBDI | Cognitive Behavioral Driver's Inventory |
| CELF | Clinical Evaluation of Language Fundamentals |
| CHSB | California Highway Safety Battery |
| COAT | Child Orientation and Amnesia Test |
| COWA | Controlled Oral Word Association Test |
| CVLT | California Verbal Learning Test |
| d2 | d2 Test of Attention |
| DRS | Disability Rating Scale |
| FAM | Functional Assessment Measure |
| FCI | Functional Capacity Index |
| FIM | Functional Independence Measure |
| LOC | Loss of Consciousness / Length of Coma |
| MMPI | Minnesota Multiphasic Personality Inventory |
| GCS | Glasgow Coma Scale |
| GOAT | Galveston Orientation and Amnesia Test |
| GOS | Glasgow Outcome Scale |
| IIS | Injury Impairment Scale |
| ISS | Injury Severity Score |
| LCFS | Rancho-Los Amigos Levels of Cognitive Function Scale |
| MVPT | Motor-Free Visual Performance Test |
| NISS | New Injury Severity Score |
| PASAT | Paced Auditory Serial Addition Test |
| PAI | Portland Adaptability Inventory |
| PIQ | Performance Intelligence Quotient |
| PTA | Posttraumatic Amnesia |
| RT | Reaction Time |

| | |
|---|---|
| SIP | Sickness Impact Profile |
| SSO | Social Status Outcome |
| STROOP | Stroop Color-Word Test |
| TBI | Traumatic Brain Injury |
| TONI | Test of Nonverbal Intelligence |
| TRF | Child Behavior Checklist - Teacher Report Form |
| TPTB | Traffic Psychological Test Battery |
| TRISS | Trauma Injury Severity Score |
| T-RTS | Triage-Revised Trauma Score |
| VABS | Vineland Adaptive Behavior Scales |
| VIQ | Verbal Intelligence Quotient |
| VTS | Vienna Test System |
| VMI | Test of Visual Motor Integration |
| WAIS | Wechsler Intelligence Scale |
| WAIS-R | Wechsler Intelligence Scale - Revised |
| WHO | World Health Organization |
| WJ | Woodcock-Johnson |
| WM | Walker-McConnell Scale of Social Competence |
| WMS | Wechsler Memory Scale |
| WMS-R | Wechsler Memory Scale - Revised |

## APPENDIX B

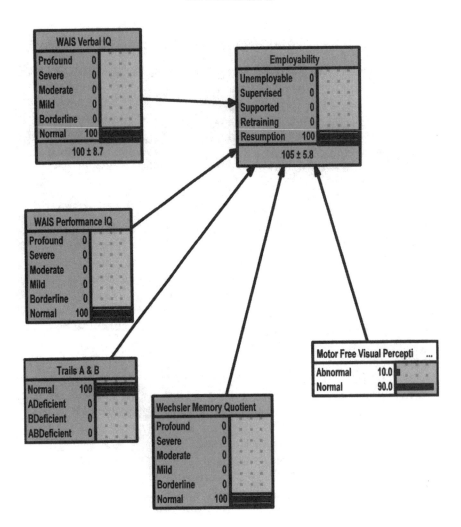

# The Prediction of Violent Behavior

**Selma De Jesus-Zayas**[1]
*Federal Correctional Institution, Miami*

**Allen B. Fleming**
*Private Practice, Miami*

Perhaps no area of psychological assessment is more controversial than the prediction of violent behavior. Members of the bar, the legislature, and the public alike seemingly expect psychologists and other mental health practitioners[2] to "read the minds" of the dangerous among us in order to protect the public. This chapter describes the apprehension produced by such views and then briefly reviews the history of violence prediction by mental health professionals as it applies to forensic settings. The chapter then blends findings from scientific undertakings with those of public policy institutes, in hopes of providing readers with a scope of information that is often missing from independent reviews of the respective sources.

The legal profession has stridently questioned the relevancy of testimony offered by mental health professionals who specialize in the area of forensics. Early critics stated that "in short, we believe there is no evidence that psychiatric opinions and terminology clarify rather than confuse the issues in a civil commitment proceeding and there is good reason to believe that judges and juries could function quite adequately in a civil commitment proceeding without 'expert testimony'". (Ennis & Litwack, 1974, p. 696). In an oft-cited work on the subject, Ziskin & Faust

---

[1] Dr. De Jesus-Zayas is Chief of Psychology Services at the Federal Correctional Institution, Miami, Fl. Opinions expressed in this article are those of the author and do not necessarily represent the opinions of the Federal Bureau of Prisons or the Department of Justice.

[2] Mental health professional implies psychiatrists and psychologists throughout this chapter unless otherwise specified.

(1988) opined that, "psychiatric and psychological evidence in the legal process, frequently does not meet reasonable criteria of admissibility and should not be admitted in a court of law, or if admitted, should be given little or no weight" (p. 1).

These critics expressed specific concerns about the testimony of mental health experts who render opinions predicting the occurrence of violent behavior. Echoing their apprehension, the American Civil Liberties Union (Ennis & Emery, 1978) concluded that mental health professionals have, "no expertise in predicting future dangerous behavior either to self or others. In fact, predictions of dangerous behavior are wrong about 95 percent of the time" (p. 20).

In *People v. Burnick* (1975), the California Supreme Court also found occasion to render negative comments regarding mental health professional evaluations. The Court stated that:

> The assumption is that predictive judgements are truly valid and that the probability of error in such judgments is significantly less than probability or error in judgment. In the light of recent studies, it is no longer heresy to question the reliability of psychiatric predictions. Psychiatrists themselves would be the first to admit that however desirable an infallible crystal ball might be, it is not among the tools of their profession. It must be conceded that psychiatrists still experience considerable difficulty in confidently and accurately diagnosing mental illness. Yet those difficulties are multiplied manifold when the psychiatrists venture from diagnosis to prognosis and undertake to predict the consequences of such illnesses. (p. 325)

## HISTORICAL PRECEDENCE

Ever since 1756 when the first mental hospitals began to appear in the United States, individuals deemed to be potentially dangerous to themselves or others were committed involuntarily (Steadman, 1981). In the early days of the Republic, the only criterion required for involuntary imprisonment or commitment was the determination that the individual was "furiously mad" and could engage in dangerous behavior toward self or others. It would not be until 1845 that the justification and limitations implicit in the common law concerning the restraint of the mentally ill first began to be spelled out. The decision in a Massachusetts court case, for the release of Josiah Oakes from McLean Asylum, stipulated that, "The question must arise in each particular case, whether a patient's own safety, or that of others, requires that he should be restrained for a certain time, and whether restraint is necessary for his restoration, or will be conducive thereto. The restrain can continue as long as the necessity continues. This is the limitation, and the proper limitation." (Deutch, 1949, pp. 422-3). Despite this ruling many states continued to involuntarily commit individuals who were not necessarily potentially dangerous to self or others but simply "mad."

By the 1970s, and partly in response to a larger movement focusing on the rights of the mentally ill that swept the United States, the criteria for the commitment of these individuals became the focus of civil rights groups. This reaction was provoked, in large measure, because a finding of "dangerousness" (to self or others) was not  a requirement for an involuntary commitment.   Instead, all that was required for an involuntary commitment was for two psychiatrists to agree that the individual was mentally ill and in need of hospitalization.   In response to the criticism put forth by civil rights groups, many states agreed to revise their civil commitment statues so that a person needed to be deemed dangerous to self or others prior to being involuntarily committed. This ruling, added to the increased involvement of mental health professionals in the legal arena, resulted in an increased frequency of dangerousness assessments,  which fell into the realms of psychiatry and burgeoning field of psychology (Otto, 1994).

**Psychiatry and Psychology's Role in Predicting Violent Behavior**

By 1975, the notion that mental health professionals could predict dangerousness to self or others was so ingrained that the California Supreme Court placed psychiatrists and psychologists on notice that they could be held liable if they failed to predict that a patient would engage in an act of violence and, consequently, failed to warn the potential victim of such attack to their person or property.   This decision (*Tarasoff v Regents of the University of California*, 1976) quickly extended beyond California and is now the standard  in many jurisdictions.

VandeCreek and Knapp (1993) explained that the innovation introduced by the Tarasoff decision was in the application of old legal principles regarding tort liability and negligence to a new concept. Anglo-American law distinguishes between injuries arising out of an action, "misfeasance," and out of noaction, "nonfeasance."    Traditionally, individuals could be held liable for injuries arising out of an action. They could not, however, be held liable for injuries arising out of nonaction. However, the practice of not providing legal remedies for nonaction gradually eroded for those in positions of "public callings." The first such public calling referred to innkeepers who had an affirmative duty to protect their guests, or public carriers who had a duty to protect their passengers. Neither could passively allow dangerous conditions to exist without warning their guests or passengers beforehand, or without removing the dangerous situation. This rule was later expanded to include any situation where a "special relationship" existed.    Courts have held that a special relationship exists when a person voluntarily agrees to assume responsibility for the conduct of another person.    For example, jailers are responsible for the conduct of their prisoners, parents for the conduct of their children, and mental health professionals for the behavior of their patients.    Consequently, mental health professionals would now be held responsible for the potential acts of violence their patients might commit against themselves or others.

### Psychiatry and Psychology's Reaction to Liability

Once mental health practitioners found themselves to be potentially liable for failing to predict dangerous behavior, or from failing to protect the potential victim, they questioned whether they could properly predict violent behavior.    The dearth of adequate research raised serious concerns. A task force of the American Psychiatric Association (1974) concluded that, "the state of the art regarding predictions of violence is very unsatisfactory. The ability of psychiatrists or any other professionals to reliably predict future violence is unproved" (p. 30).

> Likewise, a 1978 task force of the American Psychological Association stated that, "it does appear from reading the research that the validity of psychological predictions of dangerous behavior, at least in the sentencing and release situation we are considering, is extremely poor, so poor that one could oppose their use on the strictly empirical grounds that psychologists are not professionally competent to make such judgments"(p. 1110).

In a brief of *amici criae* presented by the American Psychological Association, the Michigan Psychological Association and the Michigan Psychiatric Society (*Davis v. Lhim,* 1983) summarized these issues by stating that the consistent research finding is that mental health professionals fail to predict accurately future violence in two out of three cases, and that there is no consistent professional standard for predicting violence. To support these claims, the American Psychiatric Association

Task Force reported that psychiatrist's efforts to predict violence often resulted in an unacceptably high rate of false positive predictions (i.e., violent behavior was predicted for individuals who did not demonstrate any violence within the period of study).

Despite these limitations in predicting violent behavior, the legal system continued to accept the opinions of mental health professionals. In *Barefoot v. Estelle* (1983), the U.S. Supreme Court upheld that mental health professionals could continue to testify as to issues of potential violence because the adversarial judicial system would allow for the uncovering of limitations and shortcomings of such predictions.

## Ethical and Statistical Concerns Regarding the Prediction of Violent Behavior

Beginning in the early 1970s researchers began to examine mental health professionals' ability to predict violence and the methods they employed. A seminal study was conducted by Monahan (1981) who performed a comprehensive review of the research available at the time. He concluded that there were few existing studies addressing the issue of predicting violence. He also concluded that the few studies that were available revealed that psychiatrists and psychologists were accurate only one out of three times in their prediction of violent behavior. Most important, Monahan began to identify problems within the existing research and formulated ways of correcting their deficiencies. In turn, this allowed for the speculation that new methods could be implemented and new tools constructed that would indeed enable mental health practitioners to become more accurate in their predictions.

## EMPIRICAL STUDIES

### First-Generation Studies

Monahan (1981) listed four major limitations to what he defined as the "first generations of studies," or research in the area of predicting violent behavior. He indicated that most of the studies conducted between the 1920s and 1960s shared one or more limitations. The first problem noted with these studies was that they had impoverished predictor variables in that their range of variables was so narrow that it often resulted in poorly specified study groups. Second, they had weak criterion variables, which poorly measured violent behavior. Consequently, the means of assessing the aftermath of a violent act was often inaccurate. For example, he found that these measures typically involved hospital, arrest, and/or prison incident reports that probably underestimated the true rate of violence. Third, these studies typically had  constricted validation samples.  This meant that those individuals who were at most risk for engaging in acts of violence were often not studied due, in large measure, to their hospitalization, incarceration, or other preventive measures taken against them.  By confining these individuals, the data were not an accurate prediction of how they would behave in a less restrictive setting.  Finally, research efforts were typically unsynchronized in that researchers failed to coordinate their efforts or use similar predictor variables.  This made it difficult to make comparisons across studies.

*False Positives.*  Monahan (1981, 1983) also questioned mental health professionals' propensity towards "false positives" when asked to predict dangerous behavior. ("False positives" refers to individuals who are incorrectly assessed as being at high risk for engaging in violent behavior.) In his meta-analysis of studies concerning the prediction of violence, he found a 44% average rate of false positives.  Therefore, individuals would most likely be committed unnecessarily, which raised ethical and legal concerns regarding the involuntary confinement of individuals based on an erroneous assumption.

**Second- Generation Studies**

Monahan (1981, 1983) also noted the emergence of a new generation of research that looked more closely at what mental health practitioners were able to do with regard to the prediction of violence.  This new generation of research, labeled "second generation of studies," featured an acknowledgment of the limitations of attempts to make absolute predictions about violence in favor of predictions that were more narrowly focused and situational in nature.  Instead of trying to predict who would be violent at some indeterminate point in the future, the focus changed to making probability statements as to the likelihood of a given individual becoming violent in a specific situation under specific circumstances.  This new approach infused clinicians with some optimism about their abilities to provide meaningful assistance in predicting violence while continuing to evaluate the accuracy of such predictions.

In his review of second-generation studies, Otto (1992) found that by employing criteria that were more focused and situational in nature (e.g., tighter definitions of violence, clearer time frames, etc.), "rather than one in three predictions of long term dangerousness being accurate, at least one in two short term predictions are accurate" (p. 130).  In particular, he observed that whereas Monahan's earlier meta-analysis of studies concerning false positives (those who have incorrectly been predicted to engage in violent behavior) yielded an average of 44%, his own research showed an average of 26%, suggesting improved criteria in the prediction of dangerousness. Some have opined, however, that Otto's optimistic claims were overstated. In their review of Otto's and Monahan's studies, Hart, Webster, and Menziesl (1993) found that Otto defined false positives in a statistically and conceptually different manner than Monahan, which had resulted in the differential outcome. Specifically, Hart et al. found that the striking discrepancy was not a result of improved predictive ability, but of different methodology. Whereas Otto employed false positive "rates" (the ratio of false positives to false positives plus true negatives, or, the proportion of nonviolent people who were inaccurately predicted to be violent), Monahan's method emphasized the probability that a prediction of violence was incorrect.

A more current study (Mossman, 1994) involved the meta-analysis of 58 studies examining the predictive abilities of first- and second-generation mental health professionals. In this study it was concluded that clinicians were in a position to predict violent from nonviolent patients with an accuracy that was slightly higher than chance. In addition, it was determined that (a) second-generation studies had better predictive abilities than did the first-generation studies, (b) past behavior was a strong indicator of future violent behavior, but (c) short-term predictions were no more accurate than long-term predictions.

These criticisms resulted in a modified way of conceptualizing and communicating opinions regarding violence potential. Instead of trying to maximize "true positives" while minimizing "false negatives," a goal that proved to be elusive, clinicians began to speak in terms of risk management. From this perspective, violence assessment began to be viewed as an analysis of the likelihood of a specific individual becoming violent under certain circumstances as opposed to a black-and-white prediction of future violence.

**Recent Developments**

In recent years, the Research Network on Mental Health and the Law of the John D. and Catherine T. MacArthur Foundation has been reviewing and expanding upon the body of literature concerning the prediction of dangerousness. The MacArthur Violence Risk Assessment Study (1998) was designed to improve the validity of clinical risk assessment, enhance the effectiveness of clinical risk management, and provide information on mental disorders and violence that would be useful in reforming mental health law and policy. This group reviews past studies and generates new research approaches by isolating and addressing the weaknesses found in prior research and proposing solutions. Their research identified risk factors for violence as generally falling into four domains: dispositional, clinical, historical, and contextual.

### Dispositional Factors

Dispositional factors refer to the individual's innate tendencies to engage in dangerous behavior out of anger, deficits in impulse control, and psychopathy. Novaco (1994) demonstrated that it is important to evaluate those mediating factors that might decrease the person's propensity to engage in acts of violence in reaction to anger. For example, factors such as *impulse control* (the ability to modify or control thoughts and actions) have been proven to influence an individual's propensity to engage in violent behavior. Individuals with good impulse control will be able to contain an impulse to engage in violent behavior, whereas an individual with poor impulse control is more likely to become violent.

A second dispositional factor, *psychopathy*, was defined by Meloy (1988) as a "sub-type of narcissistic personality disorder, albeit an extreme and dangerous variant" (p. 17). He preferred the term *psychopathy* over the term antisocial personality disorder, which is employed by the *Diagnostic Statistical Manual of Mental Disorders*, (4th ed. [DSM-IV]; American Psychiatric Association [APA], (1994). His argument against employing the *DSM-IV* term is that it is "too descriptive, inclusive, criminally biased, and socio-economically skewed to be of much clinical or research use" (p. 6). For Meloy the term *psychopathy* better describes those individuals who, from adolescence or early childhood, are prone toward impulsivity and pathological egocentrism, with little response to kindness. Such individuals display a callous unconcern for others, are unaffected by punishment, lack a sense of responsibility and, do not experience guilt.

Meloy also believed that acts of violence with these individuals should further be classified as falling in either the "affective" or "predatory" realm. When he referd to *affective aggression* he meant the acts that follow a threatening situation (external or internal, real or imaginary) that are accompanied by threatening vocalizations and attacking or defending postures. *Predatory aggression*, on the other hand, refers to the destruction of prey. Unlike affective aggression, this other form of violence involves minimal or no autonomic arousal, vocalization, or elaborate behavioral displays. Furthermore, it is not associated with increased irritability or conscious experience of emotions, and the acts of violence are planned and purposeful. Meloy (1992) contended that "predatory aggression is the hallmark of the psychopathic individual, whether it is a primitive act of violence against a stranger or a technically sophisticated act of revenge against a business associate" (p. 25)  He concluded that, "the psychopathic process is particularly suited to predation. It is my hypothesis that the psychopathic process predisposes, precipitates, and perpetuates predatory violence by virtue of its structural and dynamic characteristics. (p. 236).

### Clinical Factors

The MacArthur Violence Risk Assessment Study (1998) defined the second domain, clinical risk factors for violence, as the propensity for an individual with a mental disorder (along with substance abuse, psychosis, or a personality disorder) to engage in violent behavior.

The possibility that a relationship exists between mental illness and violence is an emerging concept given that for many years it was assumed that after factoring in such variables as drug abuse, poverty, gender, age, and victimization, there would be no causal relationship between the presence of mental illness and acts of violence.    However, new studies suggest that mental disorder may be a robust risk factor in accounting for the occurrence of violence (Borum, 1996).   Otto (1992) found that when violent behavior was defined narrowly (i.e., physical assaults), data showed that between 15% and 28% of psychiatric patients engaged in violent behavior.   When adopting a broader definition (i.e., physical assaults and threats), between 40% and 50% of hospital patients engaged in some type of violent behavior.

*Mental Illness.*    Meyer (1996) noted that individuals with diagnoses of schizophrenia, paranoid type, and mood disorders (i.e., major depressive disorder, bipolar disorder) are at greater risk of being influenced to commit acts of violence by their hallucinations, delusions, or poor reality testing.   More specifically,  Shapiro (1996) indicated that there are a number of active psychiatric diagnoses (e.g., obsessive-compulsive disorder; panic disorder; major depression with grief, mania, or bipolar disorder; schizophrenia or schizophreniform) that raise the frequency of violent behavior from 2% to anywhere from 10% to 12%. He indicated that the presence of two or more clinical diagnoses approximately doubles the risk for dangerous behavior, with the highest risk being for substance abuse plus schizophrenia or a mood disorder.   Furthermore, simply ascertaining that an individual has required treatment for a mental disorder increases the prevalence of aggression an average of 1.5 to 4 times over that of someone who has never been treated. Link & Steuve (1994) found that it is not the specific diagnosis that is the issue so much as a particular subset of psychotic symptoms. They found that paranoid delusions and delusions of thought control by external forces appear to increase the risk for violence.

*Deviant Personalities.* The *DSM-IV* (APA, 1994) defined a personality disorder as a relatively enduring and inflexible set of personality traits that usually surface during adolescence or early adulthood, and that deviate markedly from the expectations of the individual's culture. Some personality disorders also fall under the category of dispositional factors that may contribute to dangerous behavior. For example, the *DSM- IV* notes that individuals with a diagnosis of antisocial personality disorder (APD) are prone to repeated acts of violence. It further indicates that, "the essential feature of this disorder is a pervasive pattern of disregard for, and violation of, the rights of others that begins in childhood or early adolescence and continues into adulthood" (p. 645). These individuals view themselves as being above social mores and are not affected by the emotional or moral restraints that curtail the behaviors of most people. They fail to be empathic and most often are perceived as being callous and arrogant. They are also cocky with some superficial charm they employ to exploit others. Oftentimes they are reckless with their own life and the lives of others, are typically irresponsible, and have poor impulse control. People frequently refer to these individuals as being self-centered, manipulative, and deceitful. When individuals with poor impulse control begin to feel victimized, picked on, or stop thinking in a logical manner, they are at a higher risk than most for engaging in acts of violence. Furthermore, these individuals are often at a higher risk than the general population to die prematurely by violent means (e.g., suicide, accidents, and homicides).

The relationship between a diagnosis of borderline personality disorder (BPD) and violence is limited to two main studies (Snyder, Pitts, & Polerny, 1986; Stone, 1990), neither of which clearly indicates that a diagnosis of BPD itself suggests a predilection toward violence against others. However, individuals with BPD tend to be unstable in interpersonal relationships, erratic, markedly impulsive, and have fluctuating emotions of great intensity. In times of crises, these individuals have difficulty differentiating between reality and their own internal processes. While in this state of emotional deterioration, they are at risk of behaving violently toward themselves (i.e., self-mutilative behaviors, suicidal threats, and general recklessness). Therefore, in the course of such experiences violent acts toward others can also occur.

Schulte (1994) found that a subset of individuals whom he described as having a "pathological narcissism" are at a higher risk for violence. Narcissism refers to one's need for admiration and a tendency to greatly overestimate one's own value and abilities. Individuals at an enhanced risk for engaging in violent behavior are those whose narcissistic traits are particularly severe and those who have suffered a recent "narcissistic injury." (A narcissistic injury refers to an event that severely wounds the individual's self-esteem.) Because these individuals have an inability to acknowledge painful or angry feelings, Schulte found that they are prone to impulsive behaviors. He also found that if weapons are available to them, the risk of engaging in violent behavior increases significantly.

*Neuropsychological.* Research in the burgeoning field of neuropsychology has produced numerous studies examining the effect neuropsychological factors have on violence. In their review of the literature Golden, Jackson, Peterson-Rohner, and Gontkovsky (1996) found that brain trauma, particularly in the prefrontal area of the brain (along with their connections to the subcortical areas of the brain), damage to the temporal lobes (with their associated limbic structures), and global damage to the brain (as seen in dementia and delirium), is most commonly associated with incidents of aggression.

A caveat is in order. Brain trauma itself does not imply propensity for aggression. Although brain damage might make impulsive behavior and aggression likely to occur, it does not imply that it will be an inevitable phenomenon. In fact, Golden et al. determined that individuals with brain injuries prior to age 25 are more prone than older patients to exhibit violent behavior in moments of stress. They opined that this might be the case because the brain injury occurred prior to the individual's ability to develop a full set of internal controls that would allow them to modulate their behavior appropriately. They also found that aggression appears to be more likely in a subgroup of individuals with a prior history of violent behavior.

*Drugs and Alcohol.* Data included in the most recent MacArthur studies pertaining to violence by the mentally disordered emphasized the role drug and alcohol use plays in determining whether or not a mentally disordered individual will engage in an act of violence. Otto (2000) believed that a diagnosis of substance abuse or dependence is probably the single greatest risk factor for threatening or assaultive behaviors directed towards other unless the individual had a history of violence in the absence of drug or alcohol use. His finding reflects Swanson et al.'s (1990) study, which found that individuals with a history of substance abuse or dependency are 14 times more likely to engage in threatening or assaultive behavior than those with no diagnosis or history of substance abuse. Likewise, this figure increased to 17 times more likely for persons with a history of mental disorder that is accompanied by the use of a substance.

In another study with a sample of approximately 10,000 respondents who were queried pertaining to their history of substance abuse, violence, and psychiatric diagnosis, Swanson (1994) found that rather than being synergestic, the interactions between these variables are additive. He explained this to mean that individuals with dual diagnoses had only a "slightly" greater risk of engaging in acts of violence when compared with individuals with substance abuse alone. He concluded that "substance abuse" is a higher risk variable associated with violence, than is "mental disorder."

More specifically, it appears that alcohol, as opposed to other substances, is associated with higher incidents of violent crime among incarcerated felons. Franklin, Allison, & Sutton (1992) and Franklin, Sutton, & Harrop (1992) found that intoxication with nonalcoholic substances actually corresponded with lower incidents of violence. They did suggest, however, that drug-seeking behavior, as opposed to the actual effect of nonalcoholic substances, may result in high risks for violence.

### *Historical Factors (Factors That Predispose Violent Behavior)*

The third domain that needs to be explored in the prediction of violent behavior is historical in nature. Monahan and Steadman (1994) define these historical factors as those events that have been experienced in the past and that may predispose a person to act violently in the future. In fact, a history of violent or criminal behavior is probably the single greatest risk factor for future violence (Otto, 2000).

Studies have increasingly supported the view that modeling of violent behavior by role models contributes to violence in children (see Bandura's early work on aggression, 1973). The viewing of violent TV programs and latter aggression has also been reported by Lefkowitz, Eron, Walder, and Huesmann (1977) and Huesmann (1986). Observations of parental violence have been shown to correlate with later violence in their children (Lewis, Shanok, Pincus, & Glaser, 1979); whereas Rosenbaum and O'Leary (1981) found that abusive husbands witnessed more parental abuse than did control groups.

Modeling also appears to occur when a child is a victim of violence (Climent, Rollins, Ervin, & Plutchik, 1973; Klassen and O'Conner, 1988; Lewis et al. 1979) as does rehearsal. The latter is suggested by studies that indicate acts of violence as an adolescent correlates with acts of violence as an adult (Cocozza & Steadman, 1974).

*Context*

The last domain, context, refers to aspects of the current environment that may be conducive to the occurrence of violent behavior. In their study of 169 individuals, Estroff and Zimmer (1994) explored the possibility that what might predispose patients with severe, persistent mental disorder to engage in acts of violence is the unavailability (or absence) of mental health services, and the lack of emotional and instrumental support. Although further research is needed, they found some support for the notion that individuals who were more prone to acts of violence were those with networks composed of a higher percentage of relatives and with a low percentage of mental health professionals.

## SPURIOUS VIOLENCE

There is nothing more difficult to predict than an act of violence from an individual who has never displayed signs of violence or does not meet the traditional demographics of those who engage in this type of behavior. Acts of violence by these individuals can be against persons, institutions (e.g., federal government), or organizations (e.g., abortion clinics). These individuals often strike randomly, depending on victim accessibility and how well a potential victim represents a targeted group. In addition, these individuals often feel that they are on a mission requiring that their actions be dramatic enough to call attention to their "cause." This will often result in actions whose sole purpose is to victimize the largest number of individuals with the least number of strikes (e.g., the Oklahoma City bombing) although this is not always the case (e.g., White supremacists targeting ethnic minorities).

Moffatt (1994) proposed a format to help discern which individuals with no prior history of violent behavior and who do not appear to meet the demographics associated with violence will be at a high risk for displaying this type of comportment. He reported that these individuals possess some characteristics in common, such as low self-esteem, depressive traits, possibly some suicidal ideation, a history of parental discord, and minimal social networks. These individuals appear to lose control and give in to their aggressive impulses under heightened situational stress because of an absence of strong social networks. In fact, he stated that situational stress overwhelms these individuals psychologically in large measure due to the absence of friends and social skills.

## PSYCHOLOGICAL TESTS USEFUL
## IN THE PREDICTION OF VIOLENCE

Psychologists have evaluated data elicited by second-generation studies to explore how previous measures of personality (e.g., the MMPI and Rorschach tests) address those risk factors found to correlate with violent behavior. They are also developing new tests that they hope will enable them to be more accurate in their prediction of violent behavior.

### Objective Personality Tests

*Psychopathic Check List - Revised.*    Psychological tests are commonly used to identify and quantify various personality components of relevance to the prediction of violence, although none will predict violence in and of themselves. One of these, the Psychopathic Check List - Revised (PCL-R), developed by Robert Hare, is based on the classic construct of "psychopathy" as developed by Cleckley (1976). This test has been found to have a high predictability rate for a variety of antisocial behaviors including criminal violence, recidivism following release from a prison or hospital, and response to correctional treatment programs. A large body of research has demonstrated the validity and reliability of the PCL-R. Interrater reliabilities range from .88 to .92 whereas test-retest reliabilities range from .85 to .90 (Butcher, 1995).

The PCL-R is composed of a twenty-item, forty-point scale, which is completed following a structured clinical interview of the patient and a review of independent historical data. Each item is scored on a three-point scale: zero (the item does not apply); one (some elements apply); two (there is a reasonably good match). Items are not scored if there is no available information. Meloy and Gacano (cited in Butcher, 1995) stress the importance of reviewing background records as an "absolutely necessary" aspect of the PCL-R. They even encouraged the clinician to postpone the administration of the PCL-R until the background data become available. Background data, as has been discussed previously, are essential in determining the historical and environmental factors that might provoke an individual to engage in acts of violence.

Klosson et al. (1997) reported that the PCL-R has two underlying factors or components. Factor 1, which is often referred to as the "affective" or "aggressive narcissism" aspect of the disorder, describes a callous and manipulative approach. Factor 2 refers to a "socially deviant" or "chronic antisocial behavior." Whereas Factor 2 predicts poor educational achievement, low socioeconomic status, and frequent antisocial behavior, Factor 1 refers to the manner in which the person relates to others. Although both factors may provide significant information on the individual's personality structure, it is Factor 1 that best predicts violent recidivism (Serin, 1996).

Regression analysis on data obtained from the administration of the PCL on 231 inmates in a study conducted by Hart, Krop, and Hare (1988) determined that this test contributed to the prediction of outcome. Following release, the offenders who scored in the top third of the PCL were almost three times more likely to violate the conditions of their release, and almost four times more likely to commit a violent crime, than were those in the lower third. These findings were supported by a long-term follow-up study conducted by Harris, Rice, and Cormier (1991) with 169 male patients released from a maximum psychiatric hospital. The researchers found that the PCL-R scores were strongly correlated with violent recidivism ($r = .42$). More specifically, the violent recidivism rate of the psychopaths was almost four times that of the other releases and that 78% of the predictions were accurate. They also found that once the PCL-R was added to other sources assessing violent behavior, it raised their correlation with violent outcome from .31 to .45.

Serin (1996) compared the predictive validity of the PCL-R with three other actuarial measures (Base Expectancy Score, Recidivism Prediction Scale, and the Salient Factor Score) in a sample consisting of 81 offenders. Seventy-five percent of the sample consisted of individuals who had engaged in violent crimes such as assault, robbery, manslaughter, sexual assault, and murder. The results of this study determined that psychopaths were more likely than nonpsychopaths to recidivate, and to do it sooner. Furthermore, the results reported a violent recidivism rate of 10%. Most significant, however, is that multiple regression analysis indicated that of the four measures used, only the PCL-R provided concordance with violent recidivism ($R = .28$, $p < .05$).

***Minnesota Multiphasic Personality Inventory - 2.*** The most widely used psychometric measure in clinical settings (Greene, 1991), is the Minnesota Multiphasic Personality Inventory - 2 (MMPI-2). First constructed in 1940 by Hathaway and McKinley, the MMPI-2 provides "an objective means of assessing abnormal behavior." (Green, 1991, p. 1). This is accomplished by comparing an individual's responses to 567 items, with the responses of both a psychiatric and a normal population. In this manner, the MMPI-2 reveals the presence of clinical symptoms, deficiencies of inhibitions and controls, conflicts between expression and suppression of hostility, and cognitive strengths and weakness.

The validity and reliability of the MMPI-2 has also been analyzed extensively (Greene, 1991). Not only a robust measure, the MMPI-2 has been helpful in identifying personality factors that would suggest the likelihood of someone engaging in violent behavior. For example, it contains Scale 4, or the "psychopathy" scale, which is the clinical scale most sensitive to antisocial behavior, and which in turn correlates with violence. In and of itself, an elevation on this scale does not imply the individual will become violent, but that the individual has characteristics (traits, symptoms, etc.) that correspond with this particular behavior. Some of the characteristics that are related to elevations in Scale 4 include poor impulse control, unwillingness to adapt to society's norms, social alienation, and so on, which are correlates of violent behavior. Previous studies (McKinley & Hathaway, 1944) have offered cross validation results that have indicated that a $T$-score of $> 70$ on Scale 4 was achieved by 59% of a sample of 100 male federal prisoners. More recently, Graham (1990) noted how numerous studies of inmates reveal a fairly homogenous population with an elevated Scale 4, or a combination of elevations that include Scale 4 (e.g., 4-2, 4-9), making it the most frequent profile within this particular population.

Other scales within the MMPI-2 that may provide additional information on the potential for violence are the Over-Controlled Hostility scale, the Hysteria scale, the Ego Control scale (Sc1), and the Antisocial Practices scale (Greene, 1991). In addition, the MMPI-2 has a number of subscales that allow the assessment of the individual's ego strength, impulse control, and thought distortions that might result in acts of violence against self or others.

*California Psychological Inventory.* Whereas the MMPI-2 is often used with psychiatric populations or in clinical settings, the California Psychological Inventory (CPI) provides a good index of socialization and adherence to the values and morals of society among a normal population. This test is a self-report questionnaire that aims to assess normal personality. It accomplishes its task by targeting twenty basic features of personality referred to as "folk-concepts," thirteen special-purpose scales such as "management potential," and three structural scales of interpersonal functioning. In addition, it has three validity scales that indicate if the person has been responding in a random manner, or with a preconceived agenda. Abnormal responses, oddity in thinking, and unwillingness to abide by the morals and values established by society would place the testtaker at a higher risk for engaging in violent behavior.    More specifically, the CPI contains three scales, Empathy Scale , Sociability , and Social Presence, which help detect individuals who are unable to feel empathy toward a potential victim.    By emotionally distancing themselves from any pain they could cause a potential victim, the aggressor is at a higher risk of engaging in an act of violence.

   ***Other Tests.***    The Dangerous Behavior Rating Scheme (DBRS), the Violence Prediction Scheme (VPS),  the HCR-20 , and the Dangerousness in Psychotic Patients Scale (PAD) are among a number of instruments that have been specifically designed to assist in the clinical assessment of dangerousness. Although these tests have known psychometric properties, none have been demonstrated to be sufficiently  robust  to be used in lieu of more traditional tests and interview techniques.  The DBRS showed that it has poor longitudinal predictive validity.  The VPS combines both clinical and actuarial factors, but has yet to be proven to apply to populations other than in the prison settings where it was designed.  The HCR-20 is more of a checklist than a formal test, and validity and reliability findings  are still in the  preliminary  stages (Borum,  1996).    Bjorkly, Havik, and Loberg.(1996) indicated  that  the  PAD  demonstrated  good  interrater reliability, but required additional study to determine its predictive ability.

## Objective Personality Tests

   ***The Rorschach Inkblot.***    The Rorschach Inkblot technique is a "projective test" that is commonly employed and highly regarded.  Groth-Marnart (1990) viewed  projective test as a means to discover unconscious defenses and circumvent conscious resistances for the purpose of obtaining an accurate view of a person's internal world.  The Rorschach attempts to tap into the person's inner self by examining their responses to a set of ten bilaterally symmetrical inkblots.  The person is exposed to these inkblots and is asked to tell the examiner what he or she sees.  The test assumes that people organize their environment based on their specific needs, motives, conflicts, and characteristic ways of approaching the world.  They then rely on these characteristics to guide them in their approach to the ambiguous inkblots. The test assumes that the process by which persons organize their responses to the Rorschach is representative of how they confront other situations that require organization and judgment. These responses are then scored according to a set of specific criteria.

Of the many scoring approaches to the Rorschach, Exner's (1990) comprehensive system is the most psychometrically sound system available. Exner's scoring system gained prominence among the competing approaches due to its ability to develop clear guidelines for scoring and interpreting, and by adhering closely to empirical validation and a large normative database (Gacano & Meloy, 1994).

In Exner's system, indicators for violence typically focus on the degree to which an individual has the ability to control emotional responses as reflected in the manner the person reacts to the inkblots. Impulsive responses imply that the individual has difficulty modulating behavior and is more prone than most to engage in acts of violence. Likewise, individuals whose responses are idiosyncratic will have distorted perceptions and poor contact with reality. Such individuals are prone to misinterpret their environment and may be prone to violence. Most often, those individuals at high risk of engaging in violent behavior exhibit short reaction time in responding to the stimuli cards and more so the color cards. They also provide a low number of FormColor responses, and high Color , ColorForm, and Popular responses. Furthermore, individuals whose responses are associated with fighting (or use of weapons) or aggressive animals tend to be at a higher risk of engaging in violent behavior. If, in addition to these responses the individual renders high scores in special and content scales of Aggressive Movement, Explosion, and Morbid responses, this raises even further their potential for displaying acts of violence. In evaluating the efficacy of the Rorschach Test for the assessment of aggression, Gacono and Meloy (1994) incorporated a psychodynamic element into the psychostructural approach of Exner and provided detailed examples of Rorschach findings with a variety of aggressive and psychopathic personality styles. Their findings suggest the value of using additional or alternative scores to those used by Exner in determining violence potential. The reader is referred to their work for a more thorough exploration of the subject.

***Mental Status Examination.*** Enough cannot be said about the importance of conducting a thorough Mental Status Examination (MSE). Although not a "projective test" in the same sense as the Rorschach Test, the MSE reliance on interview (during which the clinician inquires about the individual's background, problems, and present and future concerns) also allows for limited projection by the patient. During the interview process the clinician evaluates the individual's risk factors for displaying violent behavior. This information is gathered by reviewing with the individual their background, affective reactions, behavioral style, thinking processes, and more. This information enables the clinician to generate

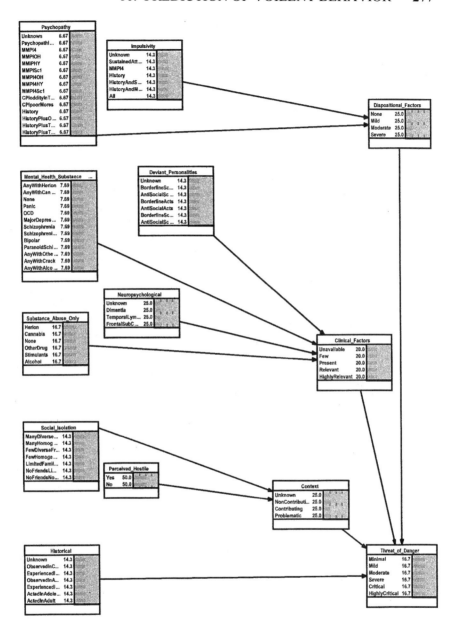

FIG. 10.1.  Bayes network proposal for predicting dangerousness.

working hypotheses that are the basis for more in-depth analysis further into the clinical relationship. Some key elements that need to be addressed during the MSE pertaining to the issue of dangerousness involve predisposition toward acts of violence, history of violence, types of internal controls, accessibility of weapons, whether the potential victim is identifiable or not, and access to the potential victim. Furthermore, the MSE would indicate whether the person has a history of mental illness, a pressing physical illness, drug/alcohol use, and fantasies that might prompt a desire to engage in an act of violence.

## CONCLUSIONS

In view of the wealth of research and data that has been generated in the past decade, how far have mental health professionals come with regard to being able to predict violence? Despite challenges, they are still expected to provide predictive services to the legal system. In response to previous criticism about their predictive abilities, a plethora of studies have been generated examining the phenomena of violence, its correlates, and risk factors associated with violent behavior. More specifically, recent research has identified key criteria for the prediction of violence by employing sociological, demographic, diagnostic, psychological, situational, and statistical methods. However, there have been no models offered for integrating findings into a single heuristic that is suitable for empirical validation.

Franklin and Allison (1992) provided a prototype for evaluating recent research findings using a Bayesian predictive model (See chapter 4, this volume.) The Bayes model is expanded to a demonstration Bayes network for predicting dangerousness in Fig. 10.1. The model is available on the Web at *http://www.geocities.com/rdfphd/index.html*.

## REFERENCES

American Psychiatric Association. (1974). *Clinical aspects of the violent individual*. Washington, DC: Author.

American Psychiatric Association. (1994). *Diagnostic and statistical manual - IV* (4th ed.). Washington, DC: Author.

American Psychological Association. (1978). Report of the task force on the role of psychology in the criminal justice system. *American Psychologist, 33,* 1099-1113.

Bandura, A. (1973). *Aggression: A social learning analysis*. Englewood Cliffs, NJ: Prentice-Hall.

*Barefoot v Estelle,* 463 U.S. 880 (1983).

Bjorkly, S., Havik, O., & Loberg, T. (1996). The interrater reliability of the scale for the prediction of aggression and dangerousness in psychotic patients (PAD). *Criminal Justice and Behavior, 23,* 440- 454.

Borum, R. (1996). Improving the clinical practice of violence risk assessment. *American Psychologist, 51,* 945- 956.

Butcher, J. N. (Ed.). (1995). *Clinical personality assessment.* New York: Oxford University Press.

Clekley, H. M. (1976). *The mask of sanity.* St. Louis, MO: The Mosby.

Climent, C., Rollins, A., Ervin, F., & Plutchik, R. (1973). Epidemiological studies of women prisoners: Medical and psychiatric variables related to violent behavior. *American Journal of Psychiatry, 130,* 985-990.

Cocozza, J., & Steadman, H. (1974). Some refinements in the measurement of prediction of violent behavior. *American Journal of Psychiatry, 131,* 1012-14.

*Davis v. Lhim,* 124 Mich. App. 291, 303;335 N.W.2d 481 (1983).

Deutsch, A. (1949). *The mentally ill in America.* New York: Columbia University Press.

Ennis, B., & Emery, R. (1978). *The rights of mental patients - An American Civil Liberties Union handbook.* New York: Avon.

Ennis, B. & Litwack, T. (1974). Psychiatry and the presumption of expertise: Flipping coins in the courtroom, *California Law Review, 62,* 693 - 752.

Estroff, S., & Zimmer, C. (1994). Social networks, social support, and violence among persons with severe, persistent mental illness. In J. Monahan & H. Steadman (Eds.), *Violence and mental disorder: Developments in risk assessment* (pp. 259-295). Chicago: University of Chicago Press.

Exner, J. E. (1990). *The Rorschach: A comprehensive system: Foundations* (Vol. 1, 2nd ed.). New York: Wiley.

Franklin, R. D., Allison, D. B. (1992). The REV: A BASIC Bayesian predictor of true test scores for IBM compatible computers. [Computer program]. *Behavior Research Methods, Instruments, & Computers, 24*(3), 491-492.

Franklin, R., Allison, D., & Sutton, T. (1992). Alcohol, substance abuse, and violence among North Carolina Prison admissions, 1988. *Journal of Offender Rehabilitation, 17,* 101-111.

Franklin, R., Sutton, T., & Harrop, A. (1992). Violent crime and substance abuse among North Carolina prisoners, 1988. *Forensic Reports, 5,* 211-213.

Gacono, C. B., & Meloy, J. R. (1994). *The rorschach assessment of aggressive and psychopathic personalities*. Hillsdale, NJ: Lawrence Erlbaum Associates.

Golden, C. J., Jackson, M. L., Peterson-Rohne, A., & Gontkovsky, S. T. (1996). Neuropsychological correlates of violence and aggression: A review of the clinical literature. *Aggression and Violent Behavior, 1*, 3 - 25.

Graham, J. R. (1990). *MMPI-2: Assessing personality and psychopathology*. New York: Oxford University Press.

Greene, R. L. (1991). *The MMPI-2/MMPI: An interpretive manual.* Boston: Allyn & Bacon.

Groth-Marnart, G. (1990). *Handbook of psychological assessment* (2nd ed.). New York: Wiley.

Harris, G. T., Rice, M. E., & Cormier, C. A. (1991). Psychopathy and violent recidivism. *Law and Human Behavior, 15*, 625-637.

Hart, S. D., Kropp, P. R., & Hare, R. D. (1988). Performance of male psychopaths following conditional release from prison. Journal of Consulting and Clinical Psychology, 56, 227- 232.

Hart, S. D., Webster, C. D., & Menzies, R. J. (1993). A note on portraying the accuracy of violence predictions. *Law and Human Behavior, 17,* 695-699.

Huesmann, L. (1986). Psychological precesses promoting the relationships between exposure to media violence and aggressive behavior by the viewer. *Journal of Social Issues, 42*, 125-139.

Klassen, D., & O'Connor, W. A. (1988). A prospective study of predictors of violence in adult male mental health admissions. *Law and Human Behavior, 12*, 143-148.

Lefkowitz, R. M., Eron, L., Walder, L., & Huesmann, L. (1977). *Growing up to be violent.* New York: Pergamon.

Lewis, D., Shanok, S., Pincus, J., & Glaser, G. (1979). Violent juvenile delinquents. *Journal of Child Psychiatry, 18*, 307-319.

Link, B. G., & Steuve, A. (1994). Psychotic symptoms and the violent/illegal behavior of mental patients compared to community controls. In J. Monahan & H. Steadman (Eds.), *Violence and mental disorder: Developments in risk assessment* (pp. 137-159). Chicago: University of Chicago Press.

McKinley, C., & Hathaway, S. (1944). The Minnesota Multiphasic Personality Inventory V. Hysteria, hypomania, and psychopathic deviate. *Journal of Applied Psychology, 28,* 153 – 174.

Meloy, J. R. (1988). *The psychopathic mind: Origins, dynamics, and treatment.* Northvale, NJ: Aronson.

Meloy, J. R. (1992). *Violent attachments.* Northvale, NJ: Aronson, Inc.

Moffatt, G. K. (1994). A checklist for assessing risk of violent behavior in historically nonviolent persons. *Psychological Reports, 74,* 683-688.

Monahan, J. (1981). *The clinical prediction of violent behavior.* Bethesda, MD: National Institute of Mental Health.

Monahan, J. (1983). *The prediciton of violent behavior: Developments in psychology and law.* Washington, DC: American Psychological Association. (The Master Lecture Series, Psychology and the Law).

Monahan, J., & Steadman, H. (Eds.). (1994). *Violence and mental disorder: Developments in risk assessment.* Chicago: University of Chicago Press.

Mossman, D. (1994). Assessing predictions of violence: Being accurate about accuracy. *Journal of Consulting and Clinical Psychology, 62,* 783- 792.

Novaco, R. (1994). Anger as a risk factor for violence among the mentally disordered. In J. Monahan & H. Steadman (Eds.). *Violence and mental disorder: Developments in risk assessment* (pp. 21-59). Chicago: University of Chicago Press.

Otto, R. (1992). The prediciton of dangerous behavior: A review and analysis of "second generation" reasearch. *Forensic Reports, 5,* 103-133.

Otto, R. (1994). On the ability of mental health professionals to "predict dangerousness." A commentary on interpretations of the "dangerous" literature. *Law and Psychology Review,18,* 43- 68.

Otto, R. (2000) Assessing and managing violence risk in outpatient settings. *Journal of Clinical Psychology, 56* (10), 1239-1262.

*People v. Burnick,* 14 Cal. 3d 306 (1975).

Rosenbaum, A., & O'Leary, K. (1981). Marital violence: Characteristics of abusive couples. *Journal of Consulting and Clinical Psychology, 49,* 63-71

Schulte, H. M. (1994). Violence in patients with narcissistic personality pathology: Observations of a clinical series. *American Journal of Psychotherapy, 48,* 610-623.

Serin, R. (1996). Violent recidivism in criminal psychopaths. *Law and Human Behavior, 20,* 207-217.

Shapiro, D. L. (1996, April). Violence prediction and risk assessment. Sixth Annual National Symposium: Mental Health and The Law, Ft. Lauderdale, Florida.

Snyder, S., Pitts, W., & Pokorny, A. (1986). Selected behavioral features of patients with borderline personality traits. *Suicide and Life-Threatening Behavior, 16*, 28-39.

Steadman, H. (1981). *Clinical prediction of violent behavior.* Washington DC: U. S. Government Printing Office.

Stone, M. (1990). Abuse and abusiveness in borderline personality disorder. In P. S. Linds (Ed.), *Family environment and borderline personality disorder*, (pp.131-48). Washington, DC: American Psychiatric Press.

Swanson, J. W. (1994). Mental disorder, substance abuse, and community violence: An epidemiological approach. In J. Monahan & H. Stedman (Eds.), *Violence and mental disorder: Developments in risk assessment* (pp. 101-136). Chicago: University of Chicago Press.

*Tarasoff v. Regents of the University of California*, 13 Cal. 3d 177, 529 P. 2d 533 (1974), *vacated*, 17 Cal. 3d 425, 551 P. 2d 334 (1976).

VandeCreek, L., & Knapp, S. (1993). *Tarassof and beyond: Legal and clinical considerations in the treatment of life-endangering patients* (rev. ed.). Sarasota, FL: Professional Resource Press.

Ziskin, J., & Faust, D. (1988). *Coping with psychiatric and psychological testimony (Vols.1-3*, 4[th]ed.). Los Angeles: Law & Psychology Press.

# Author Index

# Subject Index

## A

@TTEST, 59
Abilities Tests, 107, 108
Abbreviated Injury Scale, 244, 255
Acute Physiology, 215, 254, 255
Activities of Daily Living (*See* ADL), 218, 240, 255, 234, 237, 255
Actuarial, 4, 48, 64, 82, 171-173, 182, 273, 275
Advocacy
    Begets Advocacy, 12
    for Nonpatients, 7
    for Patients, 7
    From a Clinical Practice Treatment Perspective, 8
    Side-Oriented Advocacy, 5-7
Affective Aggression, 266
AIS, 255
Alcohol, 159, 160, 185, 187, 189, 218, 221, 241, 248, 269, 270, 277, 278
Alternate Forms, 129, 130, 145, 147
Alzheimer's disease, 75, 76, 82, 84, 150, 178, 181, 182, 247
American Medical Association (AMA), 82, 237-239, 244, 255

American Psychological Association (APA), 9, 10, 37, 119, 195, 255, 262, 268, 277, 280
Analysis of Initial Interview Information, 54
Anger, 266, 280
Antitypes, 149-153, 156-161, 163, 164, 168, 169
APA, 9, 10
APACHE, 212, 215, 254, 255
Aphasia, 53, 56, 144, 162, 186, 188, 202, 206, 222
Appropriate Advocacy, 21, 22
Are findings abnormal, 31
ASCOT, 212, 215, 246, 255
AS-NHST, 36, 53, 77
Assessment Validity, 46
Assessment, 1, 4, 6, 9-11, 14-16, 17-19, 48, 68-71, 143, 144, 18, 19, 21, 24-26, 30, 31, 33, 36, 45, 46, 63, 64, 71, 73, 74, 77, 82, 83, 93, 107, 119, 120, 123, 124, 139, 142, 144, 146, 147, 150, 164, 162, 171-178, 180, 181, 183, 185, 187, 188, 190, 193, 195-198, 210, 214-216, 218, 220, 224, 227-233, 237, 244-246, 249-251, 253, 254, 256, 259, 265, 267, 274-276, 278-281
Assessment Problems, 173, 180

# Web Index

http://www.cdc.gov/nchs/fastats, 49

http://expertpages.com/federal/federal.htm. 91

http://www.dialog.com, 49

http://www.geocities.com/rdfphd/index.html., 59,113, 277

http://www.inrets.fr/ur/ sara/Pg_simus_e.html, 228

http://www.who.int/whosis, 49